Update for the
MRCP

Update for the
MRCP

Dr Thomasin C. Andrews MRCP
Research registrar in neurology
Hammersmith Hospital

Dr Peter R. Arlett MRCP
Registrar in respiratory medicine and infectious diseases
Hammersmith Hospital

Dr Bernard T. Brett MRCP
Registrar in gastroenterology
Royal Free Hospital

Dr Rebecca L. Jones MRCP
Registrar in general medicine and gastroenterology
Bristol Royal Infirmary

Foreword by Professor R E Pounder MA MD DSc(Med) FRCP

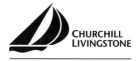

CHURCHILL LIVINGSTONE

Edinburgh London New York Philadelphia Sydney Tokyo 1996

CHURCHILL LIVINGSTONE

A Medical Division of Harcourt Brace and Company Limited

© Harcourt Brace and Company Limited 1998

ID is a registered trademark of Harcourt Brace and Company Limited

The right of Dr T. Andrews, Dr P. Arlett, Dr B. Brett and Dr R. Jones to be identified as the authors of this Work has been asserted by them in accordance with the Copyright, Design and Patents Act 1988.

First published 1996
  Reprinted 1998

ISBN 0 443 055890

British Library of Cataloguing in Publication Data

A catalogue record for this book is available from the British Library.

Library of Congress Cataloging in Publication Data

A catalog record for this book is available from the Library of Congress.

Medical knowledge is constantly changing. As new information becomes available, changes in treatment, procedures, equipment and the use of drugs become necessary. The authors and the publishers have, as far as it is possible, taken care to ensure that the information given in this text is accurate and up to date. However, readers are strongly advised to confirm that the information, especially with regard to drug usage, complies with current legislation and standards of practice.

Printed in China
NPCC/03

Foreword

It is a pleasure and privilege to introduce the first edition of *Update for the MRCP* by Thomasin Andrews, Peter A. Arlett, Bernard Brett and Rebecca Jones. Four young doctors have written a remarkable revision text of science-based medicine. Although the book purports to be for MRCP candidates, I believe all physicians – Members and Fellows – would benefit from studying it. Reading the book I have been amazed by the breadth of scholarship displayed by the authors. This book was written when they were working as registrars and research fellows. As students the authors grew up with molecular biology and immunology, and older readers will find that they make modern medicine very approachable.

The book is innovative, absolutely up-to-date, well written and easy to use. It poses 200 five-part true or false questions: one-third test the scientific basis of modern medical practice, and the remainder concern the full range of medical disciplines. In the answer section the authors score each statement as true or false, justifying their decisions by a few well-written paragraphs about each topic with the latest references. Unless the reader is already very well informed, I suspect the best way to read the book is to start at this middle section, using it as an excellent revision course, and then to attempt the questions at the beginning. The layout means that cheating is almost impossible! The book finishes with a series of random Viva questions – testing new ideas and concepts that would not be found in conventional textbooks – together with topics too new to appear in the body of the book, and a full list of references with an emphasis on review articles.

The references quoted by the authors rely heavily on *The New England Journal of Medicine, The Lancet* and the *British Medical Journal* – a practical trio because they are readily available in every medical library. They also provide a clue about how to keep up-to-date until the arrival of the book's second edition – keep reading those journals.

Finally, should we encourage books that train candidates for MRCP? The answer is, 'Yes, if they are as good as *Update for the MRCP*'. This book is not a short cut to knowledge. Readers will need a good standard of basic medicine, and they will then be rewarded by a stimulating revision of the latest trends in modern medicine. Passing

Membership should be no problem if you understand and enjoy this book. You will be more than ready for Higher Specialist Training, either as a trainee or as a trainer.

Roy Pounder MA MD DSc(Med) FRCP
Professor of Medicine,
Royal Free Hospital School of Medicine
London, United Kingdom

Preface

This book is aimed at candidates preparing for both MRCP parts 1 and 2 examinations. The fast pace of change in medicine and basic science means that textbooks quickly become out of date. Both parts 1 and 2 of the examination increasingly emphasize a knowledge of basic science and of the recent scientific and medical literature. This book reviews the new techniques of molecular and cellular biology and their application to clinical medicine. In recent years the results of large multi-centre trials have influenced changes in clinical practice and led to a drive towards evidence-based medicine. This book also reviews and references the seminal papers.

The lay-out is a series of multiple choice questions with extended answers which review the recent advances in each subject. There is also a viva section which will help candidates preparing for the part 2 clinicals. At the end of the book is an extensive list of the references we have used with which to guide your further reading.

We wish you the very best of luck.

T. Andrews   1996
P. Arlett
B. Brett
R. Jones

Contents

Questions

MOLECULAR BIOLOGY

1. Gene therapy
A. Involves insertion of genetic material into germline DNA.
B. Muscle cells are particularly susceptible to in vivo transfection, by direct injection.
C. Retroviruses used as vectors have the potential to activate cellular oncogenes.
D. Can only be used for single gene disorders.
E. Can be used for immunization.

2. Ribozymes
A. Are polypeptides.
B. Act on pre-messenger RNA to splice out exons leaving ligated introns for translation.
C. Act as enzymes.
D. Have been designed to cleave and inactivate RNA.
E. Have been designed to repair mutant RNA.

3. Antisense oligodeoxynucleotides (ODN)
A. Bind to complementary DNA strands.
B. Inhibit translation.
C. Can be used to manipulate gene expression.
D. Are lipid soluble and can cross cell membranes easily.
E. Potential side-effects result from the effects of breakdown products on cell function.

4. Transcription-factors and disease

A. A single transcription-factor can control the expression of many genes.
B. Mutation of a transcription-factor always results in loss of control of cell proliferation.
C. Li-Fraumeni syndrome results from mutation of the BRCA 1 gene.
D. In the pathogenesis of Wilm's tumours and retinoblastomas there is activation of anti-oncogenes.
E. In Burkitt's lymphoma there is translocation of the myc oncogene from chromosome 8 to 14.

5. Molecular biology

A. Transcription takes place in macromolecular complexes called ribosomes.
B. There are only 64 different codons in the human genome.
C. Adenine and guanine are purines.
D. Most people have four copies of the alpha globin gene.
E. The ALU sequence recurs 500 000 times in the human genome.

6. Human DNA

A. Adenine can only pair with thymine.
B. The genetic code is translated into functional protein within the nucleus.
C. Guanine is used instead of uracil in RNA.
D. Deoxyribose is less stable than ribose.
E. A limited number of bacterial species can translate human DNA sequences.

7. The polymerase chain reaction

A. Requires prior knowledge of the genetic sequence of the target DNA.
B. Is a useful method of identifying hepatitis C RNA.
C. Will detect even minute amounts of target DNA.
D. Requires very carefully prepared DNA in order to be accurate.
E. Is used in the tissue typing of organ transplant recipients.

8. Western blotting

A. Can be used to detect the presence of a specific DNA sequence in a complex mixture.
B. Uses an electric field applied to a nitrocellulose membrane to separate molecules based on weight and charge.
C. For the final identification of the molecule of interest, an enzyme-linked immunosorbant assay (ELISA) is required.
D. Can be used to produce the amino acid sequence of the protein fragment of interest.
E. Uses an ion exchange column to sort molecules based on charge.

9. Southern blotting

A. Can identify specific restriction fragments in a mixture of restriction fragments.
B. Specific nucleic acid fragments are identified by adding a labelled DNA probe.
C. Can give a semiquantitative estimate of the amount of a specific RNA in a mixture.
D. The nucleic acid to be analysed is first digested with a restriction enzyme.
E. Can be used to detect deletion and insertion mutations.

10. Knockout mice

A. Are produced by removing or inactivating a gene coding for a protein of interest.
B. Are produced to study the pathogenesis of autosomal dominant conditions.
C. Can be used to study the efficacy of gene therapy.
D. Always die in utero or soon after birth.
E. Can pass on their altered genes to their progeny.

11. Transgenic animals

A. Mice are the only animals in which transgenic lines have successfully been produced.
B. Transgenic animals are produced by mating two animals of different species.
C. Transgenic animals express the transgene in all their cells as the means to express selectively genes in different tissues cannot yet be transferred.
D. Transgenic founders, the first generation produced by the technique, are homozygous for the transgene.
E. Transgenic animals do not contain the transgene in their germ line and so give birth to non-transgenic animals.

12. Mitochondrial DNA

A. Is only transmitted paternally.
B. Has no exons.
C. Each mitochondrion has only one molecule of DNA.
D. Encodes all the important structural and functional proteins for each mitochondrion.
E. When damaged, is rapidly repaired by protein-RNA complexes.

13. The following are associated with abnormalities in mitochondrial DNA

A. Basal-ganglia calcification.
B. Diabetes mellitus.
C. The Wolff-Parkinson-White syndrome.
D. Elevated cerebrospinal fluid lactate levels.
E. The Kearns-Sayre syndrome.

14. p53

A. Is a protein.
B. Is a naturally occurring oncogene.
C. Can induce apoptosis.
D. Binds to sites of DNA damage.
E. Dysfunction is implicated in the pathogenesis of at least half of human cancers.

15. The following are correctly matched with the viruses implicated in their development

A. Adult T cell leukaemia and human T cell lymphotrophic virus-1.
B. Kaposi's sarcoma and coxsackie virus.
C. Cervical carcinoma and herpes simplex virus.
D. Hodgkin's disease and Epstein-Barr virus.
E. Hepatocellular carcinoma and hepatitis C virus.

GENETICS

16. In the genetics of Alzheimer's disease

A. Mutations of a gene on chromosome 14 are responsible for most cases of early onset familial Alzheimer's disease.
B. Possession of the E4 allele of the apolipoprotein E gene increases the likelihood of developing late onset Alzheimer's disease.
C. The apolipoprotein E gene is found on chromosome 20.
D. The B-amyloid-precursor protein gene is found on chromosome 2.
E. Patients with mutations of the chromosome 14 locus suffer systemic amyloidosis.

17. The risk of breast cancer is increased

A. Five fold if a first degree relative has been affected.
B. In women with a mutation of the BRCA1 gene, which occurs in 25% of all breast cancers.
C. By use of the oral contraceptive pill.
D. By breast feeding.
E. In women of higher socio-economic class.

18. Ataxia telangiectasia
A. Is an autosomal dominant disorder.
B. Patients have an increased frequency of lymphoreticular cancers.
C. Leads to chromosomal instability.
D. Causes premature ageing.
E. The gene responsible has been identified.

19. The angiotensin converting enzyme (ACE) gene
A. The DD genotype is associated with higher circulating levels of ACE than the ID or II genotypes.
B. The DD genotype is associated with hypertension.
C. The DD genotype is more common in myocardial infarction patients than in controls in all populations studied.
D. Is found on chromosome 14.
E. The DD genotype is associated with increased restenosis after angioplasty in all populations studied.

20. Hereditary haemorrhagic telangiectasia
A. Is an autosomal dominant condition with high penetrance.
B. Is associated with an increased incidence of stroke.
C. Is associated with epistaxis which characteristically worsens in pregnancy.
D. Is associated with liver cirrhosis.
E. Can be caused by a gene mutation on chromosome 9.

IMMUNOLOGY
21. Class II human leucocyte antigens (HLA)
A. HLA typing is useful in the diagnosis of rare diseases which are known to have strong HLA associations.
B. Virtually all patients with narcolepsy have DR2w2 antigens.
C. Possession of DRw4 antigens confers a 1 in 35 risk of developing rheumatoid arthritis.
D. Patients with rheumatoid arthritis who possess the associated HLA antigens tend to have aggressive, early onset disease.
E. The DQ3.2 HLA gene associated with insulin-dependent diabetes mellitus encodes for the part of the class II molecule which interacts with T cells.

22. Adhesion molecules

A. E and P-selectins are found on neutrophils and monocytes.
B. L-selectins are expressed on vascular endothelial cells.
C. Adhesion molecule ICAM-1 expression is upregulated by tissue injury.
D. Endothelial adhesion molecule VCAM-1 is upregulated by endotoxin, interleukin-1 and tumour necrosis factor.
E. Soluble E-selectin is elevated in the serum of patients with septic shock.

23. Common variable immunodeficiency

A. Results in a greater than 10 fold increase in the risk of developing gastric carcinoma.
B. Is the most common immunodeficiency in populations of European origin.
C. Affects men approximately three times as often as women.
D. Usually presents in the first 18 months of life.
E. May lead to the development of bronchiectasis.

24. Primary immunodeficiencies

A. X-linked agammaglobulinaemia presents in the second or third decade.
B. X-linked agammaglobulinaemia can be caused by a defect in a tyrosine kinase gene.
C. Hyper-IgM syndrome is usually autosomal dominant.
D. Wiskott-Aldrich syndrome is characterized by the presence of giant platelets.
E. Severe combined immunodeficiency is often clinically inapparent until the second or third year of life.

25. Autoimmune disorders

A. Antinuclear antibodies are specific to systemic lupus erythematosus (SLE).
B. Antibodies against double-stranded DNA are found in 50% of patients with SLE and are specific to the disease.
C. Grave's disease and rheumatoid arthritis are both associated with HLA DR4.
D. Immune complex mediated disease occurs when sensitized T cells react to the presence of an antigen and release lymphokines.
E. Goodpasture's syndrome is commonly associated with HLA DR2.

26. Xenotransplantation
A. Is the transplantation of tissue cultured in vitro to humans.
B. Results in IgG-mediated hyperacute rejection of the graft.
C. Results in endothelial cell activation, which is central to organ failure.
D. Genetic manipulation of donor tissue can reduce cellular rejection.
E. May result in xenozoonosis.

BASIC SCIENCE

27. Nitric Oxide
A. Inhibitors of nitric oxide synthesis block relaxation of the corpus cavernosum and prevent erection.
B. The active moiety of glyceryl trinitrate is nitric oxide.
C. Nitric oxide is a free radical with a long half life.
D. The inducible macrophage form of nitric oxide synthetase produces large quantities of nitric oxide.
E. Antioxidants protect nitric oxide.

28. Vitamin K
A. Is required for the synthesis of clotting factors II, VII, IX and XII.
B. Is required for the gamma carboxylation of glutamate residues on bone matrix proteins.
C. Is found in plants in the form of phylloquinone.
D. Is carried in the plasma mainly by low-density lipoproteins.
E. Is contained in high concentration in human breast milk.

29. Vitamin D
A. Binds to an intranuclear receptor protein.
B. Is a precursor for the steroid hormone 1,25-dihydroxycholecalciferol.
C. 25-hydroxycholecalciferol undergoes further hydroxylation in the distal renal tubule.
D. Cholecalciferol is formed by the action of ultraviolet radiation on 4-dehydrocholesterol in the skin.
E. Vitamin D receptors are transmembrane proteins which exert their intracellular effects by causing a rise in intracellular cyclic adenosine monophosphate (AMP).

30. Vitamin D

A. Receptor gene polymorphism accounts for some of the inter-individual variation in rates of osteoporosis.
B. Inhibits proliferation and promotes differentiation in a variety of cells.
C. Toxicity is a direct result of hypercalcaemia.
D. Deficiency is often secondary to inadequate oral intake.
E. Deficiency results in immunodeficiency in children.

31. Hypercalcaemia

A. Parathyroid hormone related protein has been implicated in the pathogenesis of the hypercalcaemia of sarcoidosis.
B. Osteoclast inhibitors such as the bisphosphonates take 2 to 3 days to have their effect when given intravenously.
C. Steroids are an effective treatment for the hypercalcaemia of hyperparathyroidism.
D. There is little correlation between the extent of skeletal metastases and the serum calcium concentration in malignancy-related hypercalcaemia.
E. Prostaglandins of the F series are potent stimulators of bone resorption.

32. Guanine nucleotide binding (G) proteins

A. Consist of four subunits that are non-covalently bound.
B. In the activated state the alpha subunit is bound to the nucleotide guanosine diphosphate.
C. There is altered G protein activity in pseudohypoparathyroidism.
D. G protein activity is decreased in *Vibrio cholerae* infections.
E. Abnormalities of G protein function are found in all patients with acromegaly.

33. Cell membranes and aquaporins

A. The cell membrane consists of a lipid bilayer which acts as a barrier to water and hydrophilic solutes.
B. Proteins which span the bilayer act as specific channels for the transport of substances in and out of cells.
C. Aquaporins are non-selective protein pores which allow the free passage of water across the cell membrane.
D. High resolution electron microscopy has shown aquaporins to have a tetrameric structure.
E. Physiological ligands such as hormones, immunoglobulins and neurotransmitters are first messengers that interact with specific cell surface receptors.

34. Platelet-activating factor (PAF)

A. Is a biologically active phospholipid which functions as a second messenger.
B. Is expressed only by platelets.
C. The PAF receptor protein spans the cell membrane seven times and is encoded on chromosome 1.
D. PAF receptor antagonists have been found in plants used in traditional Chinese medicine.
E. PAF-like oxidized phospholipids are generated by free-radical reactions and are less potent than PAF.

35. Copper and disease

A. Menkes' syndrome is characterized by deposition of copper in tissues.
B. Menkes' syndrome is an X-linked recessive disorder.
C. Wilson's disease may present with dystonia.
D. Wilson's disease is characterized by raised levels of caeruloplasmin.
E. Wilson's disease is caused by a mutation in the caeruloplasmin gene on chromosome 3.

36. Vascular tone

A. Noradrenaline and adenosine diphosphate act as co-transmitters in sympathetic perivascular nerves.
B. The vasodilator response to acetylcholine requires the presence of an intact endothelium.
C. Endothelium-derived relaxing factor is nitric oxide.
D. Vitamin D is a vasoconstrictor.
E. Calcitonin-gene-related peptide is a vasoconstrictor.

37. Endothelins

A. Are a group of protein hormones consisting of alpha, beta and gamma chains.
B. Interact directly with beta adrenergic receptors.
C. Exert their effect distant to their point of release.
D. Endothelin-3 predominates in the gut and kidney.
E. Plasma endothelin-1 levels correlate inversely with the severity of heart failure.

38. Natriuretic peptides

A. Atrial natriuretic peptide is the only biologically active form in humans.
B. Neutral endopeptidase is responsible for terminating their activity.
C. Are found exclusively in the heart and blood vessels.
D. Neutral endopeptidase inhibitors result in a marked fall in blood pressure.
E. Atrial natriuretic peptide causes coronary vasodilatation in angina.

39. Angiogenesis

A. Is the sprouting of new vessels from pre-existing vessels.
B. Is promoted in some tumours by basic fibroblast growth factor.
C. Is the main cause of neovascularization of the retina in response to hypoxia.
D. Can be inhibited therapeutically, which may augment cancer chemotherapy and radiotherapy.
E. Currently available inhibitors are dose limited by bone marrow suppression.

STATISTICS AND EPIDEMIOLOGY

40. Incidence, prevalence and risk

A. Incidence describes the proportion of a population that has a given disease at a point in time.
B. Measurement of prevalence is complicated by changes in the study population over time.
C. The International Classification of Diseases, Injuries and Causes of Death (ICD) assigns a six digit code to every major condition and is used to collect information on the causes of death.
D. Attributable risk is the disease rate in an exposed population minus the disease rate in the unexposed.
E. Population attributable risk is calculated by multiplying the attributable risk by the number of people exposed to the risk factor in the population.

41. Statistical terminology

A. Confounding describes a study designed to measure two independent variables.
B. Standardized rates are those which are corrected for differences in the age and sex mix of a population.
C. A study which suffers from bias has uninterpretable results.
D. Once bias is eliminated, any difference seen in the populations under study reflects true differences in the underlying populations.
E. The null hypothesis states that there is no difference in the populations under study.

42. Surveys and screening

A. A specific test is one which accurately identifies a high proportion of the positive cases.
B. A sensitive test has few false positives.
C. A test which has poor repeatability is not valid.
D. Screening is particularly useful for diseases which have a long course with no known cure.
E. Lead time describes the benefits gained in terms of patient outcome by screening and hence earlier diagnosis and treatment.

43. Mean, median, normal distribution and standard deviation

A. In a normal distribution the median equals the mean.
B. In a normal distribution approximately 95% of the values lie within one standard deviation of the mean.
C. A histogram is a good way of displaying information about a discrete quantitative variable.
D. The standard deviation is the cube root of the variance.
E. A standard deviation has the same units as the measurement it describes.

44. Statistical tests

A. A p value of 0.05 is equivalent to confidence intervals of 95%.
B. Confidence intervals are traditionally applied to the null hypothesis in statistical estimates of significance.
C. Parametric tests make assumptions about the distribution of data in the underlying population.
D. The Mann-Whitney U test is a non-parametric test.
E. Larger samples can produce narrower 95% confidence intervals.

45. Statistical power

A. Larger sample sizes reduce the probability of producing either a type 1 or a type 2 error.
B. The power of a study can be calculated retrospectively.
C. The statistical power of a study is defined as 1 minus the probability of a type 1 error occurring.
D. There is an inverse relationship between the probability of a type 1 and a type 2 error occurring.
E. The statistical power of a study is unaffected by the sample size.

46. Systematic reviews and evidence based medicine

A. GISSI-1 was the first of the trials of thrombolysis in acute myocardial infarction which was large enough on its own to confirm the effectiveness of thrombolysis.
B. A systematic review of previous small studies has shown that compression stockings fail to reduce the incidence of DVT.
C. When undertaking a meta-analysis it is important to include only trials which reached statistical significance.
D. Systematic reviews of small trials are a good substitute for large case-controlled prospective studies.
E. Evidence based medicine was designed as a means to ration health care.

47. Disadvantages of meta-analysis

A. Inclusion of all studies may let poorly conducted trials form part of the analysis.
B. Collating results may show a small and therefore insignificant difference between treatments.
C. Summarizing the results of trials reduces their statistical power.
D. Analysis may not compare homogeneous data.
E. Bias in the selection of trials included in the analysis may occur.

48. Tobacco and alcohol

A. If a smoker stops before the age of 35 his life expectancy is not significantly different from that of non-smokers.
B. Smoking accounts for one sixth of adult deaths in developed countries.
C. One quarter of regular smokers will be killed by their habit.
D. There is a positive association between smoking and death from Parkinson's disease.
E. The consumption of a moderate amount of alcohol reduces the risk of ischaemic heart disease.

49. Smoking is associated with an increased incidence of

A. Adenocarcinoma of the lung.
B. Oat cell carcinoma of the lung.
C. Crohn's disease.
D. Ulcerative colitis.
E. Obstructive sleep apnoea.

PHARMACOLOGY AND THERAPEUTICS

50. Digoxin toxicity

A. May be found with digoxin levels within the therapeutic range.
B. Is potentiated by hypercalcaemia.
C. Is increased in patients with chronic lung disease.
D. Is effectively treated with activated charcoal.
E. Most commonly causes visual disturbances.

51. In the treatment of arrhythmias

A. Amiodarone has not been shown to increase mortality in any anti-arrhythmia trial.
B. CAST showed an increase in sudden death in patients treated with flecainide, encainide and amiodarone as compared to those given placebo.
C. The BASIS trial showed that amiodarone was associated with greater survival and fewer arrhythmias compared to class I agents post myocardial infarction.
D. Amiodarone inhibits the action of warfarin.
E. Quinidine is associated with an increased mortality compared to placebo when used to treat non-sustained ventricular tachycardia.

52. Adenosine

A. Is an adenosine 1 (A1) receptor antagonist.
B. Its side-effects include facial flushing, chest pain and dyspnoea.
C. Care should be taken in heart transplant patients.
D. Dipyridamole potentiates its effects.
E. Caution should be taken in patients with bronchospasm.

53. Nicorandil

A. May be administered orally, sublingually, or intravenously.
B. No dose adjustment is required for patients with renal or hepatic impairment.
C. Does not seem to induce tolerance, unlike the nitroglycerines.
D. The commonest side-effect is headache.
E. Is not recommended in acute pulmonary oedema.

54. Angiotensin converting enzyme (ACE) inhibitors:

A. Captopril is a pro-drug which is converted by the liver to yield its active metabolite.
B. All ACE inhibitors are excreted by the kidneys and dose titration is needed in renal impairment.
C. Are contra-indicated in the over 80s.
D. Cause an increase in serum high-density lipoprotein.
E. May cause an irritating productive cough.

55. ACE inhibitors

A. Are less effective as anti-hypertensive agents in patients from the Asian sub-continent.
B. Are contraindicated in diabetic nephropathy.
C. Have been shown to be effective in the prevention of stroke and myocardial infarction in hypertensive patients.
D. Have been shown to reduce mortality after myocardial infarction.
E. Have been shown to cause regression of left ventricular hypertrophy in patients with hypertension.

56. Losartan

A. Mediates its clinically important actions through antagonism of the angiotensin receptor AT1.
B. Is subject to first pass metabolism in the liver by the cytochrome P450 system.
C. Has partial agonist activity at the AT2 receptor.
D. Can precipitate an acute attack of gout in hyperuricaemic patients.
E. Cough is a common side-effect.

57. Calcium channel blockers

A. Result in a greater reduction in the rate of myocardial infarction when used in hypertensive patients, compared to beta-blockers.
B. There is a dose dependent relationship between nifedipine use and death following myocardial infarction.
C. Reduce progression of diabetic microalbuminuria compared to beta-blockers, for the same reduction in blood pressure.
D. Of the dihydropyridine group can be used to treat atrial tachyarrhythmias.
E. Can cause cardiac failure.

58. Anti-epileptic drugs

A. Phenytoin induces the metabolism of carbamazepine, while carbamazepine inhibits the metabolism of phenytoin.
B. Sodium valproate reduces the efficacy of the oral contraceptive pill.
C. Anti-epileptic drugs should be stopped during pregnancy.
D. Using combinations of anti-epileptic drugs minimizes side-effects and provides better control than monotherapy.
E. Phenytoin toxicity may be precipitated by the concomitant use of allopurinol.

59. In the treatment of Parkinson's disease

A. Levodopa has been shown to improve significantly life expectancy.
B. Apomorphine stimulates both D1 and D2 receptors.
C. Apomorphine is given intravenously for the treatment of 'off' periods and is only licensed for in-patient treatment.
D. Domperidone can cross the blood-brain barrier and is useful for the treatment of nausea.
E. Choreoathetoid dyskinesias are common in the latter stages of Parkinson's disease and can be treated with levodopa.

60. Somatostatin and its analogues

A. Three receptor subtypes have been identified.
B. Ocreotide therapy produces tumour shrinkage in approximately 50% of growth hormone tumours.
C. Have inhibitory effects on thyrotrophin release from the pituitary gland.
D. Are of little benefit in metastatic carcinoid tumours.
E. Can improve outcome after pancreatic surgery.

61. Fibrosing colonopathy

A. Fibrosing colonopathy is a complication of Crohn's disease.
B. The first cases of fibrosing colonopathy were reported in 1983.
C. Fibrosing colonopathy was found to result from an idiosyncratic reaction to one brand of pancreatic enzyme supplements.
D. Fibrosing colonopathy is indistinguishable histologically from the strictures of Crohn's disease.
E. Adults are not at risk of developing fibrosing colonopathy.

62. Beta 2 agonists

A. There are no beta 2 receptors in the heart.
B. Can induce hypokalaemia.
C. With optimal technique only 25% of the drug is delivered to the lungs by a metered-dose inhaler.
D. Nebulizers are approximately twice as efficient at delivering drug to the lungs as metered-dose inhalers.
E. Tachyphylaxis is a severe form of anaphylaxis with rapid onset.

63. Quinine sulphate and minocycline

A. Cramp is a common side-effect of diuretics and beta agonists.
B. Quinine has been shown to be ineffective in the treatment of cramp.
C. Minocycline use is associated with cardiac arrhythmias.
D. Minocycline is safe in pregnancy.
E. Tetracycline is associated with benign intracranial hypertension.

64. The oral contraceptive pill

A. Low-oestrogen oral contraceptive pills containing gestodene have been shown to be safer in patients with a family history of venous thromboembolism than the second generation pills.
B. Third generation pills have been shown to reduce significantly the risk of myocardial infarction.
C. Pill users who smoke have 10 times the risk of myocardial infarction.
D. Hypertension may develop as a result of therapy.
E. Patients taking rifampicin will need an alternative contraception because it is a powerful enzyme inducer.

65. Retinoic acid

A. All-trans retinoic acid (ATRA) can induce remission in acute pro-myelocytic leukaemia.
B. Is the reduced form of vitamin A.
C. Is only effective when given intravenously.
D. ATRA causes regression of skin squamous-cell carcinoma.
E. Acts by inducing apoptosis of leukaemic cells.

66. Metformin produces the following effects in patients with non-insulin dependent diabetes mellitus (NIDDM)

A. It inhibits hepatic gluconeogenesis.
B. It decreases appetite and can lead to weight loss.
C. It enhances insulin secretion.
D. It lowers plasma LDL and triglyceride concentrations.
E. It frequently causes lactic acidosis.

67. Low-molecular-weight heparins

A. Inhibit the activity of anti-thrombin III.
B. Have a longer half-life than unfractionated heparins.
C. Bind to, and enhance the activity of antithrombin III.
D. Are as safe as traditional heparin therapy in the treatment of proximal deep vein thrombosis.
E. Can be used safely on an out-patient basis in selected patients with proximal deep vein thromboses.

HAEMATOLOGY

68. Blood products

A. Red cell transfusions resuspended in optimal additive solutions lack platelets.
B. White cell transfusions do not need to be cross-matched.
C. Standard human immunoglobulin intramuscular injection provides lasting immunity against rubella in non-immune pregnant women exposed to rubella.
D. All donated blood is screened for syphilis in the United Kingdom.
E. Heat treating Factor VIII will not prevent transfusion related parvovirus infection.

69. Disseminated intravascular coagulation (DIC)

A. A gram positive septicaemia is the commonest cause.
B. Haemorrhage is a common presentation.
C. Elevated plasma concentrations of fibrinogen degradation products are a prerequisite for the diagnosis.
D. Red cell fragmentation on the blood film is pathognomonic of the disease.
E. Heparin is useful in the treatment of patients with DIC secondary to adenocarcinoma.

70. Colony stimulating factors (CSF)

A. Have been shown to reduce mortality after bone marrow transplantation.
B. Granulocyte macrophage-CSF (GM-CSF) results in a rise in neutrophils and monocytes in peripheral blood.
C. GM-CSF may cause pericardial effusions.
D. CSF are used in the harvesting of peripheral blood progenitor cells.
E. May be used as a treatment for thrombocytopenia.

71. Thrombophilia

A. A specific primary hypercoagulable state can be identified in over 50% of patients with thrombophilia.
B. Most individuals identified as having a prothrombotic mutation will suffer from recurrent thrombotic complications.
C. A single gene mutation is responsible for the majority of clinically apparent hypercoagulable states.
D. The protein C/protein S complex acts by inactiving factor Xa.
E. Heparin acts as an anticoagulant by binding to and enhancing the activity of antithrombin.

72. The antiphospholipid syndrome

A. Is only seen in association with systemic lupus erythematosus.
B. Is associated with spontaneous early fetal abortion.
C. Is a common cause of Budd-Chiari syndrome.
D. Commonly presents with renal vein thrombosis.
E. May be treated with high dose anticoagulant therapy.

73. Deep venous thrombosis

A. Is associated with up to a 20-fold increase in occult malignancy in patients under 50.
B. Is best treated in early stages with intravenous thrombolytic therapy to reduce the incidence of the postphlebitic syndrome.
C. If confined to below the knee, is effectively treated with warfarin from the outset without initial heparinization.
D. Can be treated as effectively with 6 weeks of anticoagulation as it can with 6 months.
E. Is associated with a point mutation on the gene coding for factor V of the clotting cascade.

74. Aplastic anaemia

A. Is characterized pathologically by a hypocellular marrow aspirate.
B. A neutrophil count of <500/ ul associated with a reticulocyte count of <1% fulfils criteria for the diagnosis of severe disease.
C. Affects twice as many men as women.
D. Is associated with pregnancy and may be cured by termination of the pregnancy.
E. May result from an idiosyncratic adverse reaction to certain non-steroidal anti-inflammatory drugs.

75. In patients who have an absent or dysfunctioning spleen

A. Live vaccines can be given safely to children and adults.
B. The incidence of life-threatening infections in adults is less than 1%.
C. Patients have an increased incidence of severe malarial infections.
D. Phenoxymethylpenicillin and amoxycillin are effective at treating *Haemophilus influenzae* infections.
E. Patients are particularly at risk from infection with *Capnocytophaga canimorsus* (DF-2 bacillus) which is transmitted by dog bites and requires treatment with co-amoxiclav.

76. In Bone marrow transplantation (BMT)

A. Allogeneic transplantation can be used in the treatment of severe-combined immunodeficiency.
B. Apheresis is used to collect and concentrate peripheral blood progenitor cells.
C. An advantage of autologous transplantation is the enhanced graft-versus-tumour effect.
D. Once the white cell count has normalized, the patient is no longer at risk of severe sepsis.
E. Graft-versus-host disease (GVHD) does not occur after autologous transplantation.

77. In chronic myeloid leukaemia (CML)

A. The Philadelphia chromosome results from a translocation from chromosome 22q to 9q.
B. The Philadelphia chromosome results in the formation of an abnormal gene, c-abl.
C. In the acute phase, survival is better with chemotherapy and interferon alpha (IFNa) than with chemotherapy alone.
D. IFNa is only of benefit in patients who lose the Philadelphia chromosome.
E. Alpha interferons are naturally occurring glycoproteins.

78. In chronic lymphocytic leukaemia (CLL)

A. Malignant T cells express CD5.
B. The Rai staging system gives an indication of prognosis.
C. There is a survival advantage in treating early disease with chlorambucil.
D. Fludarabine is the first line agent of choice.
E. There may be a Coombs' positive haemolytic anaemia.

INFECTIOUS DISEASES

79. In human plague
A. The causative organism is *Yersinia pseudotuberculosis*.
B. Meningitis can occur.
C. Rifampicin is the treatment of choice for adults.
D. The infection is spread through contaminated water supplies.
E. In bubonic cases widespread painless lymphadenopathy is characteristic.

80. Clinical features of typical Ebola virus infection include
A. Severe frontal headache.
B. Bloody diarrhoea.
C. Tonic clonic seizures.
D. Constricting chest pains.
E. Severe aching back pain.

81. In the management of *Falciparum malaria*
A. Vertigo is a complication of quinine therapy.
B. Three negative blood films exclude the diagnosis.
C. Thrombocytopenia suggests that disseminated intravascular coagulation (DIC) is present.
D. Mefloquine is safe in pregnancy.
E. Chemoprophylaxis, starting 1 week before travel and continuing for 4 weeks after, is adequate advice to give a traveller.

82. Meliodosis
A. May present clinically with a picture similar to pulmonary tuberculosis.
B. In the acute form the commonest primary presentation is with acute pneumonia.
C. Is a common cause of hepatosplenomegaly in tropical regions.
D. Is caused by a gram negative bacillus.
E. May be effectively treated with gentamicin.

83. Brucellosis
A. *Brucella abortus* is so named because it causes abortion in sheep and cattle.
B. Epididymo-orchitis is a feature of infection in men.
C. Mitral valve endocarditis is the commonest cardiac complication of infection.
D. A 2-week course of tetracycline is adequate treatment in most cases.
E. Is a cause of splenic abscess.

84. Tick-borne diseases

A. Human ehrlichiosis is a tick-borne disease caused by *Ehrlichia chafeensis.*
B. Babesiosis is transmitted by *Ixodes* ticks.
C. Amoxycillin is the treatment of choice for human ehrlichiosis.
D. Lyme disease is the most commonly reported vector-borne disease in the USA.
E. Wood ticks and dog ticks can both transmit Rocky Mountain spotted fever.

85. In Lyme disease

A. The causative organism is the bacillus *Borrelia burgdoferi.*
B. A tender nodular erythematous rash is characteristic of early infection.
C. Acrodermatitis chronica atrophicans is seen early in the disease process.
D. Treatment is not recommended for stage I disease.
E. Erythromycin is the antibiotic of choice.

86. In the treatment of early, asymptomatic HIV infection

A. Zidovudine leads to a rise in CD4 cell count.
B. Zidovudine does not result in a significant survival benefit at 3 years follow-up.
C. Zidovudine given early compared to delaying treatment results in significantly more adverse drug events.
D. Zidovudine gives a survival benefit 1 year after commencing therapy.
E. Using two reverse transcriptase inhibitors improves prognosis compared to single agent therapy in patients who have not previously received these agents.

87. Vertical transmission of HIV infection from mother to child

A. Occurs mainly in late pregnancy and during delivery.
B. Can be reduced by up to two thirds by giving zidovudine to the mother and her infant.
C. Is more likely to occur during a caesarean than vaginal delivery.
D. Zidovudine has been demonstrated to be safe in pregnancy.
E. Should be prevented by termination of pregnancy in HIV infected mothers.

88. Human immunodeficiency virus (HIV) and the central nervous system

A. HIV dementia is seen commonly at seroconversion.
B. The CSF of patients with HIV dementia is typically acellular.
C. HIV dementia may respond to zidovudine therapy.
D. Space occupying lesions which enhance with contrast on computed tomography scans are consistent with cerebral lymphoma.
E. Cerebral lymphoma is usually of T cell origin.

89. Infections of the central nervous system in HIV infection

A. Cerebral toxoplasmosis which is due to reactivation of quiescent disease.
B. Cerebral toxoplasmosis may be treated with pyrimethamine and sulphadiazine.
C. Progressive multifocal leucoencephalopathy resulting from human papillomavirus infection.
D. Cytomegalovirus encephalopathy which characteristically affects the temporal lobes.
E. Cryptococcal meningitis which is unresponsive to fluconazole therapy.

90. In streptococcal throat infections

A. Symptom-free carriers are at much lower risk of developing complications such as rheumatic fever.
B. *Streptococcus pyogenes* can be isolated from about 55% of patients presenting to their doctor with an acute sore throat.
C. The typical features of streptococcal sore throat are present in only 40% of cases.
D. Cephalosporins are more effective than penicillin in eradicating the organism from the pharynx.
E. Treatment should be continued for 10 days.

91. The following are caused by Group A streptococcal infection

A. Rheumatic fever.
B. Erysipelas.
C. Necrotizing fasciitis.
D. Gas gangrene.
E. Pneumococcal meningitis.

92. Human parvovirus B19

A. Is the cause of sixth disease.
B. Asymmetrical small joint arthritis is the most common arthropathy seen.
C. Aplastic crisis may occur in hereditary spherocytosis.
D. Infection during pregnancy is associated with a significant increase in the rate of spontaneous abortion.
E. Chronic infection in AIDS patients may be successfully treated with human immunoglobulin.

93. Meningococcal infection

A. Is more commonly seen in the UK in the winter months.
B. Presents as septicaemia in 40% of cases.
C. Most cases in the UK are due to Group C strains of meningococcus.
D. Has an overall mortality of 30%.
E. Is readily prevented in the UK by childhood vaccination.

94. Influenza

A. Influenza A pandemics are caused by antigenic drift resulting in new virus haemagglutinin and neuraminidase antigens.
B. Rapid diagnosis of influenza A is facilitated by serological complement fixation tests.
C. Influenza epidemics are associated with an increased incidence of meningococcal infections.
D. Amantidine is equally effective against influenza A and B.
E. Allergy to eggs is a contraindication to influenza vaccination.

95. *Clostridium difficile*

A. Is a spore forming, gram positive, anaerobic bacillus.
B. Can produce three pathogenic toxins.
C. In *Clostridium difficile* diarrhoea, treatment failure is usually due to metronidazole resistance.
D. Is more effectively treated with vancomycin than metronidazole.
E. Toxigenic strains do not usually produce symptoms in neonates.

RHEUMATOLOGY

96. Paget's disease of bone

A. Has a prevalence of up to 10% in the elderly.
B. Has a greater prevalence in women than men.
C. There is a primary abnormality of osteoblasts.
D. Bone deformity is the most common presenting feature.
E. Facial palsy is the most common cranial nerve palsy.

97. In the diagnosis of Paget's disease of bone

A. Looser's zones are characteristic.
B. Areas of mixed lysis and sclerosis are characteristic.
C. Low serum phosphate is characteristic.
D. Serum osteocalcin measurement is the gold standard test.
E. Urinary hydroxyproline measurement is helpful.

98. In osteoporosis

A. The most common sites to be affected are the spine, proximal femur and distal forearm.
B. The rationale for long-term bisphosphonate use for the prevention of osteoporosis is based primarily on their effect on bone mineralization.
C. Bisphosphonates reduce the incidence of osteoporosis related vertebral fractures.
D. In post-menopausal women osteoporosis affects trabecular bone more than cortical bone.
E. Hormone replacement therapy as treatment for osteoporosis in women is indicated when lumbar spine bone density is more than one standard deviation below the mean for age related density.

99. In rheumatoid arthritis

A. There is an association with the MHC class 1 antigen DR4.
B. Monozygotic twins show a concordance rate of 75%.
C. Oestrogens are thought to protect against the severe form of the disease.
D. Anti CD4 antibody has been shown to be an effective treatment.
E. Cyclosporin A is effective in severe rheumatoid arthritis.

100. In the management of gout

A. Demonstration of positively birefringent urate crystals in synovial fluid is diagnostic.
B. The severity of the attack can be predicted by the serum urate concentration.
C. Uricosuric drugs increase the risk of an acute attack of gout by a direct action on the distal tubular urate secretory function.
D. Non-steroidal anti-inflammatory drugs are the treatment of choice for an acute attack.
E. Hyperlipidaemia predisposes to an acute attack.

101. In Raynaud's phenomenon

A. An underlying autoimmune rheumatological disease will be found in 25% of patients.
B. The presence of abnormal nail fold capillaries are helpful in predicting the onset of rheumatological disease.
C. The classical syndrome is of cold-induced digital colour change from blue (cyanosed) to white to red (erythematous).
D. A prostacyclin infusion is used for digital ulceration or gangrenous complications.
E. The underlying pathophysiology may be related to depletion of perivascular nerve fibres containing calcitonin gene related peptide (CGRP).

RENAL MEDICINE

102. Adult polycystic kidney disease

A. Has autosomal recessive inheritance.
B. Presents with end stage renal failure by the age of 30 years in the majority of cases.
C. Is associated with subarachnoid haemorrhage in 10% of patients.
D. Is associated with mitral valve prolapse.
E. May cause anaemia.

103. Haemodialysis associated amyloidosis

A. Is seen exclusively in patients on long-term haemodialysis.
B. Rarely affects visceral organs.
C. Is commonly manifest by the carpal tunnel syndrome.
D. Rarely resolves after renal transplantation.
E. Can be readily diagnosed by rectal biopsy.

104. *Escherichia coli* O157:H7

A. Can cause asymptomatic infection.
B. Outbreaks have largely been due to contaminated ground beef.
C. Almost 50% of cases develop either the haemolytic-uraemic syndrome (HUS) or thrombotic thrombocytopenic purpura (TTP).
D. Sigmoidoscopy may reveal a pseudomembrane.
E. Prompt antibiotic therapy with ciprofloxacin has been shown to reduce the risks of major complications.

105. Haemolytic uraemic syndrome (HUS)
A. May result in hypertension.
B. The commonest causative agent is *Escherichia coli* serotype O157: H7.
C. A prolonged prothrombin time and a normal kaolin cephalin time distinguishes HUS from disseminated intravascular coagulation associated with septicaemia.
D. The characteristic histological features on renal biopsy are intra-arteriolar and intra-glomerular thrombosis.
E. Heavy proteinuria (>4g/24 hrs) is common.

106 Renal disease in diabetes mellitus
A. Renal failure may develop more rapidly if autonomic neuropathy is present.
B. Good glycaemic control delays the progression of diabetic nephropathy in insulin-dependent patients.
C. Proteinuria in the absence of retinopathy suggests diabetic glomerulosclerosis.
D. Bilateral small kidneys are the hallmark of end stage diabetic nephropathy.
E. Diabetic nephropathy is more common in non-insulin compared to insulin-dependent diabetics.

107. In the management of diabetic nephropathy
A. Microalbuminuria may herald the onset of clinically overt proteinuria.
B. The rate of progression to overt proteinuria in insulin-dependent diabetics with microalbuminuria may be delayed with ACE inhibition.
C. The reduction in decline of renal function in insulin-dependent diabetics treated with ACE inhibitors is solely dependent on their anti-hypertensive effect.
D. Renal artery stenosis is an absolute contraindication to ACE inhibitors.
E. The anti-hypertensive agent of choice is hydrochlorthiazide.

108. Membranous glomerulonephritis
A. Is the commonest type of glomerulonephritis in adults.
B. Is the commonest cause of nephrotic syndrome in adults.
C. Progresses to end stage renal failure in 50% of patients unless treated with corticosteroids.
D. Is commonly associated with lymphoma in elderly patients.
E. Is characterized histologically by a thickened glomerular basement membrane and subepithelial deposits of IgG and C3.

ENDOCRINOLOGY

109. In the pathogenesis of insulin-dependent diabetes mellitus (IDDM)
A. IDDM is more common in patients with the HLA DR15 antigen.
B. Children are more likely to inherit IDDM from a mother with the disease than a father.
C. Identical twins have concordance rates of 33%.
D. At least an 80% reduction in beta cell population is needed to produce symptomatic IDDM.
E. Autoantibodies directed against the enzyme glutamate decarboxylase predict the onset of IDDM in high risk individuals.

110. Human insulin
A. Is genetically encoded on the short arm of chromosome 11.
B. Is released from beta cells of the pancreas as proinsulin.
C. Consists of two polypeptide chains linked by three disulphide bonds.
D. And C-peptide are secreted in equimolar amounts.
E. Differs from porcine insulin by only 12 amino acids.

111. In the treatment of insulin-dependent diabetes mellitus, tight diabetic control
A. Reduces the progression of macrovascular disease.
B. Can reduce the risk of retinopathy by 76%.
C. Has no significant adverse effects.
D. Can initially worsen diabetic retinopathy.
C. May reduce the occurrence of neuropathy by 90%.

112. In pregnancy, patients with insulin-dependent diabetes mellitus (IDDM)
A. Have a fetal mortality rate of 3%.
B. Have higher rates of spontaneous abortion compared to non-diabetic mothers, irrespective of their glycaemic control.
C. Develop pyelonephritis in 20% of cases.
D. Have higher rates of pre-eclampsia compared with non-diabetic mothers.
E. Have a greater risk of progression of retinopathy than non-pregnant diabetics.

113. Aldosterone
A. It is synthesized in the zona fasciculata of the adrenal cortex.
B. Primary hypoaldosteronism is characterized by subnormal plasma renin to aldosterone ratios.
C. Adrenoleucodystrophy has X-linked inheritance.
D. Salt wasting in congenital adrenal hyperplasia often improves with age.
E. Congenital adrenal hyperplasia is associated with Duchenne muscular dystrophy.

114. In Cushing's syndrome
A. Small cell carcinoma of the lung accounts for three quarters of cases of ectopic corticotrophin secretion.
B. In Cushing's disease there is increased adrenocorticotrophic hormone (ACTH) secretion from pituitary corticotroph tumours.
C. Patients with Cushing's disease usually have an exaggerated response to corticotrophin releasing hormone (CRH).
D. Petrosal venous sampling and CRH stimulation tests are useful for determining the site of a pituitary microadenoma.
E. Enhanced high resolution magnetic resonance imaging can accurately locate the site of a pituitary microadenoma in approximately 80% of cases.

115. In the diagnosis of thyrotoxicosis
A. A high titre of thyroglobulin antibodies is suggestive of Grave's disease.
B. A normal thyroid stimulating hormone (TSH) level is incompatible with a diagnosis of hyperthyroidism.
C. A low TSH with a normal free thyroxine level is characteristic of the sick euthyroid syndrome.
D. The radioisotope scan in thyroiditis characteristically shows increased uptake.
E. The radioisotope scan in toxic nodular goitre characteristically shows increased uptake.

116. In the management of hyperprolactinaemia
A. Selective dopamine antagonists are the medical treatment of choice.
B. Bromocriptine treatment may cause retroperitoneal fibrosis.
C. Surgery is always indicated if the cause is a prolactinoma more than 1 cm in size.
D. Nausea due to drug side-effects can be safely treated with domperidone.
E. Vigilant monitoring of tumour size is required in pregnancy because of the risk of rapid tumour involution and resultant cerebrospinal fluid leak.

117. Human chorionic gonadotrophin

A. Is normally increased during pregnancy.
B. Is raised in 50% of patients with choriocarcinoma.
C. When associated with choriocarcinoma can cause hyperthyroidism.
D. Is elevated in about 50% of patients with metastatic breast cancer.
E. Is a glycoprotein.

118. The following are associated with gynaecomastia

A. Hyperthyroidism.
B. Hypoparathyroidism.
C. Pompe's syndrome.
D. Digoxin therapy.
E. Captopril therapy.

NEUROLOGY

119. Atrial fibrillation (AF) as a risk factor for stroke

A. Paroxysmal AF confers a lower risk than chronic AF.
B. In patients under 60 years of age AF does not increase the risk of stroke if there are no other risk factors.
C. The use of warfarin in older patients with chronic AF has consistently been shown to reduce the risk.
D. The annual risk in patients with AF under the age of 65 without previous thromboembolism or other risk factors is 10%.
E. Warfarin will reduce the annual risk of stroke in patients with AF who have had previous thromboembolism, from 12 to 5%.

120. Acute stroke

A. Aphasia may follow from infarction in the anterior circulation.
B. Amaurosis fugax can occur in carotid artery stenosis.
C. The lateral medullary syndrome results from infarction of the posterior cerebral artery.
D. Weber's syndrome consists of sixth nerve palsy and contralateral hemiplegia.
E. Loss of consciousness is a feature of anterior circulation infarction.

121. Treatment of acute stroke and myocardial infarction

A. In ischaemic stroke thrombolytic drugs speed the recanalization of intracerebral arteries.
B. In the Multicentre Acute Stroke Trial-Italy (MAST I) streptokinase was associated with an excess 10-day case-fatality.
C. In myocardial infarction thrombolysis given within 6 hours reduces mortality by 30 per 1000 patients treated.
D. In acute myocardial infarction aspirin given early reduces the mortality rate from 13 to 10%.
E. There is no excess of haemorrhagic transformation in stroke patients treated with thrombolysis.

122. Carotid endarterectomy for ipsilateral carotid artery stenosis

A. Reduces the risk of ipsilateral stroke by 14% in symptomatic patients with 70–99% stenosis.
B. Produces a small but significant survival benefit in symptomatic patients with less than 30% stenosis.
C. Should be carried out in all otherwise fit patients with an asymptomatic stenosis of greater than 60%.
D. Results in a 2–5% perioperative mortality rate in specialist centres.
E. Should be offered to an asymptomatic patient with 50% stenosis.

123. In vascular dementia

A. Vascular dementia is characterized pathologically by the presence of amyloid plaques and neurofibrillary tangles.
B. Diabetes mellitus is a risk factor for vascular dementia.
C. Vascular dementia is diagnosed by finding white matter disease on CT scan.
D. Sub-cortical dementias classically present with agnosia, aphasia and apraxia.
E. Symptomatic stroke increases the risk of dementia more than nine fold.

124. Dementia

A. Parietal lobe tumours commonly present with dementia.
B. The presence of visual hallucinations is incompatible with the diagnosis of dementia.
C. Progressive supranuclear palsy is characterized by paralysis of upward and or downward gaze.
D. Pseudodementia may be treated with anti-depressant medication.
E. 600 000 people in England and Wales suffer from dementia.

125. Prion diseases

A. Characteristically cause vacuolar degeneration of the central nervous system.
B. Fatal familial insomnia is an example of a prion disease.
C. Have been transmitted to humans via blood products.
D. Have been transmitted to humans during neurosurgery.
E. Are associated with renal amyloid.

126. Huntington's disease

A. The genetic defect in Huntington's disease is an expanded trinucleotide repeat on chromosome 7.
B. The longer the CAG repeat sequence, the earlier the onset of the disease.
C. The Huntington's disease gene is expressed only in those tissues which are affected by the disease.
D. Huntington's disease exhibits the phenomenon of anticipation.
E. The direct test for the Huntington's disease gene, which measures the number of CAG repeats, has obviated the need for pre-test counselling.

127. The following are associated with trinucleotide repeats

A. Fragile X syndrome.
B. Turner's syndrome.
C. Myotonic dystrophy.
D. Ataxia telangiectasia.
E. Spinocerebellar ataxia.

128. Motor neurone disease

A. Orthopnoea is a common symptom of motor neurone disease.
B. Mutation of the copper/zinc superoxide dismutase gene is found in up to 30% of cases.
C. Emotional lability is associated with pseudobulbar and not bulbar palsy.
D. Characteristic electromyographic findings include a reduction in the number and an increase in the amplitude and duration of motor action potentials.
E. Fasciculation occurs when reinervation of denervated motor units creates large motor units with visible resting contractions.

129. Muscular dystrophies

A. Duchenne muscular dystrophy is an autosomal-recessive disease.
B. Duchenne muscular dystrophy is caused by the absence of dystrophin protein.
C. One third of cases of Duchenne muscular dystrophy are due to spontaneous mutations.
D. Gower's sign describes the hypertrophy seen in the calf muscles of affected children.
E. Female carriers of Duchenne muscular dystrophy usually have a myopathic pattern on EMG.

130. Clinical features of multiple sclerosis (MS) include

A. Internuclear opthalmoplegia.
B. Myokymia.
C. Symptoms which are worse in hot weather.
D. Median nerve palsy.
E. Vertigo.

131. In the diagnosis and management of patients with multiple sclerosis

A. Analysis of the cerebrospinal fluid characteristically shows oligoclonal bands which are not present in the serum.
B. Primary progressive MS is a relatively benign form of the disease.
C. Interferon was shown in a double blind randomized controlled trial to reduce relapse rates in patients with primary progressive MS.
D. The majority of patients will not suffer from long-term disability.
E. There is an increased incidence of MS in the first degree relatives of patients with the disease.

132. Guillain-Barré syndrome (GBS)

A. Has a case mortality of 20%.
B. Has been reported to have occurred following immunization with the measles/mumps/rubella vaccine.
C. Is characterized by acute weakness and absent tendon reflexes, without sensory signs.
D. In the majority of cases there is an acute purely motor axonal neuropathy.
E. The Miller Fisher syndrome consists of ophthalmoplegia, anosmia and urinary incontinence.

133. In myasthenia gravis

A. Anti-acetylcholine receptor antibodies are shown to be present on immunoassay in all patients and form part of the definition of the disease.
B. Patients present with areflexia and a distal pattern of limb weakness.
C. Patients with thymic hyperplasia classically have high titres of anti-striated muscle antibody.
D. Patients with thymomas tend to be males who are over 40 and this group show little improvement after thymectomy.
E. Electromyography shows a decremental response in the amplitude of the evoked muscle action potential with repetitive stimulation.

134. In functional neuroimaging

A. Functional MRI (fMRI) has the advantage over positron emission tomography (PET) and single photon emission computerized tomography (SPECT) of not using ionizing radiation.
B. PET can compute spatial information by detecting pairs of photons which are produced when a positron collides with an electron.
C. PET can produce spatial resolution of 3–5 mm.
D. fMRI techniques have produced spatial resolution of 0.1 mm
E. SPECT has the best spatial resolution of the various neuroimaging techniques.

135. Epilepsy and driving

A. People with epilepsy who drive have the same rates of road traffic accidents as the average driver.
B. Seizures not associated with loss of consciousness or myoclonic jerks are treated by the Driver and Vehicle Licensing Agency (DVLA) in the same way as epilepsy.
C. Following a seizure the holder of a group II licence is banned from driving buses and goods vehicles for life.
D. In order to hold a driving licence a person must be fit-free for 2 years.
E. Approximately 5% of men and 4% of women will have at least one epileptic seizure during their life-time.

136. The persistent vegetative state

A. Describes a state of reduced consciousness where the patient is fully aware of his or her surroundings but is unable to communicate except by opening and closing his eyes.
B. To diagnose the 'persistent' vegetative state the patient must be in a vegetative state for at least 4 weeks.
C. Patients may require ventilatory support.
D. Patients must show cycles of eye opening and closure simulating waking and sleep.
E. The patient characteristically exhibits nystagmus in response to ice water caloric testing.

137. In the diagnosis of brain stem death

A. An EEG is required to confirm absence of cerebral activity.
B. Criteria for children over 2 months are the same as those for adults.
C. Hypothermia must be excluded.
D. The presence of diabetes insipidus precludes a diagnosis of brain stem death.
E. The diagnosis can be made by any two doctors as long as they have full medical registration.

CARDIOLOGY

138. Hypertension in the elderly

A. Hypertensive patients tend to have peripheral insulin resistance with resulting hyperinsulinaemia.
B. Hypertension suspected of being secondary to atherosclerotic renovascular disease is best diagnosed using renal ultrasonography.
C. 80% of elderly hypertensives have coexisting postural hypotension.
D. Lowering elevated blood pressure in the elderly, either systolic or diastolic, reduces cardiovascular morbidity and mortality.
E. Beneficial side-effects of alpha-blockers include relief from the symptoms of prostatism, improvement of the lipid profile, and improvement of insulin sensitivity.

139. Hypertension

A. Is defined by the World Health Organization as a blood pressure of greater than 140/90 mmHg.
B. Hypertensive treatment should be initiated if a single blood pressure recording is greater than 190/105 mmHg.
C. Can be treated safely in the elderly with a long acting ACE inhibitor.
D. Results exclusively from arteriolar smooth muscle contraction.
E. Should be brought rapidly into the normal range once the diagnosis has been established.

140. Hyperlipidaemia

A. Type 1 hyperlipidaemia consists of chylomicronaemia plus raised very low density lipoproteins (VLDL).
B. Hypertriglyceridaemia is associated with alcoholism.
C. Hypercholesterolaemia is associated with hypothyroidism.
D. Diabetes is associated with type IIa and type IV hyperlipidaemia.
E. Hypercholesterolaemia is a common cause of pancreatitis.

141. Hyperlipidaemia

A. Raised high-density lipoprotein cholesterol levels are a known risk factor for coronary heart disease.
B. Pravastatin is an ion exchange resin which can cause constipation, indigestion and nausea.
C. Reducing the level of high-density lipoprotein (HDL) cholesterol in patients with coronary artery disease improves survival.
D. Reduction of cholesterol levels in the West of Scotland Coronary Prevention Study was associated with an increased incidence of suicide and violent death.
E. The West of Scotland study showed that lowering cholesterol levels reduced mortality rates in middle-aged men who had had a previous coronary event.

142. Peroxidation of low-density lipoprotein (LDL)

A. Prevents its recognition by the LDL receptor.
B. Renders the molecule highly cytotoxic to endothelial cells.
C. Results in the formation of immune complexes in the arterial wall.
D. Can be prevented by vitamin E.
E. Is implicated in the pathogenesis of coronary heart disease.

143. In the management of acute myocardial infarction (MI)

A. Aspirin reduces mortality in acute MI by 50% compared to placebo.
B. The use of beta-blockers significantly increases the risk of conduction defects in inferior MI.
C. There is a significant survival benefit over 35 days with the use of 12 500 units of heparin given subcutaneously twice daily in addition to aspirin and thrombolytic therapy.
D. A 3-hour tissue plasminogen activator (tPA) infusion has significant survival benefit over streptokinase in the management of acute anterior MI.
E. tPA is associated with a lower reinfarction rate following acute MI compared to streptokinase.

144. ISIS-2 showed that in the management of acute myocardial infarction

A. There was an excess of non-fatal reinfarction in the group treated with streptokinase alone compared with placebo.
B. The use of streptokinase was associated with an overall increase in cerebrovascular events post infarction.
C. Hydrocortisone prophylaxis reduced the incidence of allergic reactions to streptokinase.
D. Patients over 75 years do not benefit from thrombolysis.
E. The greatest reduction in deaths occurred in those patients presenting within 4 hours of symptom onset.

145. Contraindications to streptokinase include

A. Surgery within the previous 10 days.
B. Gastrointestinal bleeding within the previous 6 months.
C. Background diabetic retinopathy.
D. Acute pancreatitis.
E. Parturition within the previous 4 weeks.

146. In ISIS-4

A. Captopril was started 12 hours after thrombolysis.
B. Magnesium therapy only showed a significant increase in survival amongst those who presented very early (< 2 hours).
C. Nitrates showed no increase in survival and are no longer considered useful in acute myocardial infarction.
D. In patients with a previous history of myocardial infarction captopril therapy saved 18 lives per 1000 patients treated.
E. The captopril dose was gradually increased from the 6.25 mg starting dose to 25 mg three times a day over 72 hours.

147. Left ventricular remodelling, post myocardial infarction (MI)

A. Involves the process of infarct expansion.
B. Often affects parts of the ventricular wall remote from the infarcted segment.
C. Results from myocyte regeneration.
D. Results in near-normal left ventricular function if completed prior to a further vascular insult.
E. Cannot be modified with current therapies.

148. Coronary artery bypass grafting (CABG)

A. Improves prognosis when compared to medical therapy for left main stem disease.
B. Improves prognosis when compared to medical therapy for triple vessel disease.
C. Improves prognosis when compared to medical therapy in patients with coronary heart disease and impaired left ventricular function.
D. Improves prognosis when compared to angioplasty in all patient groups.
E. Results in a lower requirement for anti-anginal drugs compared to angioplasty.

149. Hibernating myocardium

A. Is the term used to describe the myocardial dysfunction which follows a temporary interruption in coronary blood flow.
B. Results in left ventricular dysfunction, which may be restored to normal by revascularization.
C. Is found in a greater proportion of patients with unstable compared to stable angina.
D. Is rare after myocardial infarction.
E. If it becomes chronic, it is associated with deposition of myocardial amyloid.

150. Angina in patients with syndrome X

A. Indicates a poor prognosis with accelerated coronary vascular disease.
B. Occurs only in patients with a single X chromosome.
C. Is characterized by a normal exercise tolerance test but an abnormal coronary angiogram.
D. Usually resolves with investigation and reassurance.
E. Is caused by an X-linked disorder with abnormal endothelin receptors.

151. Hypertrophic cardiomyopathy (HCM)

A. Is the most common cause of sudden death in the young.
B. Is an X-linked disease typically affecting young men.
C. The gene responsible encodes a protein which causes myocytes to hypertrophy.
D. Death is most commonly a result of outflow tract obstruction.
E. Beta-blockers are contraindicated because they are negatively inotropic.

152. In the diagnosis and management of cardiac tumours

A. Metastatic tumours are twice as common as primary heart tumours.
B. Pulmonary embolism occurs in 40% of patients with myxomas.
C. Myxomas typically arise in the right atrium.
D. M-mode echocardiography is efficient at demonstrating the shape, size and attachment of tumours prior to surgery.
E. The 'tumour plop' is characteristically heard in early systole.

153. Heart valve replacement

A. Is indicated in patients with asymptomatic aortic regurgitation with left ventricular dysfunction.
B. Is indicated for asymptomatic patients with mitral stenosis because sudden death is common.
C. Should be considered in asymptomatic patients with aortic stenosis who undergo exercise stress tests indicating reduced exercise tolerance.
D. Is the only method of restoring function to a regurgitant mitral valve causing symptoms.
E. May be avoided in symptomatic mitral stenosis if the valve anatomy renders it suitable for valvotomy.

154. Atrioventricular nodal re-entry tachycardia

A. Is probably the most common regular paroxysmal supraventricular tachycardia.
B. Patients usually present in the fourth or fifth decades of life.
C. Is more common in men.
D. The P waves are negative in the inferior ECG leads.
E. Are terminated by a 12 mg dose of intravenous adenosine in 90% of cases.

DERMATOLOGY

155. In paraneoplastic syndromes, the following cutaneous disorders are correctly paired with their associated solid tumours

A. Clubbing and non-small cell lung cancer.
B. Erythema marginatum and glucagonoma.
C. Trousseau's syndrome and carcinoma of the tail of the pancreas.
D. Erythema gyratum repens and lung cancer.
E. Acanthosis nigricans and abdominal adenocarcinoma.

156. In paraneoplastic syndromes

A. Multi-centric reticulohistiocytosis is a known cause of arthritis mutilans.
B. Hypertrophic pulmonary osteoarthropathy does not respond to vagotomy.
C. Trousseau's syndrome involves the rapid increase in size and number of solar keratoses.
D. Tylosis is caused by elevated tyline levels which stimulates hyperkeratosis.
E. Hypertrichosis lanuginosa acquisita is associated with cancers of the lung.

157. Basal cell carcinoma (BCC)

A. The incidence has risen by 15% in the last decade in the UK.
B. The wavelengths of ultraviolet light responsible for the development of BCCs are known.
C. Can be effectively treated with phototherapy.
D. Brain metastases are common in patients who are not treated early.
E. Melanomas are more frequent in patients who have had BCC.

158. Erythema multiforme, Stevens-Johnson syndrome and toxic epidermal necrolysis

A. Herpes simplex infection is responsible for a third of cases of erythema multiforme.
B. Erythema multiforme is characterized by target lesions and mucous membrane ulceration.
C. Systemic corticosteroids are the mainstay of treatment for Stevens-Johnson syndrome.
D. Sulphonamide antibiotics commonly cause Stevens-Johnson syndrome.
E. Toxic epidermal necrolysis has a mortality rate of 80%.

159. Dermatological treatments

A. Topical vitamin D is an effective treatment for eczema.
B. The tricyclic anti-depressant doxepin has anti-histaminic activity making it a good treatment for pruritis.
C. Topical doxepin can cause drowsiness.
D. Calcipotriol acts by raising extracellular calcium concentrations.
E. Topical steroids are the treatment of choice for psoriasis.

160. Urticaria

A. The pathogenesis may be autoimmune.
B. Angio-oedema may occur.
C. Pressure on the skin can trigger an attack.
D. Corticosteroids frequently trigger an attack.
E. Plasmapheresis has been shown to be an effective treatment for some patients.

161. Malignant melanoma

A. The incidence of melanoma in New South Wales has decreased in the last 3 years.
B. Women with lesions at the same site and of the same depth as men have a better prognosis.
C. Patients with a tumour less than 1 mm deep have a 5-year survival of 90%.
D. Patients with lesions on their upper arms have a worse prognosis than those with lesions on their legs.
E. Individuals with high continuous exposure to the sun have lower rates of malignant melanoma than those exposed intermittently.

RESPIRATORY MEDICINE

162. Pulse oximetry

A. Detects carboxyhaemoglobin as oxyhaemoglobin.
B. Compares the ratio of absorption spectra of oxygenated to reduced haemoglobin to calculate oxygen saturation.
C. A sine waveform is indicative of a good signal.
D. Is a sensitive method of detecting hyperoxia.
E. Should be used in bright ambient light.

163. Physiological responses to prolonged hypoxaemia include

A. Increased ventilatory drive.
B. Vasodilation in peripheral vascular beds.
C. Vasodilation in pulmonary vascular beds.
D. Reduced heart rate.
E. Reduced cardiac output.

164. Indications for long-term oxygen therapy in chronic obstructive pulmonary disease (COPD) include

A. A resting PaO_2 less than or equal to 7.3 kPa.
B. The exclusion of patients with hypercapnoea.
C. A forced expiratory volume in 1 s (FEV1) of less than 1.2 l.
D. Current evidence of cor pulmonale.
E. Being a non-smoker.

165. Nasal intermittent positive pressure ventilation (NIPPV)

A. Reduces mortality in type II respiratory failure from an acute exacerbation of chronic obstructive pulmonary disease (COPD).
B. Bulbar palsy is a relative contraindication.
C. When given overnight for chronic type II respiratory failure, frequently improves daytime blood gases.
D. The main disadvantage is precipitation of upper airway collapse.
E. Is unsuitable for patients with restrictive ventilatory defects from chest wall disease.

166. Features of obstructive sleep apnoea include

A. Excessive daytime sleepiness.
B. Apnoea without respiratory effort.
C. 70% of patients are cured by uvulopalatopharyngoplasty.
D. Occurrence in 10% of acromegalic patients.
E. Increased prevalence in patients with Marfan's syndrome.

167. The British Thoracic Society guidelines for acute severe asthma state that

A. Normocapnea can be a life threatening feature.
B. Bradycardia suggests that an attack is severe.
C. Nebulized salbutamol should be given with air.
D. Patients should be commenced on inhaled steroids on discharge.
E. Discharge is usually appropriate when the peak expiratory flow rate is above 50% predicted.

168. Asthma and the environment

A. House dust mite sensitivity is more common in children born in the autumn.
B. A causal role for viral infection in the induction of asthma has been established.
C. Studies have shown a correlation relating adult female mortality from asthma to table salt consumption.
D. Convincing evidence exists that air pollution is important in inducing asthma.
E. There is a critical period in infancy when sensitization to new allergens is high.

169. Occupational asthma

A. Most commonly occurs on first exposure to an allergen.
B. Is seen in about 10% of workers exposed to isocyanates.
C. Is diagnosed if asthma develops in workers known to be in high risk occupations.
D. Is best diagnosed by spirometry before and after work on more than one occasion.
E. Carries a poor prognosis if exposure to the responsible agent has been prolonged.

170. In cystic fibrosis

A. The cystic fibrosis transmembrane regulator acts as a potassium channel.
B. Respiratory colonization with *Pseudomonas aeruginosa* is an early manifestation.
C. Nebulized DNAase is used therapeutically to reduce sputum viscosity.
D. Diabetes mellitus is a recognized complication.
E. Pneumothorax is a common complication of advanced disease.

171. Cystic fibrosis

A. Prevalence in the UK is 1 in 2000.
B. The disease is universally fatal by the age of 27 years.
C. Males are usually infertile.
D. Diagnosis is confirmed by finding a sweat chloride concentration of >50 meq/l.
E. The genetic defect is located on the short arm of chromosome 7.

172. Tuberculosis

A. One third of the world's population have latent infection.
B. Causes 50 million new infections per year worldwide.
C. Co-infection in patients with HIV should be treated with five antibiotics.
D. Co-infection in patients with HIV may lead to progression of the HIV infection.
E. Frequently causes extrapulmonary disease in patients with HIV infection.

173. Multi-drug-resistant tuberculosis (MDRTB)

A. In patients who are not HIV positive there is a treatment failure rate of 50% when treatment is continued for 18–24 months.
B. Comprises 3% of new tuberculosis (TB) cases in the USA.
C. Resistance is defined as primary, if a patient has never had TB before.
D. Is defined as resistance to at least three drugs.
E. Patients who are sputum smear positive should be isolated for 4 weeks.

174. *Pneumocystis carinii*

A. Is a protozoa which causes pneumonia in immunocompromized individuals.
B. Pneumonia in AIDS is caused by reinfection more often than reactivation.
C. Nebulized pentamidine as treatment for pneumonia is associated with upper lobe relapse.
D. Pneumonia at seroconversion is well recognized.
E. May be carried asymptomatically by HIV seronegative individuals.

175. The adult respiratory distress syndrome (ARDS)

A. Is characterized by hypoxia in the presence of a raised pulmonary artery wedge pressure.
B. Has a mortality of greater than 50%.
C. May lead to pulmonary hypertension and the development of right heart failure.
D. Treatment with inhaled nitric oxide (NO) has been shown to reduce mortality in clinical trials.
E. May be treated with extracorporeal membrane oxygenation (ECMO).

GASTROENTEROLOGY

176. The risk of developing hepatocellular carcinoma

A. Is increased over 100 fold by being hepatitis B surface antigen (HBsAg) positive.
B. Is increased by the consumption of food contaminated with *Aspergillus flavus.*
C. Is increased in glycogen storage disorders.
D. Is increased more by hepatitis C viral infection than by excess alcohol consumption.
E. Is about 3% per annum in patients with cirrhosis.

177. In the management of hepatocellular carcinoma

A. Liver transplantation should be reserved for those with single tumours less than 3 cm in size.
B. Ethanol injection has been shown to be an ineffective treatment.
C. Resection of single tumours in patients with mild cirrhosis produces similar results to transplantation.
D. Screening of patients with cirrhosis does not alter survival.
E. The prognosis has not improved over the last 15 years.

178. In the aetiology of colorectal cancer

A. Mutations in the APC gene are found in approximately 70% of adenomatous polyps and colorectal carcinomas.
B. The hereditary polyposis syndromes account for approximately 1% of cases.
C. The familial adenomatous polyposis gene is located on chromosome 5.
D. Individuals with hereditary non-polyposis colorectal cancer are at increased risk from environmental factors which lead to genetic damage.
E. Colonic carcinoma is thought to develop from cells in adenomatous polyps in 50% of cases.

179. Familial adenomatous polyposis

A. Is autosomal recessive.
B. Has a prevalence of 1 in 5000.
C. 40% of index patients have no family history.
D. The non-steroidal anti-inflammatory agent sulindac leads to polyp regression in many cases.
E. Rectal polyps regress in approximately 60% of patients after colectomy.

180. Extra-colonic features of familial adenomatous polyposis include

A. Mandibular osteomas.
B. Polyps of the upper gastrointestinal tract.
C. An increased risk of peri-ampullary cancer.
D. An increased incidence of acromegaly.
E. Congenital hypertrophy of the retinal pigment epithelium.

181. In ulcerative colitis

A. 10% of patients with extensive colitis will develop colorectal carcinoma after 10 years.
B. The finding of persistent dysplasia on colonic biopsies during colorectal cancer surveillance is an indication for proctocolectomy.
C. There is an association with cholangiocarcinoma.
D. Anti-diarrhoeal drugs are a useful means of symptom control during an acute attack.
E. A reduction in diarrhoea may signal the development of toxic colonic dilatation in an acute attack.

182. In ulcerative colitis

A. Interstitial nephritis is a rare complication of 5-aminosalicylic acid therapy.
B. Erythema multiforme often precedes the onset of disease.
C. Smoking should be encouraged.
D. The severity of sacroiliitis reflects disease activity.
E. Infertility is a well recognized side-effect of mesalazine therapy.

183. Crohn's disease

A. Small bowel Crohn's disease may be difficult to distinguish from yersinial infection.
B. There is an increased incidence of Crohn's disease in Turner's syndrome.
C. Is associated with an increased incidence of rheumatoid arthritis.
D. Is twice as common in women as in men.
E. May be helped by giving up smoking.

184. In Whipple's disease

A. The causative organism is *Tropheryma whippelii*.
B. Oculomasticatory myorhythmia is virtually pathognomonic.
C. Peripheral blood leucocytes often contain the genomic material from the causative organism.
D. The electron microscopic appearances of the organism are highly specific.
E. Dementia occurs with increased frequency.

185. In oesophageal achalasia

A. The majority of patients can be treated successfully with nitrates or calcium channel blockers in the early stages of the disease.
B. The disease is characterized by reduced peristaltic activity in the oesophageal body, and an increased resting lower oesophageal sphincter (LOS) pressure.
C. It is now known to be caused by a single gene defect found on chromosome 4, and a variety of epigenetic factors which are required for its expression have been identified.
D. Botulinum toxin can be effective when injected into the dorsal vagal nuclei.
E. The incidence is 1 in 1000 in the UK.

186. *Helicobacter pylori* infection

A. Has a prevalence of 20–25% in European populations.
B. Produces symptoms in the majority of subjects.
C. Has been shown to be responsible for most cases of non-ulcer dyspepsia.
D. Has a low prevalence in developing countries explaining the low incidence of peptic ulcer disease.
E. Can be detected in over 95% of cases of duodenal ulceration.

187. *Helicobacter pylori* can be detected

A. Using serological tests with over 95% specificity.
B. Using the radiolabelled carbon-urea breath test with a false positive rate of less than 5%.
C. Using a urease based test which detects urea produced by the organisms.
D. In blood cultures of 20% of those with severe infection.
E. By testing for antibodies in patients' saliva.

188. In the medical treatment of gallstones

A. Controlled trials have shown significant symptomatic benefit from aloe juice therapy.
B. The presence of more than 30 stones is an indication for surgery.
C. Ursodeoxycholic acid is a suitable treatment for small non-calcified cholesterol stones.
D. Chenodeoxycholic acid is a suitable treatment for small calcified pigment gallstones.
E. Oral bile salt therapy achieves maximal stone dissolution after 6 months of treatment.

189. Primary sclerosing cholangitis (PSC)

A. Is more commonly associated with Crohn's disease than ulcerative colitis.
B. Predisposes individuals to cholangiocarcinoma.
C. Women are more commonly affected than men.
D. Usually presents in the seventh decade.
E. Can be mimicked by cryptococcal infection in the immunocompromised.

190. In the treatment of primary sclerosing cholangitis

A. Successful management of associated inflammatory bowel disease leads to a slowing of the disease process.
B. Corticosteroids are the treatment of choice in early disease.
C. Cholangiocarcinoma usually responds to combined radiotherapy and chemotherapy.
D. Liver transplantation is contraindicated because of rapid recurrence in the transplanted liver.
E. Prophylactic ciprofloxacin is indicated to prevent cholangitis.

191. Hepatitis E virus infection

A. Is caused by an enveloped DNA virus.
B. Can be transmitted by contaminated water.
C. Is transmitted principally by blood products in the UK.
D. Is associated with increased mortality amongst pregnant women.
E. Can be transmitted vertically.

192. Hepatitis C virus infection

A. Is an RNA virus.
B. Is thought to be the most common cause of non-A non-B transfusion related hepatitis
C. Leads to cirrhosis in up to 5% of infected individuals after 20 years.
D. Is found in the blood of 0.1% of prospective first-time blood donors.
E. Can be transmitted vertically.

193. In the treatment of hepatitis C virus infection

A. Women are less likely to respond to interferon alpha than men.
B. 50% of those who have undergone liver transplantation die from fulminant hepatitis C during the first 2 years post-transplantation.
C. Consumption of alcohol may lead to an improved response to treatment with interferon alpha.
D. Ribavirin is as effective as interferon alpha, as monotherapy.
E. People infected with type 2 or type 3 virus are more likely to have a sustained response to interferon alpha.

194. Significant risk factors for variceal haemorrhage in patients with cirrhosis include

A. A high Pugh's score.
B. Abstinence from alcohol.
C. A hepatic venous pressure gradient of less than 12 mmHG.
D. Small irregular varices.
E. Beta blockade.

195. In the prevention of recurrent variceal haemorrhage

A. Beta blockade is contraindicated as it may cause exacerbation of hypotension if further bleeding occurs.
B. Endoscopic oesophageal sclerotherapy reduces mortality by 25–35%.
C. Surgical portocaval shunts reduce mortality by 15–20%.
D. Transjugular intra-hepatic portosystemic shunts should be considered the gold standard therapy.
E. Sclerotherapy can lead to oesophageal strictures.

196. Transjugular intra-hepatic portosystemic shunt (TIPS)

A. Involves creating an artificial shunt from the inferior vena cava to the portal vein.
B. Is used to treat portosystemic encephalopathy.
C. Can often prevent the need for orthotopic liver transplantation.
D. Can make liver transplantation technically difficult.
E. Will require a replacement stent if stenosis occurs.

EMERGENCY MEDICINE

197. In adult advanced cardiac life support

A. Adrenaline is given in ventricular fibrillation (VF) to sensitize the myocardium to defibrillation.
B. Direct current (DC) cardioversion should only be attempted when the electrical activity of the heart is monitored.
C. Atropine is the first drug given in an asystolic arrest.
D. Because of its negatively inotropic effects, lignocaine is now contraindicated in VF.
E. The presence of unreactive pupils during an arrest is an indication of irreversible brain damage.

198. In hypothermia

A. Tissue hypoxia occurs because of a shift to the right of the oxygen haemoglobin saturation curve.
B. A raised white cell count indicates underlying sepsis.
C. Hypothermia may mask electrocardiographic changes of hyperkalaemia.
D. Normal prothrombin times exclude hypothermia related coagulopathies.
E. Extracorporeal rewarming is the most efficient method of raising core body temperature.

199. ECG abnormalities in cocaine users

A. Prolonged QT interval.
B. Atrioventricular nodal block.
C. Ventricular tachycardia.
D. ST segment elevation.
E. Broad QRS complexes.

200. In treatment of paracetamol overdose

A. Activated charcoal should be given if a patient presents up to 4 hours after overdose.
B. Intravenous N-acetyl cysteine (NAC) is the preferred antidote, as oral preparations induce vomiting which may limit their effectiveness.
C. NAC should be given before paracetamol levels are available, to all patients who have ingested >150 mg/kg of paracetamol.
D. If an adverse reaction to NAC occurs, the infusion should be stopped and anti-histamines administered before restarting the infusion.
E. NAC may continue to be an effective antidote to poisoning in patients presenting >20 hours after overdose or in those with fulminant liver failure.

Answers

MOLECULAR BIOLOGY

1. Gene therapy

A. **F**   B. **T**   C. **T**   D. **F**   E. **T**

Genetic engineering is the practice of either selectively mating animals or inserting genetic material into a parent's germline DNA in order to produce desired genetic phenotypes in the offspring. Gene therapy attempts to modify the phenotype of somatic cells in order to treat human disease. The first human trials of gene therapy started in 1990, and many trials are now in progress. Gene therapy can be regarded as a highly sophisticated form of drug delivery, delivering proteins to cells by transfecting them with the gene coding for that particular protein.

The advantages of gene therapy over traditional drug therapy are that it can be used to target specific cells and tissues thus reducing unwanted side-effects, and in addition the introduction of a gene can result in the long-term production of a protein. Eukaryotic cells have been found to be remarkably permissive when it comes to the short-term uptake of foreign DNA. Vectors can be introduced by aerosol to the respiratory tract or by direct injection into body tissues or compartments. Muscle cells are found to be particularly susceptible to transfection and intramuscular transfection has become popular following the observation that myocytes can take up 'naked' plasmid DNA whereas other tissues require DNA to be incorporated into liposomes. Alternatively cells can be transfected in vitro and then returned to the patient.

Vectors used for transfection include modified retroviruses, adenoviruses, vaccinia and plasmids. There has been concern that the use of retroviruses which integrate randomly into the DNA of dividing cells might activate cellular oncogenes, although so far this has not occurred. Another concern is that through transmission to daughter cells retroviruses may pass into the germline. One of the problems of using viral vectors is that expression of viral vector proteins can render the transfected cells immunogenic. Much effort has gone into removing the viral genes from viral vectors to minimize this.

Directed gene therapy requires an understanding of the molecular defects which cause disease, so that the gene coding for a specific protein can be incorporated into the correct cellular system and its expression can be controlled. Gene therapy which can deliver proteins whose quantity is critical or changes in response to physiological variables, such as insulin, are currently under intense investigation. Continued gene expression following transfection has been demonstrated for as long as 360 days in the muscle of mice, however the foreign DNA is gradually lost as it is rejected by the cell.

Gene therapy was initially directed at finding treatments for disorders caused by a single gene. In cystic fibrosis direct intratracheal administration of the cystic fibrosis transmembrane conductance regulator gene in an adenovirus vector has resulted in diffuse pulmonary expression of the protein in rats. In a canine model of haemophilia B, clotting time was reduced by 50% following the infusion of a retroviral vector containing the factor IX gene. In human subjects with hypercholesterolaemia due to LDL receptor deficiency, blood cholesterol levels have been reduced by transfusion with hepatocytes which have been transfected ex vivo with a retrovirus containing the LDL receptor gene.

Gene therapy is now being investigated as a possible tool for the treatment of acquired diseases. In one experiment the endothelial lining of porcine arteries were stripped and endothelial cells transfected with a gene expressing a protein acting as a label for their subsequent identification, were infused. Four weeks later the arterial segment was removed and the labelled endothelial cells had attached themselves to the arterial wall and proliferated. This technique could possibly be used to deliver anticoagulants, vasodilators or anti-angiogenic factors directly to the vessel wall in atherosclerotic patients.

Gene therapy is also being investigated for its possible role in the treatment of cancer. Transfected epithelial cells could be used to deliver high-dose chemotherapy selectively into the circulation of tumours or to deliver anti-tumour cytokines. Frequently cancer cells survive by escaping immune surveillance, and experiments have been carried out where tumour size has been reduced by transfecting the tumour cells with genes coding for immunogenic proteins. Lymphocytes have been transfected ex vivo with the tumour necrosis factor (TNF) alpha gene which is important in tumour cell killing, and infused back into patients with cancer.

Another exciting development has been the use of gene therapy in immunization. Influenza nucleoprotein has been expressed on mouse myocytes after intramuscular injection of a plasmid coding for the protein. The DNA was taken up into muscle cells and the protein expressed in association with class I MHC molecules, lead to an immune response. When the mice were subsequently challenged with influenza, considerable protection was observed.

Gene therapy is developing rapidly, and it is likely that before long it will have become standard treatment for certain diseases.

References

McDonnell W M, Askari F K 1996 DNA vaccines. New England Journal of Medicine 334; 1: 42-45

Wicks I 1995 Human gene therapy. Australian and New Zealand Journal of Medicine 25: 280-283

2. Ribozymes

A. **F**   B. **F**   C. **T**   D. **T**   E. **T**

In many disease processes mutant genes undergo transcription and then translation to form proteins which lead to abnormal cell functioning, including excessive proliferation in cancers and formation of new viruses or cell death in viral infection. The use of gene therapy to block or reverse these processes has received much publicity. An alternative approach is to target these processes at the translational level, where mRNA is translated into amino-acid sequences. The use of antisense oligonucleotides to do this is covered in the next question. Another method is to use ribozymes. These are a unique class of RNA which, in addition to storing information, also possess catalytic activity. Messenger RNA is single stranded and ribozymes match this mRNA with complementary base pairs of pre-mRNA. They are responsible for the splicing out of introns leaving ligated exons which form the mRNA for translation. Ribozymes specific for mutant or viral mRNA have been developed which, when added to affected cells, break the mRNA leading to its degradation. Ribozymes also rejoin mRNA and could potentially excise mutant stretches of mRNA leaving normal mRNA to be translated into unaffected protein.

A theoretical problem in implementing ribozymes as anti-viral and anti-cancer drugs is delivery of the molecules into the cells. Two possible solutions include their incorporation into liposomes and the insertion of ribozyme encoding genes into cells.

In oncogenesis the signal transduction pathway protein ras is frequently present in a mutated form. Experiments using human transitional cell carcinoma cells have demonstrated reduced invasion and metastasis in cell culture when a mutant H-ras specific ribozyme was added to cells. Similarly, when ribozymes directed against the mRNA for the bcr/abl protein in Philadelphia positive chronic myelocytic leukaemia are added to cell cultures, 99% inhibition of colony formation has been demonstrated. Another potential application is in combating the emergence of chemotherapy resistance in cancer. The human multidrug resistance (MDR)-1 gene encodes P-glycoprotein which decreases the influx and increases the efflux of chemotherapeutic agents from cells. Transfection of an MDR-1 RNA specific ribozyme into a human T cell leukaemia cell line resulted in a 35-fold increase in sensitivity to vincristine.

Future research will target drug delivery systems, protection of the ribozymes from degradation and the application of the new technology to a wider range of disease processes. Routine use in medical practice is not yet established, but may not be a long way off.

Reference

Kientopf M, Esquivel E L, Brach M A et al 1995. Clinical applications of ribozymes. Lancet; 345; 8956: 1027-1031

3. Antisense Oligodeoxynucleotides

A. F   B. T   C. T   D. F   E. T

The possibility of modifying gene expression to alter disease processes has received much recent interest. One possible method is to target the translational level, where messenger RNA (mRNA) is encoded into amino-acid sequences. If translation is inhibited, protein synthesis is curtailed. One approach is the use of antisense oligodeoxynucleotides (ODN). These are single stranded nucleotide stretches whose sequence is complementary to the mRNA of interest. By base pairing, a duplex is formed and the mRNA can no longer interact with the translational machinery. As a result, the production of the protein is blocked.

One of the potential problems of this therapeutic approach is the delivery of ODN across cell membranes in order that they can interact with intracellular mRNA. Some progress has been made using cationic liposomal delivery systems. Another problem is both the intra- and extracellular breakdown of the ODN to nucleosides and nucleotides. One possible solution is the chemical modification of these molecules to avoid the effects of nucleases. By improving ODN delivery and avoiding their breakdown, smaller doses can be used therapeutically, minimizing potential side-effects. Side-effects are likely to result from build-up of high doses of breakdown products which have been demonstrated to affect cell proliferation and differentiation.

Clinical trials are now in progress to evaluate the therapeutic potential of antisense ODN in human diseases, including acute myeloid leukaemia and infection by human immunodeficiency virus, cytomegalovirus and human papilloma virus.

References

Askari F K, McDonnell W M 1996 Antisense oligonucleotide therapy. New England Journal of Medicine 334: 316-319

Stein C A, Cheng Y C 1993 Antisense oligonucleotides as therapeutic agents – is the bullet really magic? Science 261: 1004-1012

Wagner R W 1994 Gene inhibition using antisense oligodeoxynucleotides. Nature 372: 333-335

4. Transcription-factors and disease

A. T   B. F   C. F   D. F   E. T.

Transcription-factors are proteins which regulate gene expression. They ensure that the right proteins are produced in the right cells, at the right time, in the right quantity, and in response to the correct signals. This is essential for embryonic development, growth and the ordered functioning of the adult organism. Transcription-factors have a modular structure with regions which bind to DNA sequences in the regulatory region of specific genes, known as DNA-binding domains, and regions which are designed to interact with RNA polymerase and thus control the rate of transcription.

Mutations of transcription-factors have been shown to be responsible for specific endocrine and developmental disorders and for the development of certain cancers. Some mutant transcription-factors may still be able to bind to their target site but are unable to activate transcription. By taking up the DNA-binding site they prevent the normal protein which is encoded by the wild-type gene from activating the target gene. This explains the dominant characteristics of some of these disorders. Dominance is also produced by haploid insufficiency, where the mutant protein does not inhibit the binding of the normal protein, but where the reduced quantity of normal protein proves insufficient to activate the gene.

Transcription-factors are classified together in families according to similarities in their DNA-binding domains. However, defects in transcription-factors of the same family often produce a diversity of diseases. Waardenburg's syndrome of deafness, heterochromia of the iris, and a white forelock has been associated with mutation of the transcription-factor PAX-3, while mutations of PAX-2 cause colobomas of the optic nerve and renal hypoplasia, and of PAX-6 cause aniridia.

Some transcription-factors are only transcribed in specific cells probably under the control of other transcription-factors. Pit-1 is produced only in the cells of the pituitary gland and controls the expression of the genes which encode proteins such as prolactin, growth hormone and thyrotrophin. Mutation of this factor results in mental retardation and failure to grow. Other transcription-factors are present in all cells in an inactive form and are activated by interactions with specific proteins such as steroid or thyroid hormones. In glucocorticoid resistance, distortion of the transcription-factor's hormone binding site prevents cortisol from activating it. In thyroid disease the mutant transcription-factor is left to exert widespread inhibitory effects as thyroid hormone is unable to bind to its mutated receptor site. This transcription-factor normally remains bound to its target gene and inhibits its expression until it is released by its interaction with thyroid hormone.

Certain cancers are known to result from the activation of oncogenes. Many oncogenes encode transcription-factors that regulate genes which produce proteins essential for cellular growth, such as DNA-directed DNA polymerase-alpha and thymidine kinase. Translocation of a gene to a position adjacent to a highly expressed gene will result in its overtranslation. This occurs in the pathogenesis of certain B and T cell leukaemias. It is by this mechanism that the myc oncogene causes Burkitt's lymphoma. It is translocated from chromosome 8 to a locus on chromosome 14 which is adjacent to that of the immunoglobulin heavy chain gene and is thus overexpressed resulting in excessive production of its protein and consequently cell proliferation. As well as producing excess amounts of normal gene products, translocation can result in fusion genes whose product is a novel protein with new unwanted effects. An example of this is in acute promyelocytic leukaemia where a gene for a retinoic acid receptor is fused with the promyelocytic leukaemia gene. Treatment with retinoic acid causes an initial improvement in the disease, but this is not sustained.

Anti-oncogenes inhibit cell growth, and their inactivation by mutation or deletion may result in cancer. Three anti-oncogenes, the retinoblastoma, Wilm's tumour, and p53 gene, encode transcription factors. Inherited germline mutations of the p53 gene result in the Li-Fraumeni syndrome, with breast, brain and bone tumours.

Cyclosporin and tacrolimus inhibit specific transcription-factors required for T cell activation. Fused DNA and corresponding RNA contain novel sequences which could be potential targets for antisense DNA or DNA binding proteins providing new therapeutic opportunities. New treatments for disorders involving transcription-factor dysfunction are still however remote.

Reference

Latchman D S 1996 Mechanisms of disease: transcription-factor mutations and disease. New England Journal of Medicine 334: 28-33

5.   Molecular biology

A. **F**   B. **T**   C. **T**   D. **T**   E. **T**

Translation occurs on macromolecules called ribosomes. Transcription produces a complementary single strand of messenger RNA (mRNA) from a DNA sequence within the nucleus. Each codon is a triplet of bases. Every DNA and complementary RNA triplet has four possible bases at each site in the triplet. This means there are 64 alternative codons (4x4x4=64).

Adenine and guanine are purines, cytosine and thymine are pyrimidines.

Most people have four copies of the alpha globin gene. Individuals with one of the alpha thalassaemias have fewer copies.

The ALU sequence is repeated about 500 000 times in the human genome. It is 300 bases in length and it does not code for a protein. Its function remains obscure.

Simple tandem repeats are sequences with repeated short lengths of bases. Any number of bases may be repeated. The greater the polymorphism in the number of repeats between individuals at a given locus, the more useful it is likely to be in linkage analysis. Loci are also selected for their proximity to the gene under study.

References

Housman D 1995 Human DNA polymorphism. New England Journal of Medicine 332: 318-321

Rosenthal N 1994 Tools of the trade - recombinant DNA. New England Journal of Medicine 331: 315-318

Rosenthal N 1994 Regulation of gene expression. New England Journal of Medicine 331: 931-934

Rosenthal N 1995 Recognising DNA. New England Journal of Medicine 333: 925-928

6.   Human DNA

A. **T**   B. **F**   C. **F**   D. **F**   E. **F**

Human DNA has certain properties which allow it to carry our genetic information with remarkable accuracy from one cell generation to the next and from one whole human organism to the next. Adenine can only pair with thymine and cytosine can only pair with guanine. This means that the sequence on one strand of DNA determines the sequence on the other strand of the double helix. This is crucial to the storage, retrieval and transfer of genetic information.

The genetic code is transcribed into messenger RNA (mRNA) in the nucleus. The translation of the mRNA sequence into an amino acid sequence occurs in ribosomes in the cytoplasm. Transfer RNA (tRNA) molecules recognize a unique three base pair sequence and they each carry a specific amino acid molecule. Ribosomal enzymes link adjoining amino acids carried by the tRNA molecules thus freeing them whilst constructing a unique protein structure.

Uracil replaces thymine in RNA. Another difference between RNA and DNA is in the sugar-phosphate backbone where ribose replaces deoxyribose.

Ribose is less stable than deoxyribose and as a consequence the proportions of different RNA sequences in the cytoplasm can change relatively rapidly in response to extracellular signals.

Remarkably, every cell in virtually every organism uses the same mRNA code to specify which amino acids are added to a growing protein chain. Recombinant DNA techniques take advantage of this to produce human proteins such as insulin and erythropoietin in bacteria.

References

Housman D 1995 Human DNA polymorphism. New England Journal of Medicine 332: 318-321

Rosenthal N 1994 Tools of the trade - recombinant DNA. New England Journal of Medicine 331: 315-318

Rosenthal N 1994 Regulation of gene expression. New England Journal of Medicine 331: 931-934

Rosenthal N 1995 Recognising DNA. New England Journal of Medicine 333: 925-928

7.   The polymerase chain reaction

A. **T**   B. **T**   C. **T**   D. **F**   E. **T**.

The polymerase chain reaction (PCR) is an increasingly used tool for the identification of DNA and RNA. It is very sensitive, allowing tiny amounts of genetic material to be amplified many times. At least part of the genetic sequence of the target DNA has to be known as the method depends on DNA primers annealing to single strands of DNA which have been split at high temperatures.

Sample DNA is obtained from a relevant source, for example, blood. It is then incubated with two single stranded DNA primers which are synthesized sequences of DNA complementary to the DNA of interest. Mixed with this is DNA polymerase and the DNA bases adenine, guanine, cytosine and thymine. The PCR reaction is set up in a temperature controlled environment using a thermocycle. Each PCR cycle starts at high temperatures (95°C) to split the double stranded DNA. It then cools to 60°C which is the optimal temperature for primer annealing and is then raised to 72°C for DNA synthesis. DNA sequences add to the primer sequence to duplicate the original DNA. The cycle can then restart with two new primers. If RNA is the genetic sequence of interest it has first to undergo reverse transcription by incubation with reverse transcriptase. After this DNA polymerase catalyses the synthesis of new double standed DNA with nucleotide bases in the incubation mixture.

The PCR is particularly useful for the detection of genetic material where more conventional methods may not be as sensitive. A disadvantage is that it is expensive to set up and the reaction may be contaminated by other DNA leading to false positive results. Practical applications of the technique include the identification of human immunodeficiency virus infection in neonates, hepatitis C infection in tissue biopsies or serum and mycobacterial infection in sputum. PCR is used for the tissue typing of organ transplant donors and recipients. Other clinical applications are the early detection of oncological markers, the detection of recurrence of malignancy in leukaemia and lymphoma and the antenatal diagnosis of cystic fibrosis.

Relatively crude preparations of DNA can be used for analysis, for example, cytology smears and skin scrapings.

Reference

Clark B, Gooi H C 1994 The polymerase chain reaction (PCR) and its clinical applications. Hospital Update 20: 278-286

8.   Western blotting

A. F   B. T   C. T   D. F   E. F

Western or immunoblotting is a three step process that can be used to detect the presence of a particular protein in a complex mixture. The first step is to separate the protein mixture on a polyacrymide gel. To the face of this gel is added a nitrocellulose membrane which binds most proteins. An electric field is applied which drives the proteins out of the gel and into the membrane. This is the part of the process which leads to the name 'blotting'. In the next step an antibody specific for the protein of interest is added and after incubation the membrane is washed to remove unbound antibody. Then an alkaline phosphatase linked antibody is added which binds to the first antibody. Finally a substrate is added and a purple precipitate is formed which marks the membrane band containing the protein of interest.

References

Lerner R A, Benkovic S J, Schultz P G 1991 At the crossroads of chemistry and immunology: catalytic antibodies. Science 252: 659-667

Lodish H, Baltimore D, Berk A et al (eds) 1995 Molecular cell biology. W H Freeman, New York

9. Southern blotting

A. T   B. T   C. F   D. T   E. T

Southern blotting, named after its inventor Edward Southern, can be used to identify specific fragments of DNA in a complex mixture. The DNA to be analysed is digested with a restriction enzyme giving restriction fragments. These fragments are separated according to size by gel electrophoresis. The separated restriction fragments are denatured with alkali and are transferred on to a nitrocellulose filter by blotting. This process preserves the distribution of the fragments in the gel, producing a replica. A radio-labelled DNA probe is then added and incubated with the restriction fragments. The DNA restriction fragment that is complementary to the probe hybridises with it and its location on the filter can be revealed by autoradiography. Southern blotting can be used to compare the restriction map of DNA isolated directly from an organism with the restriction map of cloned DNA. It can also be used to map restriction sites in genomic DNA next to the sequence of a cloned DNA fragment. This allows a comparison of the restriction maps of different individual organisms in the region surrounding a cloned fragment. Deletion and insertion mutations are readily detected, as well as sequence differences in specific restriction sites.

Northern blotting is used to detect a particular RNA in a mixture of RNAs. A RNA sample, for example the total cellular RNA, is denatured with an agent that prevents hydrogen bonding between base pairs. This gives the RNA an unfolded conformation. RNA is separated by gel electrophoresis and transferred to a nitrocellulose filter to which the denatured RNAs adhere. The filter is then exposed to a labelled DNA probe and the filter is developed by autoradiography. This process gives a semiquantitative measure of RNA allowing the amounts of particular messenger RNA in cells under different conditions to be compared.

References

Lodish H, Baltimore D, Berk A et al (eds) 1995. Molecular cell biology. W H Freeman, New York

Southern E M 1975 Detection of specific sequences among DNA fragments separated by gel electrophoresis. Journal of Molecular Biology 98: 503-515

10. Knockout mice

A. **T**   B. **F**   C. **T**   D. **F**   E. **T**

Inactivation or removal of a gene can be used to help us understand its function. The production of animals in which both alleles of a gene of interest have been removed or 'knocked out' can produce animal models of recessively inherited disease. To create an animal model of a dominant disease, a dominant gene is introduced into the genetic make-up of a fertilized oocyte to create a transgenic animal. A dominant gene need only replace one allele to produce its phenotypic effects.

The technique to produce knockout animals involves removing embryonic stem cells from the area of the blastocyst destined to become the fetus. These cells are then genetically altered and reinjected into the cavity of an intact blastocyst. The altered embryonic stem cells can populate all the tissues of the developing animal including the germ cells producing a chimeric animal. When the animal becomes an adult and breeds, some of the gametes will contain the inactivated gene and these will be passed on to the offspring. With selective breeding, animals homozygous for the inactivated gene are produced.

The process of genetically altering the embryonic stem cells is termed homologous recombination. The embryonic stem cells are incubated with a DNA vector which contains long stretches that are homologous to the DNA flanking the gene of interest. This permits the corresponding stretches of DNA to be exchanged. Homologous recombination only occurs in a small proportion of the incubated cells. These can be selected out by incorporating a gene coding for antibiotic resistance into the vector. This antibiotic resistance gene takes the place of the knocked out gene, and if the cells are incubated with that antibiotic, only those that have undergone homologous recombination will survive. The surviving cells are then injected into the blastocyst.

The deficits present in a knockout animal help us understand the function of the mutant gene and may also help us understand the mechanisms underlying a disease. In the study of embryogenesis, knockout experiments have shown that the gene coding sterogenic factor-1 is essential for adrenal and gonadal organogenesis, the Wilm's tumour locus WT-1 is essential for renal development, the myogenin gene for skeletal muscle development and the oestrogen receptor gene for sexual development. Sometimes the phenotype of the knockout animal can be predicted by prior knowledge of the gene's function. Occasionally however the phenotype is unexpected. For example when the interleukin-2 gene is knocked out in mice the animals develop an ulcerative colitis type disease. Knockout animals can be used as model systems to test new therapeutic agents including gene therapy.

The knocked out gene is inactive from the time of conception. The phenotype observed may be due to physiological adaptations to the mutation as well as the direct effects of the mutation. Some gene mutations cause embryonic or neonatal death, preventing the study of that mutation in adults. Knockout technology is being developed to allow the gene to be switched off later in an animal's development. Gene knockout as well as the production of transgenic animals promise to provide links between genetics and the pathogenesis of disease. With this knowledge we may be able to improve treatments for various human diseases.

Reference

Majzoub J A, Muglia L J 1996 Knockout mice. New England Journal of Medicine; 334: 904-907.

11. Transgenic animals

A. **F**   B. **F**   C. **F**   D. **F**   E. **F**

The ability to generate transgenic animals exploits the techniques of harvesting, manipulating and reimplanting early eggs and embryos. Recombinant DNA technology is used to isolate, characterize, and cut and paste genetic material. The aim is either to introduce exogenous DNA into a fertilized egg, which will then subsequently express its protein product, or to stop the expression of endogenous genes.

The transgene is the DNA which is transferred. It contains the nucleotide sequence corresponding to the gene of interest, as well as all the elements necessary for correct expression of the gene. An important component of this is the promoter or regulatory region that controls transcription. If a ubiquitous promoter is used the gene will be expressed in many tissues. Alternatively, selective expression can be coded for, using tissue specific promoters. Transgenic techniques have been applied to many animals including sheep, chicken and fish, but they have been most successfully used in mice.

Fertilized mouse eggs are harvested before the first cleavage from a female mouse which has been induced to hyperovulate with exogenous gonadotrophins and has then been mated. The transgenes are then injected by microinjection into the male pronucleus of each egg. They are cultured to the two cell stage and then implanted into a female mouse to complete gestation. About 20% will proceed to term and 20% of these will have incorporated the injected DNA into their genome. These transgenic pups are called founders and are identified by testing their genome for the transgene using Southern blot analysis. It is then necessary to determine whether the transgene is being expressed in the correct tissues and in the correct quantities by measuring the amount of messenger RNA or protein produced with quantitative tissue assays. The transgenic mice produced are heterozygous for the transgene in all their cells, including their germ cells, as the DNA was introduced into the male pronucleus before the first cell division.

The heterozygous founders are then mated with normal mice and the heterozygous mice produced are then mated with each other to produce homozygotes, which form the transgenic line.

Transgenic animals are used for producing models of disease and for assessing new therapies. Transgenic animals which overexpress the APP gene for the beta amyloid precursor protein develop neuropathological changes similar to those in people with Alzheimer's disease. Transgenes that express cytotoxic molecules have been used to destroy specifically brown adipose tissue. The animals produced were grossly obese, with deficient thermoregulation and exhibited insulin resistance and glucose intolerance. LacZ is a bacterial enzyme whose activity can be measured in vitro with a calorimetric assay. Transgenic animals with this lacZ transgene can be exposed to toxins and mutagens and specific tissues can then be tested to see to what extent the lacZ transgene has mutated, i.e. is no longer expressed. Transgenic animals thus provide models of disease and disease processes which can be used in biomedical research.

Reference

Shuldiner A R 1996 Transgenic animals. New England Journal of Medicine 334: 653-655

12. Mitochondrial DNA

A. **F**   B. **F**   C. **F**   D. **F**   E. **F**

Mitochondria are intracellular organelles which produce energy for cellular function in the form of adenosine triphosphate (ATP) through the process of oxidative phosphorylation. They are thought to have evolved from independent organisms which were incorporated into the cells of multicellular organisms. They have their own independent, circular, double stranded DNA molecules which are distinct from chromosomal or nuclear DNA.

They are able to replicate, transcribe and translate their DNA independently of nuclear DNA. Mitochondria and human cells are interdependent: normal cellular function requires the ATP produced by the mitochondria, and the mitochondria in turn rely on nuclear DNA to encode important structural and functional proteins including those involved in oxidative phosphorylation.

Mitochondrial DNA has many interesting features. It is inherited maternally and it does not recombine. Each cell contains many mitochondria and each mitochondrion contains 2 to 10 DNA molecules. Different mutations in mitochondrial DNA may be present in the same tissue, the same cell or even the same mitochondrion. If normal and abnormal mitochondrial DNA are present in the same cell then this is called heteroplasmy. Homoplasmy is when all the mitochondrial DNA in one cell is the same. Mitochondrial DNA has no introns, is estimated to mutate more than 10 times as frequently as nuclear DNA and has no effective repair mechanism. Many of these features are thought to contribute to its high association rate with many human diseases despite the small amount of genetic material in the mitochondria relative to the nucleus.

Reference

Johns D R 1995 Seminars in medicine from the Beth Israel Hospital, Boston: mitochondrial DNA and disease. New England Journal of Medicine 333: 638-644

---

13. Mitochondrial DNA

A. T   B. T   C. T   D. T   E. T

The mitochondrial diseases result in abnormalities of function through a variety of different genetic and non-genetic mechanisms. Some of the disorders can result from a single abnormal mitochondrial gene defect, others require epigenetic factors such as smoking before expression occurs. The same phenotype may be associated with several different genetic abnormalities and likewise the same genetic defect may lead to more than one phenotype. Specific mitochondrial syndromes have been described, but each individual case may have some of the other neurological, systemic or laboratory investigation features known to be associated with this group of disorders.

The neurological features include ophthalmoplegia, seizures, myoclonus, dystonia, stroke in young subjects, optic neuropathy, peripheral neuropathy, sensorineural hearing loss, myopathy, ataxia, dementia, psychiatric disorders and basal ganglia calcification.

The systemic manifestations include cardiac conduction defects, cardiomyopathy, diabetes mellitus, hypoparathyroidism, exocrine pancreatic dysfunction, short stature, cataract formation, lactic acidosis, pigmentary retinopathy, renal and liver abnormalities, intestinal pseudo-obstruction and pancytopenia. This wide range of defects probably reflects the fact that most tissues rely, at least to some extent, on oxidative phosphorylation. Patients will often first present with one of these non-specific systemic features before characteristic signs of their condition develop.

Possible laboratory findings associated with mitochondrial disease include elevated lactate levels in serum and cerebrospinal fluid, myopathic potentials on electromyography, axonal or demyelinating peripheral neuropathy on nerve-conduction studies, and ragged-red fibres in skeletal-muscle-biopsy specimens. These features can be helpful in diagnosing mitochondrial disorders but molecular genetic evidence will often be needed.

The encephalomyopathies are an uncommon group of disorders in which mitochondrial genetic defects were first identified. Chronic progressive external opthalmoplegia (including Kearns-Sayre syndrome), Leber's hereditary optic neuropathy and the MELAS syndrome (mitochondrial encephalomyopathy, lactic acidosis, and stroke-like episodes) are all examples of this group of disorders.

Reference

Johns D R 1995 Seminars in medicine of the Beth Israel Hospital, Boston: mitochondrial DNA and disease. New England Journal of Medicine 333: 638-644

14. p53

A. T   B. F   C. T   D. T   E. T.

p53 is a protein which acts as a potent and naturally-occurring tumour suppressor. Mutation in the gene coding for this protein results in protein dysfunction and an increased susceptibility to carcinogenesis. p53 has the ability to detect and bind to sites of primary DNA damage. This may form a focus for the assembly of proteins involved in DNA repair. By binding to damaged DNA, p53 is protected from proteolysis and induces either cell growth arrest or programmed cell death (apoptosis) depending on the type of cell. Both of these guard against replication and amplification of genetic damage.

Loss of p53 function may result from: mutation in its DNA binding sites, mutation leading to structural abnormalities in the protein or mutations of p53 cofactors and regulators. Loss of p53 function has been implicated in at least half of all human cancers. Restoration of p53 function, and therefore inhibition of cancer cell growth, has become an area of considerable interest in cancer research. Possible approaches include reintroducing the wild type p53 gene by gene therapy, restoring wild type p53 function by refolding the protein to its normal conformation or destroying the tumour cell via immunological recognition of structural mutant specific peptides.

Reference

Milner J 1995 DNA damage, p53 and anti-cancer therapies. Nature Medicine 1; 9: 879-880

15.   Viruses and cancer

A. T   B. F   C. F   D. T   E. T

It has now been established that various infectious agents are involved in the pathogenesis of certain cancers. Of these, viruses are the most important. A cell has to acquire multiple genetic changes to become malignant. Activation of oncogenes and inactivation of tumour suppressor genes by mutation are central events in oncogenesis. The latter is an almost invariable step. The prevalence of the viral infection is always much greater than the incidence of the associated cancer. Development of cancer often follows many years after initial infection and infection is only one of the many steps in oncogenesis.

Human T cell lymphotrophic virus-1 is a human retrovirus and is the cause of adult T cell leukaemia. The virus produces a possible oncogene, tax, which upregulates transcription of growth related genes.

Some of the tumours seen in human immunodeficiency virus-1 (HIV-1) infection are secondary to chronic immunosuppression as opposed to the direct oncogenic activity of the virus. Examples include lymphomas such as Epstein-Barr virus (EBV) related immunoblastic lymphoma, human papilloma virus (HPV) related anogenital cancers and Kaposi's sarcoma. The observation that Kaposi's sarcoma is much more common in patients with sexually acquired HIV-1 infection led investigators to look for a possible infectious agent in its pathogenesis. Human herpes-like virus DNA has been detected in specimens of Kaposi's sarcoma from various patient groups, raising the possibility that a new herpes virus may be involved in its pathogenesis.

DNA sequences from HPV are detectable in the majority of cervical, vulval and anal squamous cell carcinomas. Infection is usually with types 16 and 18. These types produce two proteins (E6 and E7), which act to promote tumourigenesis, E6 by promoting proteolytic degradation of p53 (important in DNA repair), and E7 by binding and inactivating the proteins of other tumour suppressor genes.

EBV is endemic in all populations. In the majority of individuals it is carried as a life long latent infection of lymphoid tissues. Some EBV encoded proteins expressed in latent infection can deregulate cell growth. Associated tumours include Burkitt's lymphoma, nasopharyngeal carcinoma, Hodgkin's lymphoma, some non-Hodgkin's lymphomas, salivary gland carcinomas, urogenital tumours, immunoblastic lymphomas in acquired immunodeficiency syndrome and lymphoproliferative disease in graft recipients. In nasopharyngeal carcinoma, EBV DNA is invariably present. A viral membrane protein LMP-1 has the ability to inhibit terminal differentiation of epithelial cells in culture, suggesting a possible role in tumourigenesis.

In chronic hepatitis B virus (HBV) infection the life time risk of hepatocellular carcinoma increases by a factor of 30 to 100 fold. In some patients it occurs without the development of cirrhosis, suggesting a specific virus-driven oncogenic process. HBV produces an antigen designated X which associates with p53 and inhibits regulation of transcription. This provides an obvious method by which HBV can lead to genomic instability and thus oncogenesis. Another possibility is that when HBV integrates into the host genome mutagenesis occurs. Hepatitis C virus (HCV) is also associated with hepatocellular carcinoma in the absence of cirrhosis, although the oncogenic process is unclear.

It can be seen that certain viruses have evolved to inactivate tumour suppressor genes and their products. These viral products may have evolved to increase host cell replication and promote viral replication, or to prevent apoptosis in response to viral infection. In the future it may be possible to reduce the incidence of cancers by vaccinating against viral infection, for example against EBV, HBV, HCV and HPV. It may be possible to interfere with the interaction of viral products with tumour suppressor gene products. It may even be possible to exploit virally encoded gene products to target cancer-cell specific gene therapy.

References

Huang Y Q, Li J J, Kaplan M H et al 1995 Human herpes virus-like nucleic acid in various forms of Kaposi's sarcoma. Lancet 345: 759-761

Morris J D H, Eddleston A L W F, Crook T 1995 Viral infection and cancer. Lancet 346: 754-758

Rady P L, Yen A, Rollefson J L et al 1995 Herpes like DNA sequences in non-Kaposi's sarcoma skin lesions of transplant patients. Lancet 345: 1339-1340

Rooney C M, Smith C A, Ng C Y, et al 1995 Use of gene-modified virus-specific T lymphocytes to control Epstein-Barr-virus-related lymphoproliferation. Lancet 345: 9-13

GENETICS
16. Alzheimer's disease

A. T   B. T   C. F   D. F   E. F

Alzheimer's disease is a syndrome of progressive cognitive failure and is the most common cause of late life dementia in developed countries. Early onset cases also occur and may present when patients are in their fifth decade. All cases develop extracellular plaques of the 40-42 residue amyloid beta-protein in the brain. Almost all develop neurofibrillary tangles which are intraneuronal bundles of abnormal filaments composed of highly phosphorylated forms of the microtubule-associated protein tau.

Chromosome 19 carries the apolipoprotein E gene (AD2). Inheritance of the naturally occurring E4 allele increases the likelihood of developing late onset Alzheimer's disease and lowers its age of onset. Conversely, inheritance of the E2 allele appears to confer a decreased risk.

Several missence mutations in the beta-amyloid-precursor protein gene on chromosome 21 (AD1) have been found in a few families with early onset Alzheimer's disease. These mutations lead to altered proteolytic processing of B-amyloid-precursor protein in a way that favours production of its amyloidogenic and potentially neurotoxic amyloid-beta fragment. These mutations on chromosome 21 account for only 2–3% of early onset Alzheimer's cases.

In 1992 a locus on chromosome 14q (AD3) was found that causes a particularly malignant form of familial Alzheimer's disease, with onset in the fifth decade, accounting for 70–80% of all early onset cases. By June 1995 the gene had been cloned. The gene, named S182, was found by collecting pedigrees of Alzheimer's-prone families in which the disease was linked to the chromosome 14 defect and then searching with DNA markers near the gene that would help narrow the search area. Once this had been achieved, individual genes were sequenced until a gene with mutations in conserved areas was found only in affected patients and not in unaffected family members and controls. From its sequence the S182 gene appears to code for a transmembrane protein. It has strong sequence analogy to a membrane protein (SPE-4) from a nematode worm. In the worm this protein is involved in transporting proteins between cellular compartments during the formation of sperm. It has been speculated that S182 may be involved in the intracellular transport and processing of amyloid-precursor protein and mutations in this gene may lead directly to B-amyloid accumulation.

A fourth locus (AD4) is found on chromosome 1 and may account for 20% of cases of early onset Alzheimer's disease. The gene product of this locus shows marked sequence analogy with S182 and is therefore also likely to be involved in beta-amyloid transport.

Discovery of genes involved in Alzheimer's disease offers hope for a diagnostic test for the disease and should lead to greater understanding of the biology of this complex syndrome.

References

Harrison P J 1995 S182: from worm sperm to Alzheimer's disease. Lancet 346: 388.

Hyman B T, Tanzi R 1995 Molecular epidemiology of Alzheimer's disease. New England Journal of Medicine 333: 1283-1284

Selkoe D J 1995 Missence on the membrane. Nature 375: 734-735

Sherrington R, Rogaev E I, Liang Y et al 1995 Cloning of a gene bearing missence mutations in early-onset familial Alzheimer's disease. Nature 375: 754-760

17. Breast cancer

A. F   B. F   C. T   D. F   E. T

In developed countries breast cancer is the most common cancer affecting women. The incidence increases with age, but the rate of increase declines after the age of 50.

A positive family history in a first degree relative results in a two to three fold increased risk. Other risk factors are early menarche, late menopause, nulliparity, obesity, prolonged use of the oral contraceptive pill, hormone replacement therapy, higher social class, high alcohol intake and high doses of ionising radiation. In addition to the reverse of the above, taking exercise in adolescence, prolonged breast feeding and oophorectomy are found to reduce the risk. Other factors whose role is yet to be clarified include dietary fat, vitamin A, carotenoids, smoking, pesticides and electromagnetic fields.

About 1 in 300 women carry the BRCA1 gene on chromosome 17 which has been cloned and sequenced. 4% of all patients with breast cancer have this gene. Women who carry the gene have an 85% chance of developing breast cancer by the age of 80 and half of these cases are likely to occur before the age of 50. This gene accounts for 25% of breast cancers in women under 40 years of age. Breast cancer occurs when the inherited mutant allele is accompanied by loss or inactivation of the wild type homologue.

Other genetic mutations which increase breast cancer susceptibility include BRCA2 (on chromosome 13), mutations of the p53 gene and polymorphisms of the oestrogen receptor gene. Ataxia telangiectasia heterozygotes are also at increased risk of breast cancer. This group has radiation sensitivity which renders mammography potentially hazardous. Identification of these genes is increasing our knowledge about cancer pathogenesis and providing preventative opportunities for young women. Screening of women with a positive family history of breast cancer for mutations of these genes is now possible. Increased surveillance with regular mammography and clinical examination allows earlier diagnosis in those identified as being at risk. The definitive preventative procedures of bilateral mastectomy and oophorectomy can still not offer 100% protection as tumours can develop in the chest wall. The role of the synthetic anti-oestrogen, tamoxifen, in primary prevention is being investigated in clinical trials.

References

Collins F S 1996 BRCA1: Lots of mutations, lots of dilemmas. New England Journal of Medicine 334: 186-189

Hulka B S, Stark A T 1995 Breast cancer: cause and prevention. Lancet 346: 883-887

18. Ataxia telangiectasia

A. **F**   B. **T**   C. **T**   D. **T**   E. **T**

Ataxia telangiectasia is a rare autosomal recessive disorder which typically presents in childhood with ataxia and progressive neuromotor degeneration. It has wide ranging effects including a propensity to lymphoreticular cancers, chromosomal instability, premature ageing, immunological abnormalities, growth retardation and hypersensitivity to ionizing radiation.

The gene responsible has recently been identified and is called the ATM gene. A region of the protein product has similarities with a known yeast DNA repair gene and another, with similarities to phosphoinositol-3 kinases, is involved with a variety of cellular transduction mechanisms such as responses to growth factors. Defects in these regions could be responsible for many of the features of the disease.

Heterozygotes have been estimated to make up for between 0.5 and 1.5% of the population. Heterozygotes appear to have an increased susceptibility for developing cancer and may account for up to 8% of breast cancer cases. They may also be more sensitive to radiotherapeutic and chemotherapeutic regimens.

References

Kastan M 1995 Ataxia-telangiectasia: broad implications for a rare disorder. New England Journal of Medicine 333: 662-663

Savitsky K, Bar-Shira A, Gilad S et al 1995 A single ataxia telangiectasia gene with a product similar to PI-3 kinase. Science 268: 1749-1753

Swift M, Chase C L, Morrell D 1990 Cancer predisposition of ataxia telangiectasia heterozygotes. Cancer Genet Cytogenet 46: 21-27

Swift M, Morrell D, Massey R B et al 1991 Incidence of cancer in 161 families affected by ataxia telangiectasia. New England Journal of Medicine 325: 1831-1836

19. Angiotensin converting enzyme

A. **T**   B. **F**   C. **T**   D. **F**   E. **F**

Angiotensin converting enzyme (ACE) is an ectoenzyme of vascular endothelial cells and plays a key part in the renin-angiotensin and kallikrein-kinin systems by activating angiotensin I to angiotensin II and inactivating bradykinin. The two peptide hormones have opposite effects on vascular tone and on smooth muscle cell proliferation. As neointimal proliferation and vasospasm may be involved in the pathogenesis of coronary heart disease, investigators have considered whether variability in ACE levels might be a risk factor for coronary heart disease.

The ACE gene has been cloned and is found on chromosome 17. Polymorphism exists at intron 16 with either an insertion (I) or deletion (D) giving II, ID or DD genotypes. Subjects with the DD genotype have circulating ACE levels twice as high as those with the II genotype. Some investigators have found that in patients suffering from myocardial infarction, the DD genotype is significantly more common than in the general population, although more recent reports have yielded conflicting results. The DD genotype is not associated with hypertension, and the exact mechanism by which it may increase cardiac risk is yet to be discovered. It is postulated that the higher resulting ACE levels might, by promoting atheroma formation, be an independent risk factor for ischaemic heart disease. Family linkage studies have indicated that the ACE insertion/deletion polymorphism is unlikely to be the locus directly influencing plasma ACE, but it could be a marker in strong linkage disequilibrium with this locus.

Animal studies have indicated that the DD genotype is a risk factor for restenosis after angioplasty. However, studies in different human populations have given conflicting results, with no clear relationship between the presence of the DD genotype and increased restenosis. The role of ACE inhibitors in the prevention of coronary heart disease is yet to be clarified.

A mutation of the angiotensinogen gene has also recently been shown to be associated with increased risk of coronary heart disease. In a large case control study comparing patients with coronary heart disease to controls, a methionine to threonine amino acid substitution at position 235 of the angiotensinogen gene was found to be significantly more common in the coronary heart disease group, particularly after other risk factors were controlled for.

References

Cambien F, Poirier O, Lecerf L et al 1992 Deletion polymorphism in the gene for angiotensin-converting enzyme is a potent risk factor for myocardial infarction. Nature 359: 641-644

Katsuya T, Koike G, Yee T W et al 1995 Association of angiotensinogen gene T235 variant with increased risk of coronary heart disease. Lancet 345: 1600-1603

Samani N, Martin D S, Brack M et al 1995 Insertion/deletion polymorphism in the angiotensin converting enzyme gene and risk of restenosis after coronary angioplasty. Lancet 345: 1013-1016

Teo K K 1995 Angiotensin converting enzyme genotypes and disease. British Medical Journal 311: 763-764

20. Hereditary haemorrhagic telangiectasia (HHT)

A. T   B. T   C. F   D. F   E. T

Osler-Weber-Rendu syndrome is now usually referred to as hereditary haemorrhagic telangiectasia (HHT). It is an autosomal dominant condition with high penetrance, and has equal sex distribution. It occurs in 1 in 25 000 of the western population. Patients usually present in childhood or early adult life with epistaxis. Examination often reveals telangiectasia on the skin and mucous membranes. Approximately 25% have gastrointestinal, 15% pulmonary and 4% cerebral involvement. Although HHT is a genetic disorder, its phenotypic expression is influenced by female sex hormones. Epistaxis is aggravated by low oestrogen states and improves during pregnancy. Oestrogen and progestogen therapy improves the epistaxis and gastrointestinal bleeding in HHT.

Pulmonary arteriovenous malformations (PAVMs) are more common in women with HHT. They may be detected by screening radiology or oximetry, and present with respiratory symptoms particularly dyspnoea and cyanosis. Hypoxia is caused by shunting of blood through PAVMs, which have a low resistance. PAVMs may also present with neurological symptoms secondary to paradoxical embolism or cerebral abscess. Paradoxical embolism occurred in 35% in one series of HHT complicated by PAVMs. Cerebral AVMs may cause symptoms secondary to pressure effects or haemorrhage. Gastrointestinal AVMs present with haemorrhage, which may be massive.

Management involves screening patients and their families for PAVMs and cerebral AVMs. Complications such as epistaxis or gastrointestinal haemorrhage are treated if recurrent or severe. PAVMs can now be successfully treated by percutaneous trans-catheter embolization with steel coils or detachable balloons, rendering surgery unnecessary in most cases. This therapy can be used in the chronic setting to improve hypoxia and prevent paradoxical embolism or acutely, to treat haemoptysis.

There has been striking progress in elucidating the cause of HHT. There is a genetic linkage on the long arm of chromosome 9. In 1994 mutations of the gene coding for endoglin were found in three families with HHT. Endoglin is a transforming growth factor-beta (TGF-beta) binding protein found in various tissues particularly endothelium and connective tissue. TGF-beta is an autocrine and paracrine growth factor, a potent angiogenic factor and mediates vascular modelling via production of the extracellular matrix. It is proposed that mutations of the endoglin gene lead to an interruption in the signal from TGF-beta to endothelial cells which in turn leads to abnormal blood vessel formation. Not all families with HHT have mutations of the endoglin gene and it is likely that mutations of other genes can give rise to the HHT phenotype. Other HHT genes may code for the TGF-beta receptor or binding proteins. As the molecular genetics of HHT is better understood, we may in the future be able to offer genetic screening as well as specific therapies which target the underlying molecular defects.

References

Hughes J M B 1994 Intra-pulmonary shunts: coils to transplantation. Journal of the Royal College of Physicians 28; 3: 247-253

McAllister K A, Grogg K M, Gallione C J et al 1994 Endoglin, a TGF-beta binding protein of endothelial cells, is the gene for hereditary haemorrhagic telangiectasia type 1. Nature Genetics 8: 345-351

McDonald M T, Papenberg K A, Ghosh S et al 1994 A disease locus for hereditary haemorrhage telangiectasia maps to chromosome 9q33-34. Nature Genetics 6: 197-204

St. Jacques S, Cymerman U, Pece N et al 1994 Molecular characterization of murine endoglin. Endocrinology 134; 6: 2645-2657

Shovlin C L, Hughes J M B, Scott J et al 1994 A gene for hereditary haemorrhagic telangiectasia maps to chromosome 9q3. Nature Genetics 6: 205-209

IMMUNOLOGY
21.   Human leucocyte antigens
A. **F**   B. **T**   C. **T**   D. **T**   E. **F**

The major histocompatibility complex (MHC) is divided, in humans, into three classes. The class I gene encodes 44 kDa transmembrane peptides associated at the cell surface with beta-2-microglobulin. These are the human leucocyte antigens (HLA) A, B and C and are present on virtually all cells in the body. They signal cytotoxic T cells. Class II molecules (HLA DR, DQ and DP) are transmembrane heterodimers, which are expressed on B cells and macrophages and signal T-helper cells. Class III products are heterogeneous but include complement components, heat shock proteins and tumour necrosis factors.

Many autoimmune and immune mediated diseases are genetically associated with specific HLA molecules. However, most individuals with these molecules do not develop disease. HLA molecules appear to have a permissive role in immune activation and therefore the development of autoimmune diseases.

Over 70 diseases are associated with HLA class II molecules, but in no case is identification of a particular HLA class II molecule diagnostic for a specific disease. In some rare diseases virtually all patients have a specific class II gene, examples being insulin autoimmune syndrome (DR4w13) and narcolepsy (DR2w2). These genes are common but demonstrate low penetrance such that more than 99% of individuals with them will not develop disease. Two-thirds of patients with the clinically and genetically heterogeneous diseases rheumatoid arthritis and type I diabetes carry a specific HLA susceptibility gene. These genes also do not show full penetrance but because these diseases are common, HLA typing can be used to predict disease onset and prognosis.

The HLA DR beta locus encodes the genotypes associated with severe aggressive erosive rheumatoid arthritis. DRw4 carries a 1 in 35 risk, DRw14 a 1 in 20 risk and possession of both a 1 in 7 risk. This final genotype (DRw4/DRw14) is associated with a particularly aggressive, early onset form of disease.

67% of patients with type 1 diabetes have the susceptibility gene DQ3.2, which is found in 27% of the normal population. However, only 1 in 60 people with this genotype will develop the disease. The risk increases to 1 in 25 if the DQ2 antigen is present in addition to the DQ3.2 antigen. The penetrance of the HLA susceptibility genes is increased by the presence of certain non-HLA genes in some families and this explains why possession of DQ3.2/DQ2, when combined with a positive family history, gives a 1 in 4 risk of developing disease.

HLA typing is not useful in population screening to predict risk of developing disease because even for the more common diseases, like rheumatoid arthritis and type 1 diabetes, the vast majority of people with the associated HLA gene will not develop the disease. However, there may be a role for HLA type identification once known HLA associated diseases have developed. In rheumatoid arthritis, patients who have the associated HLA genes usually have much more aggressive disease. These patients can therefore be targeted for more aggressive therapy. In type 1 diabetes the DQ3.2./DQ2 genotype is associated with early onset disease. Patients with this genotype, particularly if they have a positive family history and measurable autoantibodies may be targeted for immunotherapy to prevent or delay overt clinical disease.

Understanding the role of these class II molecules holds promise for the development of more specific forms of immunotherapy. In diabetes the HLA susceptibility gene encodes for the specific part of the HLA molecule which binds to the antigenic peptide. In contrast, in rheumatoid arthritis the susceptiblity gene encodes the part ot the HLA molecule which directly interacts with the T cell receptor.

As our understanding of HLA molecular interactions increases we may be able specifically to target these interactions for therapeutic intervention.

References

Klareskog L, Ronnelid J, Holm G 1995 Immunopathogenesis and immunotherapy in rheumatoid arthritis: an area in transition. Journal of Internal Medicine 238: 191-206

Nepom G T 1995 Class II antigens and disease susceptibility. Annual Review of Medicine 46: 17-25

22. Adhesion molecules

A. F   B. F   C. T   D. T   E. T

The adhesion of leucocytes to endothelium is a critical step in both the effective immune response to tissue injury and in many diseases characterized by an excessive immune response. A great deal of research attention has focused on the manipulation of the molecules responsible for these adhesions.

Selectins and the ICAM family are found mainly on endothelial cells and are upgraded by inflammatory cytokines like tumour necrosis factor (TNF) and interleukin-1 (IL-1) as well as by endotoxins. Selectins are transmembrane glycoproteins which cause adhesion of leucocytes (neutrophils, monocytes, eosinophils and some lymphocytes) by interaction with carbohydrate molecules on these cells. The ICAM family causes adhesion by interaction with the beta-2 integrins on the leucocyte surface.

E-selectin reaches maximal levels 5 hours after tissue insult. P-selectin is synthesized and stored in granules of platelets and endothelial cells. Various stimuli, including thrombin, histamine and certain complement components, lead to the rapid redistribution of P-selectin within minutes to the cell surface. IL-1 and TNF enhance the synthesis of P-selectin. L-selectin is expressed by most leucocytes and participates in the localization of lymphocytes to lymph nodes, and neutrophils and monocytes to sites of inflammation. Initial contact of leucocytes with activated endothelium requires the interaction of selectins E and P with carbohydrate molecules like tetrasaccharide sialyl Lewis x on leucocytes.

Other endothelial expressed adhesion molecules belong to the immunoglobulin (Ig) superfamily, including ICAM-1, ICAM-2, VCAM-1 and PECAM-1. ICAM-1 is a transmembrane glycoprotein with 5 Ig domains expressed on haemopoietic and non-haemopoietic cells. VCAM-1 is found on endothelial cells as well as dendritic and bone marrow stromal cells. Like ICAM-1, it is upregulated by inflammatory cytokines over several days. ICAM-2 is expressed by endothelial and non-endothelial cells and has two extracellular Ig domains. Unlike ICAM-1 and VCAM-1 its expression is not modified by inflammatory cytokines.

The beta-2 integrins contain 1 of 3 alpha chains and a common beta chain. They are activated by complement components, cytokines and lipid mediators like platelet activating factor (PAF).

During the inflammatory response E-selectin is expressed early, correlating with neutrophil influx, whereas ICAM-1 and VCAM-1 expression occurs over a more prolonged time course, correlating with monocyte and lymphocyte influx. Congenital defects of adhesion molecules are associated with frequent severe infections, reinforcing the central role of these molecules in the immune response. Because of this central role, the adhesion molecules form an obvious target in diseases where the immune system itself causes pathology. Interestingly, in addition to their effects on prostaglandins, platelet activating factor and cytokines, corticosteroids inhibit the expression of endothelial E-selectin and ICAM-1.

In both humans and in experimental animal models of human disease various adhesion molecules have been shown to be upregulated, and antibodies to these molecules have been successful in reducing inflammation and delaying disease progression. In some diseases like vasculitis, sepsis, adult respiratory distress syndrome, asthma, glomerulonephritis, rheumatoid arthritis, inflammatory bowel disease and multiple sclerosis, as well as organ graft rejection and graft-versus-host disease, an involvement of adhesion molecules in the disease process has been suggested by experimental evidence. The adhesion molecules play an important role in other conditions however, where the role of inflammation is less obvious. Atherosclerosis and haematogenous dissemination of neoplasms are two examples. In the example of tumour metastasis, tumour cells have been shown to express integrins and tetrasaccharide sialyl Lewis x leading to their adherence to VCAM-1 and E-selectin respectively.

Reference

Bevilacqua M P, Nelson R M, Mannori G et al 1994 Endothelial-leucocyte adhesion molecules in human disease. Annual Review of Medicine 45: 361-378

23. Common variable immunodeficiency

A. T   B. T   C. F   D. F   E. T

The primary immunodeficiency disorders reflect abnormalities in the development and maturation of the immune system. These defects result in an increased susceptibility to infection. Recurrent pyogenic infections occur with defects of humoral immunity, and opportunistic infections with defects in cell-mediated immunity.

Common variable immunodeficiency is a term used to designate a group of as yet undifferentiated syndromes all characterized by defective antibody formation. The diagnosis is based on the exclusion of other known humoral immune defects. Several patterns of inheritance have been noted. It is the most frequent of the primary immunodeficiencies among populations of European origin. It affects men and women equally and it usually presents in the second or third decade of life.

Presentation is usually with recurrent pyogenic sinopulmonary infections. Without early diagnosis and treatment chronic obstructive lung disease and bronchiectasis may develop. Recurrent attacks of opportunistic infections also occur.

A 50 fold increase in gastric carcinoma has been observed and the risk of developing lymphoma is also markedly increased. Diffuse lymphadenopathy, splenomegaly and nodular lymphoid hyperplasia of the gastrointestinal tract leading to a coeliac-like syndrome also occur. Inflammatory bowel disease is more common. Patients are also more prone to a variety of autoimmune disorders.

Defective antibody production leads to decreased serum IgG concentrations and usually also decreased IgA and IgM concentrations. It is thought that many patients with common variable immunodeficiency have defective interactions between T and B cells leading to reduced antibody production and a failure in B cell differentiation and proliferation.

Reference

Rosen F S, Cooper M D, Wedgwood R J 1995 Medical progress: the primary immunodeficiencies. New England Journal of Medicine 333: 431-440

---

24. Primary immunodeficiencies
A. **F**   B. **T**   C. **F**   D. **F**   E. **F**

X-linked agammaglobulinaemia is an X-linked recessive trait. It usually presents towards the end of the first year of life with recurrent pyogenic infections. Bronchiectasis and chronic obstructive lung disease can develop. Chronic meningo-encephalitis, a syndrome resembling dermatomyositis, chronic *Giardia lamblia* infestation and a large joint arthritis often caused by *Ureaplasma urealyticum* also occur. Prophylaxis with intravenous immune globulin has become the standard therapy. It is relatively safe but outbreaks of hepatitis C virus infection have occurred. A defect in a tyrosine kinase gene called btk (Bruton's or B cell tyrosine kinase) seems to be the main genetic abnormality responsible. This gene has been shown to be involved in B cell maturation.

Hyper-IgM syndrome resembles X-linked agammaglobulinaemia clinically but there is an increased incidence of opportunistic infections and autoimmune diseases. It is characterized by undetectable amounts of IgA and IgE and very low levels of IgG but normal or elevated levels of IgM. Approximately 70% are X-linked and the defect is an inability of T cells to synthesize the CD40 ligand. The CD40 ligand is normally expressed on activated T cells and it interacts with the CD40 on B cells as part of the normal switching process by which B cells convert from IgM production to the production of other immunoglobulins.

Severe combined immunodeficiency has many genetic causes. It presents as a medical emergency with profound lymphopenia in the first few months of life. Persistent candida, *Pneumocystis carinii*, herpes, varicella, adenovirus and cytomegalovirus infections all occur. Early bone marrow transplantation is the treatment of choice. It is more common in boys as 50–60% of cases are X-linked. Defects in the gamma chain of the interleukin-2 receptor have been found. The gamma chain is also an important component of the receptors for interleukins-4, 7, 11 and 15.

Other immunodeficiency syndromes include defects in the MHC class molecules and the Wiskott-Aldrich syndrome. This is an X-linked recessive disorder characterized by profound thrombocytopenia, small platelets, low serum IgM concentrations and a progressive decrease in the number of T cells. Cases are susceptible to bloody diarrhoea and pyogenic and opportunistic infections. Bone marrow transplantation is the treatment of choice.

Reference

Rosen F S, Cooper M D, Wedgwood R J 1995 Medical progress: the primary immunodeficiencies. New England Journal of Medicine 333: 431-440.

25. Autoimmune disorders

A. F   B. T   C. F   D. F   E. T

Autoimmunity is the loss of tolerance to self-antigens. Autoantibodies are produced to a wide variety of antigens. They may be organ specific like thyroid antibodies in Hashimoto's disease and intrinsic factor antibodies in pernicious anaemia, or non-organ specific like antinuclear antibodies in systemic lupus erythematosus.

Three mechanisms are involved in the pathogenesis of autoimmune disease. Firstly, immune complex mediated disease occurs when antibody-antigen complexes form and are deposited in tissues. Secondly, in cell-mediated immunity, sensitized T cells cause injury through the release of lymphokines. Thirdly, circulating autoantibodies react with antigens on the surfaces of cells stimulating the release of inflammatory mediators and inducing cell lysis. In myasthenia gravis antibodies have been shown to reduce the number of acetylcholine receptors on the post-synaptic membrane by at least three processes. There is accelerated endocytosis and degradation of the receptors, functional blockade of acetylcholine binding sites and complement mediated lysis of the receptors.

A set of five criteria define the pathogenesis of autoantibody-mediated disorders. Specific antibody must be present and be shown to interact with the target antigen, passive transfer of the antibody should reproduce features of the disease, immunization with the antigen should produce a model of the disease, and a reduction in antibody levels should ameliorate the symptoms of the disease.

Many autoimmune diseases have been shown to be more common in patients with certain human leucocyte antigen (HLA) alleles. Thus autoimmune chronic active hepatitis, Grave's disease, myasthenia gravis without thymoma, Addison's disease, Sjögren's syndrome and systemic lupus erythematosus are linked to HLA B8 DR3, Goodpasture's syndrome to DR2, rheumatoid arthritis to DR4 and Hashimoto's thyroiditis to DR5.

Reference

Drachman D B 1994 Myasthenia gravis. New England Journal of Medicine 330: 1797-1807

26. Xenotransplantation

A. **F**   B. **F**   C. **T**   D. **T**   E. **T**

Xenotransplantation is the transplantation of tissue between different species. Xenografts are concordant if they occur between species which are phylogenetically closely related and discordant if they are phylogenetically widely removed. Interest in xenotransplantation has increased as the gap between demand for donor organs and the supply of organs widens. The barriers to this form of transplantation are great. They include early and aggressive rejection, xenozoonosis (transmission of infection from the animal donor to humans), the ethical issues involved in the sacrifice of animals for human gain and whether animal tissues and organs can maintain the required physiological functions. To date animal organs have supported human life for many months. For example, chimpanzee kidneys have supported life for 9 months and a baboon heart has supported an infant for 3 weeks. In the transplantation of animal liver to humans, biochemical markers of liver failure have improved, suggesting that animal organs can perform at least some of the metabolic functions required by humans.

At present the greatest barrier to successful xenotransplantation is early and aggressive rejection which appears to be mediated by humoral mechanisms. Rejection is either hyperacute or acute. Hyperacute rejection is mediated by IgM antibodies in discordant *transplants.* Acute rejection occurs in concordant species due to the formation of IgG antibodies to donor antigens. These antibodies target the donor vascular endothelium and rejection results in an occlusive endothelialitis. Complement plays a central role in hyperacute rejection either via the classical pathway (after antibody binding) or the alternative pathway. In humoral rejection, endothelial cell activation is a central event in organ failure.

Long-term survival of xenografts requires control of cellular as well as humoral rejection. In vitro studies have suggested that the cellular response to xenotransplantation may be weaker than in allotransplantation.

A difficult issue is which patients should be offered xenotransplantation rather than allotransplantation. In view of the current poor results with xenotransplantation, this means that further studies in humans should probably not proceed until the results of xenotransplantation to non-human primates approach those of allotransplantation. Recently baboon bone marrow has been transplanted into patients with advanced acquired immunodeficiency syndrome (AIDS) because human immunodeficiency virus-1 does not infect baboon T cells. It is too early to say whether this procedure will improve survival.

Given the enhanced immune rejection of xenotransplants, new methods of immunosuppression are being developed. These include new drugs which suppress both humoral and cellular immunity, plasmapheresis, organ absorption and column absorption of antibodies and splenectomy. Genetic manipulation of donor tissue is also being investigated as a way of preventing cellular rejection.

Xenotransplantation is not yet a viable treatment option for patients with end stage organ failure. However, the enormous efforts being made in overcoming the barriers to this form of therapy promise to enrich our understanding of immunology and hopefully will one day enable more patients to receive life saving transplantation.

Reference

Steele D J R, Auchincloss Jr H 1995 Xenotransplantation. Annual Review of Medicine 46: 345-360

BASIC SCIENCE
27. Nitric Oxide
A. T   B. T   C. F   D. T   E. T

Over the past 10 years nitric oxide has been found to be an ubiquitous biological mediator. It is synthesized from arginine and regulates the activity of soluble guanylate cyclase and thus the intracellular concentration of cyclic guanosine monophosphate (c GMP) through which it mediates its cellular affects. Nitric oxide is a free radical which decomposes rapidly to nitrate and nitrite. Antioxidants protect nitric oxide by scavenging other free radicals.

Nitric oxide synthetases are large complex proteins of which three isoenzymes, endothelial, neuronal, and macrophage, have been identified. Their genes have been located on chromosomes 7, 12, and 17 respectively. The macrophage type is an inducible enzyme capable of producing large quantities of nitric oxide with local toxic effects. Unlike the other synthetases it is not expressed under normal physiological conditions.

In the cardiovascular system nitric oxide is released continuously from arterial and arteriolar endothelium causing vasodilation and regulating basal vascular tone. In contrast, veins have no basal nitric oxide synthesis. Inhibitors of nitric oxide synthesis block relaxation of the corpus cavernosum and prevent erection. Nitric oxide is also thought to inhibit platelet and white cell adhesion and aggregation. It affects cardiac relaxation during diastole and may be negatively inotropic. Nitric oxide relaxes smooth muscle and is thought to play a part in bronchodilation and in the relaxation of sphincters in both the gastrointestinal and urinary tracts.

Nerves which stain for nitric oxide synthetases have been found in the cardiovascular system, the bronchial tree, urinary tract and gut forming a putative nitrergic nervous system. In the central nervous system nitric oxide is thought to be involved in memory, cortical arousal and the modulation of pain perception.

Human cells express inducible nitric oxide synthetase in response to exposure to endotoxins and cytokines. In mice nitric oxide has been shown to be important in killing pathogens, mediating non-specific immunity and in killing tumour cells. It has been suggested that nitric oxide may be responsible for the cerebral damage seen in stroke, Parkinson's disease, acquired immunodeficiency syndrome (AIDS) and dementia. The enzyme is induced in the joints of patients with rheumatoid arthritis, the colons of patients with ulcerative colitis and the ventricles of patients with cardiomyopathy.

The pharmacological applications and interactions of nitric oxide are myriad. Nitric oxide has been found to be the active moiety of nitrodilators. Their particular effectiveness at reducing preload might be explained by upregulation of nitric oxide receptors in the venous system in response to low nitric oxide basal concentrations. This would make the venous system more sensitive to exogenously administered nitric oxide in the form of nitrodilator agents. Angiotensin converting enzyme inhibitors are found to inhibit the degradation of bradykinin which stimulates endothelial cells to produce nitric oxide. Glucocorticosteroids and antifungals such as imidazole inhibit the induction of the macrophage isoenzyme and methotrexate inhibits the synthesis of an essential cofactor for nitric oxide synthesis.

Inhibition of nitric oxide synthetases with substrate analogues such as N-monomethyl-L-arginine have been shown to reverse the local vasodilation associated with inflammation and the hypotension seen in patients with septic shock. Selective inhibitors of the inducible isoform of nitric oxide synthetase are being developed as possible anti-inflammatory drugs.

References

Burnett A L, Lowenstein C J, Bredt D S et al 1992 Nitric oxide: a physiological mediator of penile erection. Science 257: 401-403

Moncada S, Higgs A 1993 Mechanisms of disease: the L-arginine-nitric oxide pathway. New England Journal of Medicine 329: 2002-2012

Vallance P, Collier J 1994 Biology and clinical relevance of nitric oxide. British Medical Journal 309: 453-457

28. Vitamin K

A. F   B. T   C. T   D. F   E. F

Vitamin K is a fat soluble vitamin which is required for the synthesis of clotting factors II, VII, IX and X. Vitamin K has several molecular forms. Phylloquinone is the only important form in plants, whereas bacteria synthesize a number of menaquinones. Dietary vitamin K comes mainly from green leafy vegetables and vegetable oils and in smaller amounts from fish, red meat and cereals. It is probable that vitamin K is also partly derived from the large pool of menaquinones synthesized by the gut microflora. Vitamin K is stored mainly in liver and bone. It is transported in the plasma by triglyceride-rich lipoproteins rather than low-density lipoproteins, and fasting plasma phylloquinone concentrations are strongly influenced by apolipoprotein E polymorphism.

Non-iatrogenic vitamin K deficiency resulting in bleeding is very rare in adults. In the neonate it is a well recognized cause of spontaneous haemorrhage in the first 6 months of life. Interestingly, exclusive breast feeding is associated with an increased incidence of haemorrhagic disease of the newborn because the concentration of vitamin K in breast milk is low. To help prevent haemorrhagic disease of the newborn, routine vitamin K prophylaxis was introduced in the 1950s. An epidemiological study which suggested an association between intramuscular vitamin K prophylaxis and the later development of childhood cancer spurred much debate. Further studies failed to confirm these results but many centres are now giving vitamin K prophylaxis orally rather than by the intramuscular route. Concerns about the bioavailability of the oral form and the fact that many infants are not completing the whole course are causing continuing debate.

A diverse group of proteins not involved in the clotting cascade has been found to be dependent on vitamin K. Vitamin K acts to promote the conversion of glutamate residues to gamma-carboxyglutamate (Gla) on these proteins. Osteocalcin is a Gla-containing protein in bone and the Gla residues facilitate calcium binding to the hydroxyapatite matrix of bone. Osteocalcin and matrix Gla protein, another vitamin K-dependent bone matrix protein, are synthesized by osteoblasts. It is unclear whether the normal functions of these proteins, and therefore of bone, are affected by vitamin K status. Experimental vitamin K deficiency and short-term warfarin therapy have not been shown to affect bone healing and structure. Markers of uncarboxylated osteocalcin are strongly correlated with the subsequent risk of hip fracture in women and low circulating levels of phylloquinones have been found in patients sustaining either spinal crush fractures or fractures of the neck of the femur. It is not known whether long-term deficiency of vitamin K or warfarin therapy impairs skeletal integrity in mature bone, but there is substantial evidence that vitamin K deficiency has toxic effects on rapidly growing bone.The fetal warfarin syndrome is well recognized and results in excess calcification of the epiphyses and irregular growth of the facial and long bones.

References

Golding J, Greenwood R, Birmingham K et al 1992 Childhood cancer, intramuscular vitamin K, and pethidine given during labour. British Medical Journal 308: 341-346

Shearer M J 1995 Vitamin K. Lancet 345: 229-234

29. Vitamin D
A. T   B. T   C. F   D. F   E. F

30. Vitamin D
A. T   B. T   C. F   D. F   E. F

Cholecalciferol (vitamin D3) is formed by the action of ultraviolet radiation on 7- dehydrocholesterol. This is converted to 25-hydroxycholecalciferol in the liver and transported to the proximal renal tubule. Here it is further hydroxylated to 1,25-dihydroxycholecalciferol (1,25 (OH)D), the active form, which is classified as a steroid hormone. Like other steroid hormones,1,25 (OH)D binds to an intranuclear receptor. The vitamin-receptor complex then directly affects the transcription of specific proteins responsible for the cellular functions of vitamin D. It does this by binding to regulatory sequences of DNA. The interaction of the vitamin D receptor and DNA is influenced by a number of factors. Interleukins, interferons and c-myc downregulate receptor function, and prolactin and fibronectin upregulate receptor function.

The traditional role of vitamin D is in calcium homeostasis. Vitamin D helps to maintain a constant extracellular calcium concentration by its effects on bone turnover, renal tubular function and gut calcium absorption. However, vitamin D is probably involved in many other physiological processes. In vitro studies have demonstrated that 1,25 (OH)D can inhibit proliferation and promote differentiation in a variety of cells. A synthetic analogue of 1,25 (OH) D, calcipotriol, has equal effects on cell differentiation but much less potent effects on calcium homeostasis. Calcipotriol has found clinical use as a topical agent in the treatment of psoriasis, a disorder characterized by excess proliferation of skin epithelial cells. The muscle weakness of vitamin D deficiency suggests it has a role in regulation of skeletal muscle cells. Increased susceptibility to infection in children with rickets may reflect an influence of vitamin D in regulating immune function.

Epidemiological studies have linked vitamin D status with risk of cardiovascular disease and colon cancer. In vitro studies have shown an action of 1,25 (OH) D on myocytes, large vessel intimal cells and colonic mucosal cells and it may be that any effect of vitamin D in these diseases is mediated by the cellular effects of 1,25 (OH) D.

Infants, adolescents and the elderly are particularly vulnerable to vitamin D deficiency. This usually results from inadequate exposure to sunlight. It is unusual for a diet to be deficient in vitamin D. However, diets deficient in calcium are common and this leads to increased clearance of 25 (OH) D by hepatocytes and secondary vitamin D deficiency. The same situation occurs in chronic malabsorption. Vitamin D deficiency causes rickets in children and osteomalacia in adults (with a biochemical profile of low phosphate, low or low normal calcium and high alkaline phosphatase).

The ingestion of large amounts of synthetic vitamin D results in toxicity. Affected individuals have hypercalcaemia and metastatic microcalcification of soft tissues, but the toxic action is probably independent of the effects on calcium homeostasis. In rats ingestion of large amounts of vitamin D produces death before hypercalcaemia develops suggesting a direct toxic effect on essential cellular functions by a vitamin D metabolite. It is thought that the toxic effects are mediated directly by 1,25 (OH) D. After excessive ingestion, large amounts of 25 (OH) D are produced which have high affinity for the plasma binding protein, resulting in displacement of 1,25 (OH) D and therefore toxic tissue concentrations of this form.

Osteoporosis is characterized by normal bone mineralization but a reduction in total bone mass. Although it does not correlate directly with vitamin D status, bone loss in the elderly is related to osteocalcin concentration which is partly regulated by vitamin D. Osteocalcin is a protein secreted by osteoblasts and levels in blood reflect bone metabolic function. Variation in osteocalcin concentration and levels of bone loss in the elderly are genetically determined. Osteocalcin production is induced by binding of 1,25 (OH) D and its receptor complex to promoter regions of the osteocalcin gene. The 1,25 (OH) D receptor is a protein with genetically determined polymorphism and a particular allelic variant of this is related to increased bone loss in old age. A study of dizygotic and monozygotic twins found a significant association between receptor genotype and bone mineral density. It is possible that the genotyping of individuals will help identify those at risk of osteoporosis and help target preventative therapy.

References

Fraser D R 1995 Vitamin D. Lancet 345; 8942: 104-108

Spector T D, Keen R W, Arden N K et al 1995 Influence of vitamin D receptor genotype on bone mineral density in postmenopausal women: a twin study in Britain. British Medical Journal 310: 1357-1360

31. Hypercalcaemia
A. F   B. T   C. F   D. T   E. F

90% of patients with hypercalcaemia have either hyperparathyroidism or malignancy. Evidence of ectopic calcification such as renal stones usually points to the former diagnosis, while most patients with malignancy will have overt signs or symptoms of their underlying disease at presentation. Some patients who are found to have hypercalcaemia while being investigated for malignancy have concomitant hyperparathyroidism. A relatively new parathyroid hormone assay based on the double antibody method gives accurate parathyroid hormone levels and can be used to differentiate between the two most common causes of hypercalcaemia. In malignancy the level will be low.

The incidence of hyperparathyroidism is 0.5 per 1000 in the general population but it is especially common in post-menopausal women. It is caused by an adenoma in 90% of patients, of which 50% are diagnosed on routine blood tests and are asymptomatic at presentation.

10–15% of patients with lung cancer have hypercalcaemia. It is also commonly found in patients with cancer of the breast and kidney and in patients with myeloma and lymphoma. It was traditionally thought that the development of hypercalcaemia was due to a direct destructive effect of the tumour on bone resulting in calcium mobilization.

Parathyroid hormone related protein has been implicated in the humoral hypercalcaemia which occurs in squamous cell carcinoma of the lung and kidney, where there is hypercalcaemia with hypophosphataemia. A parathyroid hormone related protein has been identified which competes with parathyroid hormone for its receptor. It has been shown to stimulate cyclic AMP production and cause bone resorption in vitro. It can also induce hypercalcaemia in test animals.

In patients with lymphoma, high levels of vitamin D have been implicated in the development of hypercalcaemia; whether these are due to ectopic production or an increase in 1-alpha hydroxylase activity at the kidney is not known. In breast cancer prostaglandins of the E series are found to be potent stimulators of bone resorption. Other bone resorbing factors such as tumour necrosis factor, interleukin-1 and osteoclast activating factor may also play a role in the hypercalcaemia of certain malignancies.

In sarcoidosis the cause of hypercalcaemia is excess vitamin D. It is thought that there is ectopic synthesis of 1,25-dihydroxycholecalciferol in macrophages and that this is not under parathyroid hormone control. Normocalcaemic patients with sarcoidosis have unregulated production of 1,25-dihydroxycholecalciferol in response to vitamin D loading and so should be advised to avoid direct sunlight or excess oral intake of vitamin D.

Patients presenting with hypercalcaemia have a gross sodium and water deficit. The initial management is rehydration with normal saline. Loop diuretics depress tubular reabsorption of calcium. Osteoclast inhibitors like the bisphosphonates take 2 to 3 days to have their effect. The most potent is pamidronate which is given intravenously. Glucocorticoids decrease calcium absorption from the gut and cause a negative skeletal calcium balance. They are of no benefit in hyperparathyroidism but are used in the treatment of vitamin D related hypercalcaemia including sarcoidosis and in the hypercalcaemia of malignancy. Calcitonin reduces skeletal release of calcium, phosphates and hydroxyproline within minutes of injection and increases the renal clearance of calcium and phosphates. However, escape from the drug's action occurs in 12–24 hours.

In young patients with hypercalcaemia secondary to hyperparathyroidism a diagnosis of multiple endocrine neoplasia (MEN) must be considered. MEN 1 or Werner's syndrome consists of hyperparathyroidism and tumours of the pancreatic islet cells and pituitary, while MEN IIa consists of hyperparathyroidism, phaeochromocytoma and medullary carcinoma of the thyroid.

Reference

Martin T J, Grill V 1995 Hypercalcaemia. Clinical Endocrinology 42: 535-538

32. G proteins

A. F   B. F   C. T   D. F   E. F

The 1994 Nobel Prize in physiology or medicine was awarded to Alfred G. Gilman and Martin Rodbell for the discovery of G (guanine nucleotide binding) proteins and their role in cellular signal transduction. These proteins link a large array of receptors to intracellular secondary messengers.

They consist of three subunits: alpha, beta and gamma. In the unactivated state the alpha subunit is bound to the nucleotide guanine diphosphate(GDP). When a membrane receptor is activated, for example by the binding of a hormone, it interacts with the G protein causing the GDP to dissociate. It is rapidly replaced by guanine triphosphate (GTP) which leads to a dissociation of the G protein complex into an alpha-GTP unit and a beta-gamma unit. Either or both of these units in a given cell can then act as effectors. Effectors can generate elevated levels of second messengers such as cyclic AMP (cAMP) which allow the first messengers, such as hormones or adrenaline, to alter intracellular function. The alpha unit is a GTPase and it therefore inactivates itself allowing the alpha-GDP unit to reassociate with the beta-gamma unit. This inactivates the intracellular effectors, turning the G protein switch to the 'off' position.

In Albright's hereditary osteodystrophy there is a generalized resistance to the action of a variety of hormones combined with dysmorphic characteristics. Most patients with this disorder have a 50% reduction in the activity of one of the G proteins which activates adenylate cyclase in response to hormones such as parathyroid hormone, thyrotrophin and gonadotrophins.

In *Vibrio cholerae* infection G protein activity is increased. The bacteria secrete an exotoxin that catalyses adenosine diphosphate ribosylation. This chemically alters a specific arginine in the alpha subunit and drastically reduces the GTPase activity leading to prolonged activation of adenylate cyclase. The resultant increase in cAMP levels in turn leads to the increased water and electrolyte transport that causes secretory diarrhoea.

Up to 40% of patients with acromegaly due to pituitary somatotroph tumours have mutations in G proteins leading to reduced adenylate cyclase activity.

Reference

Lefkowitz R L 1995 G proteins in medicine. New England Journal of Medicine 332: 186-188

33. Cell membranes and aquaporins
A. T   B. T   C. F   D. T   E. T.

Each eukaryotic cell has a cell membrane that separates it from the environment, and compartmentalizes its many specialized organelles. The cell membrane consists of a lipid bilayer with proteins and carbohydrates inserted in it. It acts as a barrier to water and hydrophilic solutes. The cell membrane contains protein channels whch transport selective ions and molecules in and out of the cell. Other proteins act as specific receptor molecules which interact with physiological ligands. When activated, these protein receptors interact with an enzyme system which produces a second messenger. This, in turn, triggers a chain of intracellular events which are the desired response to the first messenger.

The aquaporins are a large family of recently discovered membrane water-transport proteins which are thought to play a key role in the transport of water across permeable mammalian cell membranes. High resolution electron microscopy has shown them to have a tetrameric structure. Many different studies have shown that aquaporin 1 (AQP1) and several homologous proteins are freely permeated by water but not by ions or other small uncharged molecules. This selectivity is intriguing. Separate water and urea transporters are known to exist in both red cells and the renal medulla. It may be that the aquaporin channels are too small to let urea through, but evidence that water molecules cross the bilayer in single file suggests that the orientation of the charged residues within the aqueous pore also restricts permeability to ions.

AQP1 has been identified in cell membranes throughout the body, including red cells, corneal endothelial cells, in the choroid plexus, hepatobiliary duct and gall bladder. Investigators have attributed a large variety of tissue water movement to AQP1 but interestingly, patients who lack the Colton blood group antigens and have deletion mutations in AQP1, show marked delay in osmotic water permeability of red cells but do not seem to suffer from any pathophysiological disorders in the other organ systems which usually express AQP1.

The first identified aquaporin, major intrinsic protein (MIP), is found only in the membrane of lens fibre cells and is vital for maintaining lens transparency. A murine model for congenital cataracts has been produced from mutations in the MIP gene.

AQP2 is expressed exclusively in kidney collecting ducts and is believed to be the predominant vasopressin-regulated water channel. Some patients suffering from a severe form of nephrogenic diabetes insipidus have mutations in the AQP2 gene which produces a protein with abnormal folding. Reduced levels of AQP2 have also been found in lithium-induced nephrogenic diabetes insipidus.

AQP3 and AQP4 are both expressed in the basolateral plasma membrane of collecting duct principal cells. It is known that these two proteins, although selectively permeable to water, also transport other compounds to a limited degree, but why they should both be expressed within the same membrane is not yet clear. AQP4 is predominantly expressed in the brain and in situ hybridization has detected a particularly strong signal in the paraventricular and supraoptic nuclei of the hypothalamus, which project axons to the neurohypophysis and contain osmoreceptors involved in the release of vasopressin. It is thought that AQP4 is the osmoreceptor in the central nervous system responsible for triggering antidiuresis.

AQP5 has been isolated in salivary and lacrimal glands, corneal epithelium and lung tissues. It is thought to play a major role in the secretion of tears, saliva and sputum and it has been hypothesized that an autoimmune process recognizing some extracellular antigenic domain may be responsible for some forms of Sjögren's syndrome.

It is likely that many more aquaporins will be identified and that there is much more to be discovered about the role they play in cellular functions and disease processes. Their discovery has answered the long-standing biophysical question of how water crosses plasma membranes.

References

Agre P, Brown D, Nielsen S 1995 Aquaporin water channels: unanswered questions and unresolved controversies. Current Opinion in Cell Biology 7: 472-483

Connolly D L, Shanahan C M, Weissberg P L 1996 Water channels in health and disease. Lancet 347: 210-212

34. Platelet-activating factor

A. **F**   B. **F**   C. **T**   D. **T**   E. **T**

Platelet-activating factor (PAF) is a phospholipid signalling molecule. It was originally identified as a factor which when released from stimulated rabbit basophils, activated platelets. It is now known to be produced by a large number of different human cells including endothelial cells, polymorphonuclear leucocytes (PMN), eosinophils, macrophages, monocytes, platelets, mast cells and spermatozoa. It acts at very low concentrations and is believed to cause a myriad of actions in its effector tissues. It causes platelet adherence and aggregation, and results in the activation of PMNs, eosinophils, monocytes and macrophages, resulting in aggregation and the production of leucotrienes, cytokines and chemotactic agents. It plays a role in glycogenolysis in the liver, in uterine contraction, in bronchoconstriction, in alterations of cardiac rhythm and output and in increased glomerular filtration.

PAF can be produced de novo or by the acetylation by acetyl coenzyme-A of lyso-PAF, a metabolite of arachidonic acid. PAF acts via a specific receptor whose gene is located on chromosome 1. The complementary DNA (cDNA) for the receptor has been cloned and the predicted structure produces a protein which spans the cell membrane seven times. Binding of PAF to the receptor induces intracellular signalling mediated through G proteins. There are several powerful mechanisms which control the biological activity of PAF under physiological conditions, including regulation of expression and activity of the receptor, as well as the tightly controlled production and degradation of PAF itself. The PAF receptor is also able to recognize and be activated by phospholipids with a similar structure to PAF. These PAF-like oxidatively fragmented phospholipids are generated by free radical reactions and may be important in syndromes of inflammatory tissue damage in which oxidants are produced.

Excess synthesis and accumulation of PAF is thought to occur in some pathological processes and contribute to tissue injury. The administration of exogenous PAF to experimental animals induces hypotension mimicking endotoxic and anaphylactic shock, cerebral ischaemia, gastric erosions and ischaemic bowel necrosis. Neither PAF nor PAF- like oxidized lipids have been shown to be the sole mediator in any human disease, but evidence that they may play a pivotal role in a number of disease processes is mounting.

Patients with sepsis have increased PAF activity in the blood, decreased PAF acetylhydroxylase activity in plasma and evidence of downregulation of PAF receptors on platelets. These facts could suggest that there is production of PAF or a PAF-like lipid in response to the presence of bacterial endotoxin. Reports that a PAF receptor antagonist BN52021 decreased mortality in patients with gram-negative septicaemia lends further support to this theory.

PAF has been implicated in the pathoaetiology of various inflammatory joint and collagen-vascular diseases. In systemic lupus erythematosus there is again increased PAF-like activity with reduced PAF acetylhydrolase activity.

PAF may play a central role in the pathogenesis of bronchial asthma. It induces the contraction of smooth muscle in the airways, increases airways resistance and hyper-reactivity, stimulates the accumulation of eosinophils, enhances the generation of prostaglandins and leucotrienes and alters lung morphology. Initial trials of PAF receptor antagonists in patients with asthma have not, however, produced therapeutic benefits. Interestingly, PAF receptor antagonists have been found to be constituents of various plants used in Chinese traditional medicines.

Alterations in PAF metabolism have also been found in association with systemic hypertension and pregnancy-induced hypertension with elevated PAF acetylhydrolase activity. It is not known if this is a primary or secondary phenomenon. PAF has also been implicated in the pathogenesis of cardiovascular and cerebrovascular diseases as well as diabetes, renal disease and gastrointestinal and liver diseases.

Cigarette smoking is a risk factor for atherosclerosis, gastric ulcer disease and asthma. Cigarette smoking has been shown to increase levels of PAF-like lipids in plasma lipoproteins, and to increase plasma PAF acetylhydrolase activity. It may be that it is through alterations in PAF metabolism and the production of PAF-like oxidized phospholipids that smoking induces or amplifies these disease processes.

Reference
Imaizumi T, Stafforini D M, Yamada Y et al 1995 Platelet-activating factor: a mediator for clinicians. Journal of Internal Medicine 238: 5-20

35. Copper and disease
A. F   B. T   C. T   D. F   E. F

Copper is an essential trace element. The main storage organ is the liver, but it is found in most body tissues. It is a constituent of a number of enzymes including dopa beta-hydroxylase, superoxide dismutase, tyrosinase and cytochrome oxidase. It is also a component of caeruloplasmin and is necessary for the formation of myelin and haemoglobin. Ionic copper is readily absorbed from the stomach and small intestine. After storage in the liver, it is either excreted in the bile or incorporated into caeruloplasmin. Some is loosely bound to albumin and is readily available for uptake by the tissues.

Copper metabolism is under the control of at least three genes located on chromosome 3 (caeruloplasmin), chromosome 13 (Wilson's disease) and the X chromosome (Menkes' syndrome). Both the Wilson's and Menkes' syndrome genes code for copper containing P-type ATPases which show marked homology. Variability in the site and type of mutation of the Wilson's disease gene on chromosome 13 leads to the variability in phenotype seen in the disease, although different phenotypes between identical twins suggests that environmental factors are also important.

Menkes' syndrome is characterized by severe copper deficiency. The condition is X-linked recessive and presents soon after birth with failure to thrive, peculiar hair, cerebral and cerebellar degeneration and death within a few years. Copper deficiency probably results in these clinical features through the dysfunction of essential enzyme processes. The results of therapy, including parenteral copper, are disappointing.

Wilson's disease is characterized by excess copper deposition in the liver and brain. In the tissues copper is toxic to the membrane ATPase and with chronic exposure it poisons mitochondrial enzymes. Wilson's disease has an incidence of about 30 per million and presentation may occur from childhood into middle life, with liver dysfunction, cirrhosis, psychiatric disturbance or neurological dysfunction including parkinsonism, dystonia and choreiform disorder. The rate of progression is variable, from rapid progression with spasticity, dementia and death to a slower decline over many years. Interestingly the sensory nervous system always escapes damage. Patients often have characteristic Kayser-Fleischer rings.

The role of caeruloplasmin in normal physiology and in Wilson's disease is unclear. It is a protein containing six atoms of copper and is encoded by a gene on chromosome 3. Although low levels of caeruloplasmin are characteristic of Wilson's disease some patients have near normal levels. Penicillamine, a copper chelating agent, is the treatment of choice. If started before the onset of symptoms it can delay or even prevent their onset, and in patients with established tissue damage some reversal has been observed on initiation of therapy.

Side-effects can be serious and include induction of pyridoxine deficiency by the D-isomer, various immunologically mediated disorders including lupus, and an initial clinical worsening on commencement of therapy. Other agents which can be considered include zinc, which reduces copper absorption, and other chelating agents. Liver transplantation cures the condition by removing the site of the metabolic lesion. It is indicated for end stage cirrhosis or acute severe hepatitis, but its role in the treatment of predominantly neurological disease is controversial. A significant implication of the discovery of the Wilson's disease gene is that family members can now be screened and offered therapy before the onset of clinical symptoms.

Reference

Walshe J M 1995 Copper: not too little, not too much, but just right. Journal of the Royal College of Physicians London 29; 4: 280-288

36. Vascular tone
A. F   B. T   C. T   D. F   E. F

Historically it was thought that peripheral vascular tone was under the control of the autonomic nervous system. Sympathetic nerves released noradrenaline which acted on alpha receptors producing constriction. Parasympathetic nerves released acetylcholine which acted on muscarinic receptors producing dilation. Over recent years it has become clear that the situation is much more complex. The regulation of blood vessel tone involves both perivascular nerves at the adventitial-medial border and the endothelium. Many new chemical messengers have been identified, including monoamines, purines, polypeptides and nitric oxide. Many nerves synthesize, store and release more than one transmitter.

In sympathetic nerves noradrenaline and adenosine triphosphate (ATP) are released from the same nerves as co-transmitters. Neuropeptide Y has important neuromodulatory actions in that it alters synaptic function without directly causing synaptic transmission. In other sympathetic nerve endings dynorphin acts as a principal neuromodulator. In parasympathetic perivascular nerves, vasoactive intestinal peptide is a co-transmitter with acetylcholine in some fibres, whilst ATP is found in others.

Sensory-motor perivascular nerves are non-sympathetic, non-parasympathetic nerves that have a motor as well as sensory function with ATP, substance P and calcitonin-gene-related peptide (CGRP) acting as vasodilators.

The vasodilator response to acetylcholine requires the presence of an intact endothelium. Endothelial receptors exist, that when occupied, lead to the release of endothelium-derived relaxing factor (now known to be nitric oxide) and constricting factors (of which endothelins are important examples).

Endothelium-dependent vasodilation occurs in response to acetylcholine, ATP, ADP, arachidonic acid, substance P, 5-hydoxytryptamine and various other compounds. The endothelium and smooth muscle have different receptors, so that the same substance can produce opposite effects. For example ATP released from perivascular nerves acts on smooth muscle receptors resulting in vasoconstriction, while ATP released from endothelial cells acts on different receptors of the same endothelial cells to produce vasodilation. Various vasoactive substances have been found in endothelial cells including acetylcholine, substance P and angiotensin II, supporting the concept that they are produced by, as well as act on, the endothelium.

The endothelium is involved in vasoconstriction as well as vasodilation. In response to mechanical and chemical stress endothelial calcium channels open, raising intracellular calcium and leading to release of endothelially-derived vasoconstrictors such as endothelin-1. Stressors include thrombin, high extracellular potassium, hypoxia and stretch. It seems likely that endothelium-mediated release of vasoactive substances is most important in control of the local environment, whereas perivascular nerves are more concerned with the integrated control of blood pressure.

Another recently discovered vasodilator is CGRP. It is found in nerve fibres around cerebral, mesenteric and skin vessels and also circulates in the plasma. It can produce endothelium dependent and independent vasodilation. The endothelium independent dilation is associated with an increase in intracellular cyclic-AMP in smooth muscle cells, whereas the endothelium dependent mechanism is associated with a rise in both cyclic-AMP and cyclic-GMP. It is likely that for endothelium dependent vasodilation, CGRP acts on endothelial receptors, activating adenylate cyclase and raising cyclic-AMP. This activates nitric oxide synthase, nitric oxide then diffuses to the smooth muscle, stimulates guanylate cyclase, increasing cyclic-GMP which stimulates vasodilation.

References

Ong A C M 1996 Surprising new roles for endothelins. British Medical Journal 312: 195-196

Report of a meeting of physicians and scientists, University College Medical School, London 1995 Raynaud's phenomenon. Lancet 346: 283-290

37. Endothelins

A. F   B. F   C. F   D. F   E. F

The endothelins are a group of peptides, each 21 amino acids in length which are produced in a variety of tissues where they modulate vasomotor tone, cell proliferation and hormone production. The three members of the family (endothelin-1, endothelin-2, and endothelin-3) interact with two identified receptor types (type A endothelin receptor and type B endothelin receptor).

Endothelin-1 is produced in endothelial cells and vascular smooth muscle cells. Approximately 75% of endothelin-1 released from endothelial cells is thought to be secreted towards the vascular smooth muscle cells rather than into the lumen of the vessel. It should be regarded as a paracrine rather than an endocrine hormone. Endothelin-2 is produced predominantly in the intestine and kidney. Endothelin-3 is found in high concentration in the brain.

Both endothelin receptor types are bound to guanine-nucleotide-binding (G) proteins, which when activated, stimulate phospholipase C. This leads to the formation of inositol trisphosphate and diacylglycerol. These in turn cause an increase in intracellular calcium concentration and stimulate protein kinase C.

Endothelin-1 is the most potent vasoconstrictor so far identified. It is 100 times more potent than noradrenaline on a molar basis. It also has mitogenic activities on vascular smooth muscle and myocardial cells. It is probably involved in the pathogenesis of a wide variety of conditions such as myocardial damage after infarction and reperfusion, heart failure, cyclosporin induced renal failure, post-ischaemic renal failure and vasospasm following subarachnoid haemorrhage.

Endothelin-A receptor antagonists have been successfully used to reduce the extent of experimentally induced myocardial infarction in dogs, and endothelin-1 antibodies produced a similar effect in rats. Plasma endothelial levels correlate well with the severity of heart failure, and levels 3 days after a myocardial infarction correlate well with prognosis. High plasma levels in heart failure could induce bronchospasm through interaction with the endothelin-A receptors on bronchial smooth muscle cells. In experimental subarachnoid haemorrhage in rats the associated vasospasm is almost completely abolished by pre-treatment with endothelin receptor antagonists.

Experiments using 'knockout mice', and genetic analysis of members of the Menonite sect in the US suggest that endothelins are important in the development of tissues derived from the neural crest.

Endothelins may prove to be very useful as prognostic markers and their manipulation will hopefully lead to the development of novel agents to treat cardiovascular disease. Their importance in development needs further investigation.

References

Levin E R 1995 Mechanisms of disease: endothelins. New England Journal of Medicine 333: 356-363

Ong A C 1996 Surprising new roles for endothelins. British Medical Journal 312: 195-196

38.   Natriuretic peptides

A. F   B. T   C. F   D. F   E. T.

Atrial natriuretic peptide was discovered in 1981 and has been the focus of much research attention. Three peptides have been isolated: A, B and C. Atrial or A natriuretic peptide is stored mainly in the right atrium and causes natriuresis and vasodilatation. Type B is largely stored in the cardiac ventricles and has similar physiological effects to type A. Type C is stored mainly in vascular endothelial cells and its main effect is vasodilation, predominantly venodilation. Both types B and C were first discovered in brain. Study of the natriuretic peptide receptors is still in its early stages. So far, three receptors have been discovered. Receptors A and B appear to be active in signal transduction, whereas receptor C binds the peptides thereby terminating their effects.

Neutral endopeptidase breaks down the natriuretic peptides as well as other endogenous peptides such as bradykinin, substance P and angiotensin II. Oral neutral endopeptidase inhibitors have now been developed. Animal and human studies suggest that these agents may have a therapeutic role. In hypertension they may reduce atheroma formation and in combination with angiotensin converting enzyme inhibitors they cause a profound fall in blood pressure. Because of their potentiating effects on angiotensin II, their effect on blood pressure when given alone is small. Other potential therapeutic uses include the treatment of heart failure, myocardial ischaemia, cor pulmonale, left ventricular hypertrophy and cyclosporin toxicity.

Diagnostic uses for these peptides are also being investigated. In the future their measurement may be used to detect mild heart failure, myocardial ischaemia and left ventricular hypertrophy. Their measurement may also be used to optimise diuretic therapy.

Reference

Struthers A D 1994 10 years of natriuretic peptide research: a new dawn for their diagnostic and therapeutic use? British Medical Journal 308: 1615-1619

39. Angiogenesis
A. **T**   B. **T**   C. **T**   D. **T**   E. **F**

Angiogenesis is the sprouting of new vessels from pre-existing ones, whereas vasculogenesis is the appearance of new vessels. It is fundamental to reproduction, development and repair. Angiogenesis requires tight control allowing vessel sprouting to be rapidly switched on and off.

Tumour hypervascularity results from angiogenesis when chemical signals from tumour cells shift resting endothelial cells into a phase of rapid growth. Most human tumours persist for months or years without neovascularization. At this stage they are usually small, asymptomatic and clinically undetectable. The tumour becomes more vascular when a subgroup of cells in the tumour switches to an angiogenic phenotype.This switch results from a change in the equilibrium between the positive and negative regulators of angiogenesis. Vascular endothelial growth factor (VEGF) and basic fibroblast growth factor (bFGF) are the most commonly found angiogenic proteins in tumours.

Neovascularization augments tumour growth by improved perfusion and paracrine effects. Perfusion delivers nutrients and removes waste more efficiently than simple diffusion. Endothelial cells produce paracrine growth factors like bFGF, platelet derived growth factor, insulin-like growth factor and granulocyte colony-stimulating factor which promote tumour growth. Neovascularization permits tumour growth and metastasis and heralds the onset of symptoms. Tumours do not outgrow their blood supply but eventually compress it. This results from increased interstitial pressure from leaky vessels in the relative absence of lymphatics. Angiogenesis therefore gradually reduces a tumour's accessibility to chemotherapeutic drugs and eventually central tumour necrosis occurs.

Retinal neovascularization is an important cause of blindness and is triggered by hypoxia. VEGF is thought to be the major mediator of this form of angiogenesis. The formation of heart collateral vessels and the neovascularization of atherosclerotic plaques probably also occur in response to angiogenic factors following hypoxia. In haemangiomas of infancy the expression of both VEGF and bFGF is excessive. Panus formation in rheumatoid arthritis may result from angiogenesis promoted by release of angiogenic factors from inflammatory cells. In the hypervascular skin lesions of psoriasis the angiogenic polypeptide interleukin-8 has increased expression and thrombospondin-1, an angiogenesis inhibitor, has reduced expression. Certain aspects of the reproductive cycle like ovulation, repair of the menstruating uterus and formation of the placenta depend on angiogenesis, and disorders of angiogenesis may underlie reproductive disorders like menorrhagia and some cases of infertility. Abnormal angiogenesis (excessive or inadequate) may also explain various developmental abnormalities such as vascular malformations, haemangiomas and bowel atresia.

The clinical applications of angiogenesis fall into three areas: diagnostic, angiogenesis acceleration and angiogenesis inhibition. The density of microvessels in tumour biopsy specimens provides a valuable predictor of metastasis and quantification of angiogenic proteins in body fluids provides indirect evidence of the presence of tumour. Potentiating angiogenesis may have a role in the healing of gastric ulcers where bFGF is deficient, and in animal models of gastric ulceration, ingestion of acid-stable bFGF accelerates healing. Interestingly, sucralfate probably acts by protecting endogenous mucosal bFGF from degradation by acid. The inhibition of angiogenesis has applications for cancer, haemangioma, arthritis and retinal neovascularization therapy. Haemangiomas are most common in premature infants and occasionally need treating because they cause serious tissue damage or interfere with a vital organ. 30% respond to steroid treatment but occasionally steroids actually make them expand. Interferon alpha-2a is anti-angiogenic and has been successfully used to treat haemangiomas. This effect is probably through the suppression of bFGF. Both thalidomide and interferon alpha-2a are being evaluated for the treatment of retinal neovascularization because of their anti-angiogenic effects. In rheumatoid arthritis minocycline, which has anti-angiogenic activity, is being investigated. In cancer therapy several agents with anti-angiogenic properties are currently undergoing phase 1 and 2 clinical trials including TNP-470, platelet factor 4, interleukin-12 and thalidomide.

Studies to date have established that anti-angiogenic agents do not suppress the bone marrow, cause hair loss, or cause severe gastrointestinal disturbances like cytotoxics. They need to be administered over many months to be of benefit and the development of resistance has not been observed. A combination of anti-angiogenic and cytotoxic therapy may work better than either alone by attacking both the tumour cell and vascular compartments of the cancer.

Angiogenesis is clearly a fundamental process both in health and disease and there appear to be only subtle differences in the mechanisms of pathogenic angiogenesis between very different diseases. The manipulation of angiogenesis holds promise for the future therapy of these diseases.

References

Folkman J 1995 Angiogenesis in cancer, vascular, rheumatoid, and other diseases. Natural Medicine 1: 27-35

Folkman J 1995 Clinical applications of research on angiogenesis. New England Journal of Medicine 333; 6: 1757-1763

STATISTICS AND EPIDEMIOLOGY
40. Incidence, prevalence and risk
A. F   B. F   C. F   D. T   E. T.

Epidemiology is the study of how often a disease occurs in a population and why. A key feature of epidemiology is the measurement of disease outcomes in a defined population at risk. The incidence of a disease is the rate at which new cases occur in a population during a specific period, usually a year. Measurement of incidence can be complicated by changes in the population under study due to births, deaths and migrations. This is overcome by relating the number of new cases to the person years at risk. The prevalence of a disease is defined as the proportion of a population with the disease at a point in time. It is a snap-shot of the number of people with the disease in a given population and is only appropriate as a measure of chronic stable conditions. The mortality is the incidence of death from the disease. In studies of aetiology incidence is the most appropriate measure of disease frequency.

The International Classification of Diseases, Injuries and Causes of Death (ICD) assigns a three digit numerical code to every major condition. The system is used for coding death certificates, hospital discharges, and is used in the Registrar General's report. The classification is revised and updated periodically. When this happens, disease rates may not be directly comparable and some aggregation of categories is needed when analysing the results.

Attributable risk is the disease rate in exposed persons minus the disease rate in unexposed persons. Relative risk is the ratio of the disease rate in the exposed to that in the unexposed. Attributable risk gives a better indication of the risk to the individual of a certain action like smoking on the chance of developing, for example, lung cancer. The relative risk of two diseases may be doubled by smoking but if one is much more common than the other the attributable risk reflects this. In practice, relative risk is more commonly used because it can be estimated from a larger number of trial designs, in particular from case-control studies. Population attributable risk measures the potential impact of control measures in a population. It is the rate of disease in a population minus the rate that would apply if all of the population were unexposed. It is calculated by multiplying the attributable risk by the number of people exposed to the risk factor in the population, and is used to calculate the possible effect of public health campaigns.

41. Statistical terminology
A. F   B. T   C. F   D. F   E. T

A confounder is a hidden variable which causes or contributes to the differences observed in a study independently of the exposure under investigation. It may give rise to spurious associations or obscure a true association. Two common confounders are age and sex. Standardized rates allow for differences in the age and sex structure of the populations under study. Direct standardization involves the comparison of weighted averages of age and sex specific disease rates, weighted in proportion to the size of each age and sex group in a standard known population. Indirect standardization is used to compare the disease rate in an age/sex group with the expected rates from reference data. The standardized mortality ratio (SMR) is used by the Registrar General in summarizing time trends, and regional and occupational differences in death rates.

Bias is a systematic tendency to under or overestimate the parameter of interest because of a deficiency in the design or execution of the study. There are many sources of potential bias in epidemiological studies. Selection bias occurs when the subjects selected for a study are not representative of the population. This is a common problem when questionnaires are used, as non-responders may have different characteristics to responders. Information bias arises from errors in measuring exposure or disease. Bias cannot usually be totally eliminated from epidemiological studies, but it should be identified wherever possible and its impact taken into account when interpreting results.

Even if biases can be eliminated the study samples may be unrepresentative just by chance. An indication of such chance effects is provided by statistical analysis. This is often done by calculating the probability (p) of obtaining the result by chance if there were in fact no difference between the study sample and the target population (the null hypothesis). The lower the calculated p value the more one is inclined to reject the null hypothesis. Usually a p value of less than 0.05 is deemed to be statistically significant, but this is arbitrary.

42. Surveys and screening
A. **F**   B. **F**   C. **F**   D. **F**   E. **F**

When a survey technique or test is used to define patients as cases or non-cases, its validity is analysed by classifying subjects as positive or negative by the method of the study or test under investigation, and again by a standard reference test. The information is displayed in a two-by-two table and from this sensitivity, specificity, systematic error, and predictive value can be determined. The proportion of cases correctly diagnosed by a test is known as its sensitivity and it is calculated from the number of true positives correctly identified by the test divided by the total number of true positives. The proportion of non-cases correctly classified by a test is termed the specificity and this is calculated from the number of true negatives correctly identified by the test divided by the total number of true negatives. Systematic error is a measure of the ratio of the total numbers of positives in the survey to those in the reference test. The predictive value is the proportion of positive test results that are truly positive.

When there is no satisfactory standard against which to assess the validity of a measurement technique, then examining its repeatability is helpful. Consistent findings do not necessarily imply that a technique is valid, but poor repeatability indicates either poor validity or that the characteristic being measured varies over time, and in either case the results must be interpreted cautiously.

Common study methods include longitudinal studies where subjects are followed over time with continuous or repeated monitoring of risk factors and outcomes, case-control studies where patients who have developed the disease are identified and their past exposure to possible aetiological factors compared to that of controls, and cross sectional studies which measure the prevalence of health outcomes or health determinants in a population at a given point in time.

Screening patients for preclinical disease has become an established part of medical practice. Screening is only of use where earlier treatment can be shown to improve prognosis, where there is a satisfactory and acceptable screening test available with a good predictive value, and where the yield of the test is sufficiently high to warrant the cost of the screening both financially and in terms of the discomfort and inconvenience caused to those people who do not have the disease. Assessing the benefits of early screening is not always clear and one potential source of error is lead time, i.e. with screening, a disease is diagnosed earlier than without screening and survival is thus longer from diagnosis, even without a change in the prognosis from treatment intervention.

Epidemiology can be analytical where clues to the aetiology of diseases are sought from case-control and longitudinal studies, descriptive where, for instance, information about the changing incidence of a disease in a population is sought, and experimental where interventions are assessed in terms of changing health outcomes.

Reference

Coggon D, Rose G , Barker D J P 1993. Epidemiology for the uninitiated. 3rd edn. British Medical Journal, London

43. Mean, median, normal distribution and standard deviation

A. T   B. F   C. F   D. F   E. T

The following describe techniques for analysing univariate data.

The mean describes the average of the sum of the variables. It is calculated by adding together all the individual measurements and then dividing by the total number of measurements. The median is the middle value when all the values are placed in rank order. Where there are an even number of measurements in a data set the median is the average of the middle two measurements. The mean of a discrete quantitative variable (that is a variable which consists of whole numbers in a limited range) need not necessarily take one of the discrete values of the variable. The average of 2.4 children in a family is acceptable even though it is not a whole number. The mean is strongly influenced by a single eccentrically outlying variable or a rogue result, whereas the median is much less so.

The range of a variable describes its distribution. It is usually quoted as the difference between its highest and lowest values. Like the mean, it is sensitive to any outlying results. This problem is overcome by using the interquartile range, which is produced by ranking all of the measurements in ascending order and identifying the lower and upper quartiles.

The measure of dispersion most commonly used in medical practice is the standard deviation. Firstly the mean is calculated. Next the difference between each variable and the mean is determined (its deviation); some of these numbers will be minus numbers. Each deviation is then squared. The squared numbers, all positives, are then summed for the whole data set and divided by the number of measurements minus one to obtain a quantity known as the variance.

The standard deviation is the square root of the variance. The standard deviation and variance measure the spread of a distribution. Standard deviation has the same units as the measurements from which it was calculated.

Data which is in the form of a continuous quantitative variable is often displayed in the form of a histogram. The measurements are grouped into intervals and represented by a rectangle whose width corresponds to the range of the interval, and whose area corresponds to the frequency of measurements within that interval. Unlike a bar chart the rectangles are contiguous. When a histogram is based on a large number of measurements it is possible to divide their range into relatively fine intervals and the outline of the rectangles may then approximate to a smooth curve. This curve maps out the frequency distribution of the variable. The shape of this curve can display features which describe the distribution of the variable within the population. It may show it to be unimodal or bimodal. It may be positively (to the right) or negatively skewed, or symmetrical. In a symmetrical distribution the mean is equal to the median. Some shapes of distribution occur frequently in nature; one is the normal distribution which has a symmetrical bell shape and is described by a mathematical equation. Whatever the dispersion of the data, approximately 95% of measurements will lie within two standard deviations of the mean.

References

Coggon D 1995 Statistics in clinical practice. British Medical Journal, London

Gore S M, Altman D G 1982. Statistics in practice. British Medical Journal, London

44. Statistical tests

A. T   B. F   C. T   D. T   E. T

A p value is the probability of obtaining an outcome as extreme as that observed if the null hypothesis were true, i.e. simply by chance. The derivation of the p value from first principles would be extremely complicated for most studies. It is usually done by application of an appropriate statistical test. It entails calculating a special summary statistic from the sample data, and then looking up this value in a statistics table to get the corresponding p value. This is now usually carried out by computer. The choice of the correct statistical test depends on the nature of the data, the study design and the hypothesis under investigation.

Parametric tests make assumptions about the distribution of data in a population, such as it having a normal distribution. Non-parametric tests make no such assumptions. Parametric tests allow stronger conclusions to be made provided that the assumptions can be accepted. Examples of parametric tests include Student's t-test and paired t-test, and non-parametric tests include the Mann-Whitney U test and the Wilcoxon two sample test.

Often hypothesis testing is not the most appropriate statistical technique for making informed medical decisions. A finding that is highly significant statistically may be clinically irrelevant if, for example, the effect is small. In contrast, clinically important outcomes may fail to achieve statistical significance if they are observed only in small samples. An alternative approach to statistical inference from hypothesis testing is the use of estimation with confidence limits. The concept of a confidence interval, as with hypothesis testing, should be viewed in the context of a sample derived from a larger population about which conclusions are to be drawn. If repeated sample populations are studied for the prevalence of a given condition in a population, it is likely that the point estimate obtained would differ by chance from one sample to the next. A confidence interval gives a range around a point estimate within which the corresponding population parameter is likely to lie. Most often 95% confidence intervals are quoted, and these are derived from the sample data according to set mathematical rules. A confidence interval of 95% means that 95% of samples taken repeatedly from a population will have confidence intervals that include the population parameter. The method used for calculating the confidence intervals depends on the type of data being analysed, the design of the study and the parameter that is being estimated. Probability and confidence intervals give approximately the same information but the former refers to the null hypothesis and the latter refers to an estimate of a population parameter. Because of this, p values tell us little extra when confidence limits are known. In general the larger the size of the sample the narrower the confidence interval that will be obtained.

References

Coggon D 1995 Statistics in clinical practice. British Medical Journal,
    London

Gore S M, Altman D G 1982 Statistics in practice. British Medical
    Journal, London

45. Statistical power

A. T   B. T   C. F   D. T   E. F

The power of a study is its ability to minimize the uncertainties that
arise because of chance variation between samples. Once a study
has been completed, confidence intervals provide the most
convenient and easily interpreted measure of power, but in
planning a study the usual approach is to base power calculations
on the hypothesis testing approach to statistical inference.

The null hypothesis is subject to two types of error. Type 1 error is
when the null hypothesis is wrongly rejected, while in a type 2
error the null hypothesis is not rejected when in fact it is incorrect.
There is an inverse relationship between the probability of
producing type 1 or type 2 errors. For any given sample size, the
stricter the requirements are for rejecting the null hypothesis, the
higher the probability of a type 2 error occurring. The statistical
power of a study is defined as 1 minus the probability of a type 2
error and thus studies with greater power have a lower probability
of type 2 errors. The power of a study depends on the sample size,
the magnitude of the difference being measured and various
features of the study population. It is important to conduct a study
with a sample large enough to give adequate power. Studies which
are too small are extremely common and their failure to produce
statistically significant results can be argued as unethical in their
use of patients and resources.

When a sample size large enough to give the study the required
power has been calculated, it is then necessary to choose the
right method for sampling the population under study. Data from a
sample of individuals used to extrapolate information about a
population must be representative if statistical inferences are to be
valid. Even with random sampling many potential sources of bias
remain. The electoral register or the doctors list are often used to
provide a list of the whole population, but these are frequently out
of date and often under-represent certain groups in society who
may have quite different features to the population at large. Using
questionnaires has the same problem, with non-responders
probably forming a distinct group from responders; non-
responders should be chased up and questionnaires kept short
and simple to reduce the non-responder rate. Case-control studies
of hospital patients are often used to study the relationship
between a particular disease and exposure to a suspected causal
agent. If the hospital admission rates for exposed and unexposed

individuals are found to differ from the exposure rate in the population as a whole, the results could be severely biased in either direction. Results from these studies should be supported by evidence from prospective studies. Not all of these sources of bias can be eliminated but an awareness of their existence helps when analysing the clinical significance of statistical inferences.

References

Coggon D 1995 Statistics in clinical practice. British Medical Journal, London

Gore S M, Altman D G 1982 Statistics in practice. British Medical Journal, London

---

46. Systematic reviews and evidence based medicine

A. T   B. F   C. F   D. F   E. F

Archie Cochrane (1909–88) was a respiratory epidemiologist and clinical trialist, who believed that treatments that had been shown to do more good than harm should be encouraged, while those where the benefits were unproven should only be practised within the confines of a clinical trial. He was particularly critical of the inability of the medical profession to review in a critical and statistically accurate way data from all relevant randomized controlled trials in order that it might act on the evidence and change its practice. The enormous number of publications printed every week makes it impossible for an individual to digest and analyse the new facts, make a systematic review of all previous studies and then alter practice accordingly. Often physicians practise what they believe to be beneficial from their own experience and from unsystematic reviews, even in the face of contrary evidence from well conducted randomized controlled trials and systematic reviews.

Undertaking a clinical trial without also reviewing the data from all previous trials both published and unpublished, may have harmed and may continue to harm many patients. It has been argued that if systematic reviews of the evidence from trials of thrombolysis in acute myocardial infarction had been undertaken earlier, proof of its effectiveness would have been established by the late 1970s, 10 years before GISSI-1. A systematic review of small studies which had failed to reach significance showed that compression stockings reduced the incidence of DVT post surgery.

The usefulness of a systematic review depends on the quality of the design and methodology of the original trials. One of the problems is that trials with insignificant or negative results are often not written up or not published, and this is a major source of bias in meta-analysis. A register of all trials started is useful for monitoring and eliminating publication bias. The United Kingdom Cochrane Centre in Oxford was set up in 1992 to coordinate systematic reviews of treatments in all specialities. There is now international collaboration with an international trials register being established. Systematic reviews are not a substitute for large randomized controlled trials, but may help to direct the design of these trials to ensure they can provide a definitive answer to a given question. The drive towards evidence based medicine should result in increased interest in the work and results of the various Cochrane collaborative groups, and encourage clinical trialists to consult with and cooperate with the groups when planning research.

References

Counsell C E, Fraser H, Sandercock P A G 1994 Archie Cochrane's challenge: can periodically updated reviews of all randomized controlled trials relevant to neurology and neurosurgery be produced? Journal of Neurology, Neurosurgery, and Psychiatry 57: 529-533

Sackett D L, Rosenberg W M C, Muir Gray J A et al 1996 Evidence based medicine: what it is and what it isn't. British Medical Journal 312: 71-72

47. Disadvantages of meta-analysis

A. **T**   B. **F**   C. **F**   D. **T**   E. **T**

Meta-analysis has been defined as a statistical summary of the numerical outcomes of a group of studies. It is a form of systematic review which attempts to include all trial evidence on a subject whether published or not, and in so doing avoid bias in data collection. Using individual patient data from trialists allows the statistician to check and correct the original data, obtain further information on the timing of outcomes in the trials, and allows more powerful subgroup analysis. To improve the quality of the analysis unrandomized participants should be excluded, intention to treat should be included in the analysis, all subgroups and subanalyses should be included and complete follow-up data should be obtained.

Potential problems with meta-analysis are, amongst others, the inclusion of poorly conducted studies, loss of important subgroup results, no attempt to analyse why differences occur and inclusion of non-homogeneous studies. Most of these problems can be overcome by collecting individual patient data and by attention to detail in experienced hands, but this is time consuming and in many meta-analyses these guidelines are not or cannot be met.

The subject has become very topical following the publication of ISIS 4, where with reference to magnesium in acute myocardial infarction, a large, prospective, well-conducted trial has contradicted the results of previous widely quoted meta-analyses on the subject.

References

Clarke M J, Stewart L A 1994 Obtaining data from randomized controlled trials: how much do we need for reliable and informative meta-analysis? British Medical Journal 309: 1007-1010

Eysenck H J 1994 Meta-analysis and its problems. British Medical Journal 309: 789-792

Flournoy N, Olkin I 1995 Do small trials square with large ones? Lancet 345; 8952: 741-742

48. Tobacco and alcohol
A. **T**   B. **T**   C. **F**   D. **F**   E. **T**

49. Smoking and disease
A. **F**   B. **T**   C. **T**   D. **F**   E. **F**

One in six adults in the developed world die from a smoking related illness.

In 1951 Austin Bradford Hill set up a study of the smoking habits of 40 000 British doctors. Their habits were reviewed occasionally and in 1978 the drinking habits of a proportion (12 321) of those still alive were collated. Smoking and drinking habits were compared to death rates from different causes of death.

With regard to smoking, a 40-year follow-up of the cohort revealed that half of all regular smokers would be killed by their habit. A positive association with smoking was found for death from 24 different diseases, the only negative association being with Parkinson's disease. The study also revealed that giving up smoking before the age of 35 resulted in an expectation of life not significantly different from life-long non-smokers.

Results correlating alcohol consumption with death rates were equally revealing. The cohort had a mean age of 60 and were followed up for 13 years, by which time almost a third had died. There was a U-shaped relation between all-cause mortality and the average amount of alcohol drunk. Above 21 units a week all-cause mortality rose progressively. Consumption of one to two units a day was associated with significantly lower all-cause mortality than the consumption of no alcohol or the consumption of large amounts. The consumption of alcohol appeared to reduce the risk of ischaemic heart disease, largely irrespective of amount.

A recent Danish study examining the association between alcohol consumption and mortality in 13 000 subjects found the relative risk of dying fell from 1 to 0.51 when comparing drinking no red wine with drinking three to five glasses per day. This effect was independent of other drinks consumed or other possible confounding factors. The fall in relative risk of death from moderate red wine intake was the same for stroke and cardiovascular disease as from all causes. A summary of published reports from epidemiological, case-control and cohort studies has contradicted the previously held belief that reduced cardiovascular risk is peculiar to red wine drinkers. This analysis concluded that reduced cardiovascular risk was independent of type of beverage drunk and therefore likely to be an effect of alcohol itself rather than some other constituent of the drink. Further evidence has revealed that the cardioprotective effects of alcohol are greatest in patients with high circulating low density lipoprotein, suggesting that the protective effect may result from lipid lowering. In response to the recent figures suggesting a health benefit from moderate alcohol intake, the British government has now increased the maximum recommended weekly alcohol intake to 28 units for men and 21 units for women.

References

Doll R, Peto R, Wheatley K et al 1994 Mortality in relation to smoking: 40 years' observations on male British doctors. British Medical Journal 309: 901-911

Doll R, Peto R, Hall E et al 1994 Mortality in relation to consumption of alcohol: 13 years' observations on male British doctors. British Medical Journal 309: 911-918

Gronbaek M, Deis A, Sorensen T I et al 1995 Mortality associated with moderate intake of wine, beer, or spirits. British Medical Journal 310: 1165-1169

Hein H O, Suadicani P, Gyntelberg F 1996 Alcohol consumption, serum low density lipoprotein cholesterol concentration, and risk of ischaemic heart disease: 6 year follow up in the Copenhagen male study. British Medical Journal 312: 736-741

Rimm E B, Klarsky A, Grobbee D et al 1996 Review of moderate alcohol consumption and reduced risk of coronary heart disease: is the effect due to beer, wine, or spirits? British Medical Journal 312: 731-736

PHARMACOLOGY AND THERAPEUTICS

50.   Digoxin toxicity

A. T   B. T   C. T   D. T   E. F

Digoxin is a cardiac glycoside acting on the Na/K ATPase pump on myocardial cells, producing a positive inotropic effect on the heart and causing prolongation of the refractory period of the atrioventricular node, thereby slowing conduction through this node. It is useful in heart failure and atrial fibrillation.

Digoxin has a narrow therapeutic index. Digoxin levels will not always correlate with toxicity. The diagnosis of digoxin toxicity should therefore be based on clinical grounds. Despite normal digoxin levels, several conditions will predispose to toxicity. Congestive heart failure, renal failure and old age reduce the volume of distribution of the drug. Renal failure also impairs elimination of digoxin. Cardiac amyloidosis, hypothyroidism and chronic lung disease are all associated with increased myocardial sensitivity to digoxin. Verapamil and amiodarone interfere with digoxin binding to plasma proteins and hypomagnesaemia, hypokalaemia and hypercalcaemia all potentiate digoxin toxicity.

Nausea, vomiting, headache, confusion, lethargy and anorexia are all symptoms of digoxin toxicity. Visual disturbance is less common. All types of cardiac dysrrhythmia can be seen in serious toxicity including heart block, bradycardias and tachycardias. Digoxin can cause minor electrocardiographic changes including ST depression and T wave inversion. A hockey stick deformity of the ST segment is a classical abnormality.

The management of digoxin toxicity depends on its presentation. For mild symptoms the drug can simply be stopped. Non-serious cardiac effects can be managed by drug withdrawal and correction of any electrolyte abnormalities. Severely symptomatic patients with or without cardiac toxicity can be effectively treated with activated charcoal, especially if the last dose was taken shortly before presentation. This both moderates gastrointestinal absorption of digoxin and reduces enterohepatic circulation thereby increasing elimination. Colestipol and cholestyramine are also effective agents. Life threatening arrhythmias are treated best by rapid reversal of digoxin toxicity with digoxin specific fab antibody fragments. This is expensive and can be complicated by anaphylactoid reactions and serum sickness.

Reference

Lip G Y H, Metcalfe M J, Dunn F G 1993 Diagnosis and treatment of digoxin toxicity. Postgraduate Medical Journal 69: 337-339

51. The treatment of arrhythmias

A. T   B. F   C. T   D. F   E. T

Several studies have highlighted the risks of pharmacological therapy for cardiac arrhythmias. CAST (the Cardiac Arrhythmia Suppression Trial) compared the effect of placebo with the class 1 anti-arrhythmic agents flecainide, encainide and moricizine in patients with ventricular premature beats post myocardial infarction (MI). These agents were associated with an increase in sudden cardiac deaths. In a meta-analysis of quinidine in the treatment of non-sustained ventricular tachycardia (VT) and prevention of atrial fibrillation, drug therapy was associated with an increased mortality compared to placebo. In contrast, none of the studies in patients treated with amiodarone has shown an excess mortality.

Amiodarone is a vasodilator and a negative chronotrope. It has class III activity, prolonging the action potential and repolarization time. This increases the refractory period of the conduction system. It is also a weak calcium channel blocker and has some class I activity. Amiodarone directly reduces automaticity of the sinus and atrioventricular node and has beta and alpha blocking properties. It is a peripheral and central vasodilator and will therefore reduce afterload. It has a vast volume of distribution. It also has a half-life of 7 to 8 weeks and a loading dose is required to achieve an anti-arrhythmic effect. The most important side-effects are heart block, pulmonary fibrosis, dermatitis, neuropathy, tremor, corneal microdeposits and gastrointestinal disturbance. Although thyroid function tests are commonly affected, clinically significant derangement occurs in only about 10% of patients. Despite these side-effects, at low dose the drug is usually well tolerated. It should be noted that amiodarone potentiates warfarin and raises digoxin levels.

Amiodarone is effective in the prevention and cardioversion of atrial fibrillation and flutter. In a trial comparing it with quinidine alone and quinidine combined with verapamil, amiodarone achieved the highest rates of chemical cardioversion (60%).

Beta-blockers reduce mortality and sudden death post MI. BASIS (Basel Anti-arrhythmic Study of Infarct Survival) showed that in patients with ventricular arrhythmia post MI, amiodarone led to improved survival and reduced arrhythmias compared to placebo and various anti-arrhythmic agents. This effect was not seen in patients with an ejection fraction below 40%. Beta-blockers remain the anti-arrhythmic treatment of choice post infarction, but if non-sustained ventricular tachycardia still occurs it is reasonable to substitute amiodarone. This agent may also be preferred in patients who have suffered ventricular tachycardia or fibrillation.

40% of deaths in patients with cardiomyopathy and congestive heart failure result from ventricular arrhythmias. Conventional anti-arrhythmic drugs may cause increased cardiac toxicity in these patients with worsening heart failure and aggravation of arrhythmias. Trials have shown, however, that amiodarone is successful at suppressing ventricular arrhythmias in this group. It reduces cardiac mortality and mortality from sudden death. The GESICA (Grupo de ettudio de la sobrevida en la insuficienca cardiaca en Argentina) trial compared amiodarone to placebo in patients with symptomatic congestive heart failure and showed a significant reduction in all cause mortality and hospital admissions in the amiodarone group. CHF-STAT (Veterans Affairs Congestive Heart Failure Anti-arrhythmia Trial) randomized patients with ischaemic and non-ischaemic cardiomyopathy with heart failure and more than 10 ventricular premature beats per hour to receive either amiodarone or placebo. Amiodarone significantly suppressed arrhythmias but did not reduce all cause mortality. For patients resuscitated from sustained ventricular arrhythmias amiodarone reduces mortality compared to conventional anti-arrhythmics (CASCADE) and produces mortality results equivalent to implantable defibrillators (CASH).

References

Burkart F, Pfisterer M, Kiowski W et al 1990 Effect of anti-arrhythmic therapy on mortality in survivors of myocardial infarction with asymptomatic complex ventricular arrhythmias: Basel anti-arrhythmic study of infarct survival (BASIS). Journal of the American College of Cardiology 16: 1711-1718

Doval H C, Nul D R, Grancelli H O et al 1994 Randomized trial of low dose amiodarone in severe congestive heart failure. Grupo de ettudio de la sobrevida en la insuficienca cardiaca en Argentina (GESICA). Lancet 344: 493-498

Green H L, Roden D M, Katz R J et al 1992 The cardiac arrhythmia suppression trial: first CAST... then CAST-II. Journal of the American College of Cardiology 19: 894-898

Kendall M J, Lynch K P, Hjalmarson A et al 1993 Beta-blockers and sudden cardiac death. Annals of Internal Medicine 123: 358-367

Podrid P J 1995 Amiodarone: re-evaluation of an old drug. Annals of Internal Medicine 122: 689-700

Siebels J, Cappato R, Ruppel R et al 1993 Preliminary results of the cardiac arrest study Hamburg (CASH). CASH investigators. American Journal of Cardiology 72: 109F-113F

Singh S N, Fletcher R D, Fisher S et al 1993 Veterans affairs congestive heart failure anti-arrhythmic trial. CHF STAT Investigators. American Journal of Cardiology 72: 99F-102F

The Cardiac Arrest in Seattle: conventional amiodarone drug evaluation study (CASCADE) investigators 1993 Randomized anti-arrhythmic drug therapy in survivors of arrest (the CASCADE study). American Journal of Cardiology 72: 1295-1300

52. Adenosine

A. **F**   B. **T**   C. **T**   D. **T**   E. **T**

Adenosine is an adenosine receptor agonist, and is a useful agent in the treatment and diagnosis of supraventricular tachycardias. It is particularly useful in the treatment of nodal re-entrant tachycardias, and is an agonist with rapid onset and a brief duration of action.

Its side-effects include facial flushing, dyspnoea and chest pain. They tend to be short lived, but can be very distressing and patients should therefore be warned in advance. Certain patients are at increased risk of unwanted effects. Cardiac transplant patients tend to be very sensitive probably due to denervation hypersensitivity. Dypirimadole potentiates its effects. There is a theoretical risk of inducing bronchospasm in asthmatics but this has yet to be firmly established in clinical practice.

New agents in this class are being developed, and the function of adenosine receptors in the rest of the body is being studied in the hope of new therapeutic options in the future.

Reference

Ganz L I, Freidman P L 1995 Supraventricular tachycardia. New England Journal of Medicine 332: 162-174

53. Nicorandil

A. T   B. T   C. T   D. T   E. T

Nicorandil was introduced into the UK in 1994. It is the first of a new class of anti-anginal drugs, and combines the properties of an organic nitrate with those of a potassium-channel activator. It relaxes vascular smooth muscle, particularly venous, and so reduces ventricular filling and myocardial work. Nicorandil also dilates coronary arteries and arterioles. It activates ATP-dependent potassium channels increasing the efflux of potassium ions, which hyperpolarizes the cell membrane and thus inhibits calcium entry causing arteries and arterioles to dilate. In vitro nicorandil has been shown to open ATP-dependent potassium channels in ischaemic cardiac myocytes. This hyperpolarization reduces electrical and contractile activity in ATP-depleted cells. In animal models of ischaemia, nicorandil has been shown to limit the infarct size.

Plasma concentration bears little correlation with the drug's physiological effects. Nicorandil can be administered orally, sublingually or intravenously. After oral administration there is 75% absorption by the gut. Rapid elimination by the liver clears 96% of the dose. No dose adjustment is required in patients with hepatic or renal impairment or in the elderly.

In trials, both a decrease and an increase in cardiac output have been demonstrated but in patients with cardiac failure most studies show an improvement of 17–55%. Nicorandil does not affect atrioventricular conduction and has no clinical effect on the contractility of non-ischaemic myocardium.

Side-effects include headache, dizziness, nausea, palpitations and flushing. Oedema and tachycardia, which are seen with calcium channel blockers, are not commonly reported and it does not cause bronchospasm or heart failure.

In contrast to treatment with nitroglycerine, the reduction in total peripheral resistance produced by nicorandil is maintained with long-term treatment, and the anti-anginal effects are maintained for at least a year. These sustained effects are thought to be due to potassium channel activation, as experimental evidence suggests that tolerance develops to the nitrate component just as it does with conventional nitrates. This would explain why the headache, which is such a common side-effect of both these drugs usually disappears with continued treatment. In practice careful timing of nitrate dosing can minimize tolerance, and in a 6 week trial of the two drugs, both were as effective at reducing angina and in preventing exercise induced changes on ECG. The available data are insufficient to date to say whether nicorandil's dual mechanism of action has any clinical advantage. There is little information on its use with other anti-anginal drugs. Nicorandil should be avoided in patients with hypovolaemia, low systolic blood pressure, pulmonary oedema or acute myocardial infarction with left ventricular failure.

Reference

Nicorandil for angina 1995 Drugs and Therapeutics Bulletin 33(12): 89-92

---

54. ACE inhibitors

A. F   B. T   C. F   D. F   E. F

55. ACE inhibitors

A. F.   B. F   C. F   D. T   E. T

ACE inhibitors are useful anti-hypertensive drugs, and when used in combination with a thiazide diuretic or a calcium antagonist are effective at controlling blood pressure in 80% of patients. Patients with low renin concentrations and patients of Afro-Caribbean origin may respond less well. All ACE inhibitors are active orally and all but two (captopril and lisinopril) are pro-drugs converted in the liver to yield their active metabolites. All ACE inhibitors are excreted by the kidneys and dose titration is needed in renal impairment.

In hypertensive patients ACE inhibitors cause regression of left ventricular hypertrophy but have not yet been shown to reduce the incidence of stroke, myocardial infarction, or affect mortality.

In severe and mild heart failure ACE inhibitors used in conjunction with a diuretic improve symptoms, and increase survival. In patients with asymptomatic left ventricular dysfunction ACE inhibitors reduce the incidence of heart failure.

After myocardial infarction ACE inhibitors reduce mortality in all patients and not just those with impaired left ventricular function, although the benefits are greatest in this group. ACE inhibitors can be started within 24 hours of an infarct.

They are the most effective drugs at slowing the decline in renal function in hypertensive patients with diabetic nephropathy.

ACE inhibitors can cause first dose hypotension, especially if the patient is already on a diuretic. They can cause impaired renal function and are hazardous in patients with renal artery stenosis. Other side-effects include hyperkalaemia and an irritating dry cough. Angio-oedema is a rare complication and ACE inhibitors are contraindicated in pregnancy.

References

The CONSENSUS trial study group 1987 Effects of enalapril on mortality in severe congestive heart failure: results of the cooperative north Scandinavian enalapril survival study. New England Journal of Medicine 316: 1429-1435

Gruppo Italiano per lo Studio della Sopravivenza nell'Infarto Miocardio (GISSI-3) 1994 Effects of lisinopril and transdermal glyceryl trinitrate singly and together on 6-week mortality and ventricular function after acute myocardial infarction. Lancet 343: 1115-1122

Kostis J B 1988 Angiotensin converting enzyme inhibitors. II. Clinical use. American Heart Journal 116: 1591-1605

The SOLVD Investigators 1991 Effect of enalapril on survival in patients with reduced left ventricular ejection fractions and congestive heart failure. New England Journal of Medicine 325: 293-302

The SOLVD Investigators 1992 Effect of enalapril on mortality and the development of heart failure in asymptomatic patients with reduced left ventricular ejection fractions. New England Journal of Medicine 327: 685-691

Treating hypertension in patients with diabetes mellitus 1994 Drugs and Therapeutics Bulletin 32: 79-80

Who needs nine ACE Inhibitors? 1995 Drugs and Therapeutics Bulletin 33: 1-3

56. Losartan

A. **T**   B. **T**   C. **F**   D. **F**   E. **F**

The angiotensin receptor antagonists are phenyl tetrazole substituted imidazoles. The best known is losartan. They are non-competitive antagonists of the angiotensin II receptors AT1 and AT2. They are 30 000 times more selective for the AT1 receptor than for the AT2. Angiotensin II binds to the AT1 receptor which is coupled to a G protein and causes vasoconstriction and aldosterone release. Angiotensin receptor antagonists have been shown to block these effects both in vitro and in vivo and are now licensed for the treatment of essential hypertension. Losartan has the advantage over its predecessors of having no partial agonist activity.

Unlike the angiotensin converting enzyme (ACE) inhibitors, losartan has no other substrates and therefore has no action on bradykinins, luteinizing hormone releasing hormone or substance P. The most common side-effect of ACE inhibitors is an irritating dry cough. This is mediated via the bradykinin system and therefore should not occur with losartan. Losartan is a pro-drug and is metabolized in the liver by the cytochrome P450 system to the more active metabolite EXP 3174. It is advised that the dose of losartan should be reduced in hepatic impairment but more data is needed regarding its safety in renal impairment. Caution should be also exercised in patients with very low creatinine clearance and it is not recommended for the treatment of renovascular hypertension. It has uricosuric activity and can be used safely in hyperuricaemic patients.

References

Bauer J H, Reams G P 1995 The angiotensin II type 1 receptor antagonists. A new class of anti-hypertensive drugs. Archives of Internal Medicine 155: 1361-1368

Johnston C I 1995 Angiotensin receptor antagonists: focus on losartan. Lancet. 346: 1403-1407

Losartan– a new anti-hypertensive 1995 Drugs and Therapeutics · Bulletin 33: 73-74

57. Calcium channel blockers
A. **F**   B. **T**   C. **F**   D. **F**   E. **T**

Calcium channel blockers inhibit the slow inward calcium current in cardiac and smooth muscle by combining with specific receptors on voltage and receptor operated calcium channels. Reduced intracellular calcium leads to vasodilation and negative inotropic, chronotropic and dromotropic effects. The dihydropyridine group, of which nifedipine is an example, act mainly on arterial smooth muscle whereas diltiazem and particularly verapamil have more direct cardiac actions. Dihydropyridines are used in hypertension and angina, and verapamil is mainly used for atrial tachyarrhythmias. The dihydropyridines frequently cause headache, flushing and palpitations; they can also cause peripheral oedema by disturbing local microcirculatory dynamics. Verapamil can precipitate cardiac failure particularly if prescribed with beta-blockers.

There has been recent controversy surrounding the role of these agents in ischaemic heart disease. In a case-control study 623 hypertensives who had suffered a first myocardial infarction (MI) were compared to 2032 hypertensive controls. In hypertensives who were free of previous cardiovascular disease, those taking calcium antagonists had 1.62 times the risk of having an MI. Some have criticized the study, stating that differences in the degree of hypertension between patients taking calcium channel blockers and those on other drugs were not adequately controlled for. However, the odds ratio for MI was still 1.57 when those on calcium antagonists alone were compared with patients on beta-blockers. The increased risk of MI was dose dependent. Although this study does not prove that calcium antagonists increase the incidence of MI, it clearly suggests that there is a potential risk which needs further evaluation.

Further evidence which has cast doubt on the safety of calcium antagonists comes from a meta-analysis of nifedipine used for secondary prevention of ischaemic heart disease. Nifedipine use was linked to death in a clear dose-dependent manner. Clearly different calcium antagonists have different therapeutic and side-effect profiles, and extrapolation of results from one drug to another is not valid. However the results of these trials has led to a re-evaluation of these agents, particularly the use of high dose nifedipine, as first-line agents in angina and hypertension.

References

Horton R 1995 Spinning the risks and benefits of calcium antagonists. Lancet 346: 586-587

Psaty B M, Heckbert S R, Koepsell T D et al 1995 The risk of myocardial infarction associated with anti-hypertensive drug therapies. Journal of the American Medical Association 274: 620-625

58. Anti-epileptic drugs

A. T   B. F   C. F   D. F   E. T

Treatment with an anti-epileptic drug is usually indicated if a patient has more than one unprovoked seizure within a year. About 30% of patients with seizures have an identifiable neurological or systemic disorder, the remainder have idiopathic epilepsy.

Carbamazepine, sodium valproate and phenytoin are all effective in reducing the frequency of both partial and tonic-clonic seizures. They all act by preventing sustained repetitive firing through voltage- and use-dependent blockade of sodium channels. Sodium valproate is often preferred to phenytoin because of the latter's saturation kinetics and unwanted cosmetic side-effects.

Carbamazepine should not be used in patients with absence or myoclonic seizures. Its common side-effects are diplopia, headache, dizziness and nausea. Peak plasma concentrations which occur about 2 hours after the dose can cause drowsiness, but by prescribing a controlled release preparation this can be avoided. Idiosyncratic reactions include a morbilliform rash which occurs in up to 10% of patients, other skin eruptions and a mild leukopenia. At high plasma concentrations carbamazepine has an anti-diuretic hormone effect which can cause hyponatraemia. Carbamazepine induces liver enzymes accelerating its own metabolism and that of other lipid soluble drugs, such as the oral contraceptive pill. Drugs which inhibit its metabolism include cimetidine, diltiazem, erythromycin, isoniazid and verapamil. It produces a neurotoxic reaction with lithium which is not related to either of their plasma concentrations.

The pharmacokinetics of phenytoin are unusual changing from first order to zero order at therapeutic doses. Phenytoin causes reversible gum hypertrophy, acne, hirsutism and coarsening of the facies. Drowsiness, tremor, slurred speech and ataxia usually occur only at high plasma concentrations, but the diagnosis of toxicity should be a clinical one. Phenytoin is an inducer of liver enzymes involved in oxidative metabolism. Drugs that inhibit its metabolism and precipitate toxicity include allopurinol, amiodarone, cimetidine, imipramine and sulphonamides.

The most common side-effects of sodium valproate are dose related tremor, appetite stimulation, hair loss and menstrual irregularities. Stupor and encephalopathy are very rare and are thought to be due to a deficiency of carnitine. 20% of patients have hyperammonaemia but only 1 in 20 000 has evidence of hepatotoxicity.

About 30% of patients with epilepsy have seizures that are refractory to monotherapy. It is important to establish patient compliance before adjusting treatment. If the seizure is due to an underlying structural lesion the addition of other drugs is successful in only 10% of cases. Patients should be controlled whenever possible on one drug. Careful introduction of a second drug until control is reached and then the discontinuation of the first is the ideal. The addition of one of the newer drugs, lamotrigine, gabapentin, vigabatrin, and clobazam may be the most appropriate second line treatment but no consensus has been reached. In severe refractory epilepsy surgical ablation of the epileptic focus may be beneficial.

Most women with epilepsy have uneventful pregnancies and their seizures remain well controlled. The risk to mother and baby from stopping treatment and inducing seizures is far greater than the risk to the foetus from the anti-epileptic drugs. There is a 3% chance of fetal malformation in mothers taking monotherapy for epilepsy compared to a 2% chance in the general population. However, the risk increases dramatically if the mother is on more than one drug. A syndrome involving palate and lip malformations, cardiac defects, digital hypoplasia and nail dysplasia was initially attributed to phenytoin use, but also occurs with carbamazepine and sodium valproate. Carbamazepine and sodium valproate are also associated with an increased risk of neural tube defects and it is practice to give 5 mg of folic acid to women taking these drugs who are trying to conceive or who are pregnant. Carbamazepine and phenytoin can cause a reversible deficiency in vitamin K dependent clotting factors in the neonate, with an increased risk of intracerebral haemorrhage. Women should be given vitamin K for the last few weeks of their pregnancy and the neonate should be given a single intramuscular dose of vitamin K.

References

Brodie M J, Dichter M A 1996 Anti-epileptic drugs. New England Journal of Medicine 334: 168-17

Engel J 1996 Surgery for seizures. New England Journal of Medicine 334: 647-652

59. Parkinson's disease
A. F   B. T   C. F   D. F   E. F.

Parkinson's disease is a progressive neurodegenerative disorder affecting 165 per 100 000 of the population. The prevalence increases with age. The clinical features are bradykinesia, a resting tremor and rigidity. In the early stages of the disease no drug treatment may be necessary but counselling and advice are vital.

None of the current treatments alters the progression of the disease process. Selegiline is a type B monoamine oxidase inhibitor which reduces the breakdown of dopamine. Early reports suggested that it might protect against oxidative stress induced neurodegeneration and improve life expectancy in Parkinson's disease. DATATOP was a large multicentre trial that showed that treatment with selegiline delayed the need to start levodopa by about 9 months. Initially this was thought to be evidence of the neuroprotective action of selegiline, but it may have been simply that selegiline was treating the symptoms of the disease as opposed to delaying its progression. A recent report found levodopa given in combination with selegiline conferred no benefit over levodopa alone and that mortality in the combination arm was significantly higher. The role of selegiline in the treatment of Parkinson's disease is now under question.

Levodopa is the mainstay of treatment. It is given in combination with a peripheral dopa-decarboxylase inhibitor, preventing the peripheral breakdown of levodopa to dopamine and reducing the systemic side-effects, as well as ensuring a sufficiently large dose of levodopa reaches the striatum. Unwanted side-effects of nausea, vomiting and postural hypotension are minimized by slowly titrating up the dose. Domperidone can be useful at reducing the nausea and vomiting without exacerbating the Parkinson's disease as it does not cross the blood-brain barrier. The dose titration usually continues over 3 to 5 years and disability disappointingly returns to pretreatment levels after 4 to 5 years. After 8 years half of the patients will have developed choreoathetoid dyskinesia and response fluctuations with end-of-dose deterioration. These fluctuations associated with changes in drug concentration may be improved by increasing the dose frequency without altering the total dose, and this is in contrast to the poor results obtained by dose manipulation in patients exhibiting the 'on-off' phenomenon characterized by the patient moving between immobility and mobility in a matter of minutes. Modified-release preparations are commonly used in combination with conventional formulations and adjusted according to the symptoms of the individual. There is some evidence that modified-release drugs used from the outset of drug treatment may delay the development of motor response fluctuations and dyskinesias.

Dopamine agonists such as bromocriptine, lysuride and the longer acting pergolide are used when levodopa alone is no longer adequate. They all cause nausea and vomiting and should be given with domperidone. Antimuscarinic agents block cholinergic receptors in the striatum reducing the relative excess of cholinergic activity and are used in the treatment of tremor in younger patients. Unwanted side-effects include dry mouth, constipation and hesitancy, and less commonly confusion and hallucinations. Amantadine is thought to have antimuscarinic effects and to act as a weak dopamine agonist.

Apomorphine is a potent D1 and D2 agonist which is given by subcutaneous injection when 'off' periods occur. This switches the patient back 'on' and lasts for about 45 minutes giving time for an oral dose of levodopa to take effect. Domperidone must be started 3 days before treatment commences and continued until tolerance occurs. Autoimmune haemolytic anaemia is a rare side-effect of this treatment.

The role of physiotherapy, speech therapy and occupational therapy remains unclear but most evidence suggests it must be on-going to provide any lasting benefit. Support for the carer, both financial and in the provision of respite care, is vital. Depression is common in patients with Parkinson's disease. Dementia occurs in anything from 20–77% of patients, and the common psychiatric side-effects of many of the drugs further complicates the assessment and treatment of these patients.

References

Drugs for Parkinson's disease reviewed 1995 Drug and Therapeutics Bulletin 33 (7): 49-52

Lees A J 1995 (on behalf of the Parkinson's Disease Research Group of the United Kingdom) Comparison of therapeutic effects and mortality data of levodopa, and levodopa combined with selegiline in patients with early, mild Parkinson's disease. British Medical Journal 311: 1602-1607

Parkinson's study group 1989 Effect of deprenyl on the progression of disability in early Parkinson's disease. New England Journal of Medicine 321: 1364-1371

Parkinson's study group 1993 Effects of tocopherol and deprenyl on the progression of disability in early Parkinson's disease. New England Journal of Medicine 328: 176-183

60. Somatostatin and its analogues

A. **F**   B. **T**   C. **T**   D. **F**   E. **T**.

Somatostatin was first detected as an agent which inhibited growth hormone release. We now know that it has a wide range of actions mediated through its interaction with at least five receptors found in a variety of tissues. It is a multigene family of peptides which are expressed in a wide range of species. It is synthesized as a large precursor molecule and then cleaved to produce a pro-hormone which undergoes further modification to produce the bioactive products such as somatostatin-14 and somatostatin-28.

Somatostatin has inhibitory actions on the release of thyrotrophin from the pituitary gland as well as on growth hormone release. It acts as a neurotransmitter in other areas of the brain as well as having wide-ranging inhibitory effects on the gastrointestinal tract. The five receptor subtypes all have seven membrane spanning regions and they have considerable sequence homology. They are all linked to adenylate cyclase by a nucleotide binding G protein.

Somatostatin has a short half-life and it has to be administered intravenously. Structural analogues have therefore been developed in an attempt to produce clinically useful drugs. The best described of these to date is ocreotide. This does not bind to somatostatin receptor subtypes 1 and 4 but has a high affinity for receptor subtypes 2 and 5.

Ocreotide has been used in a variety of clinical settings. In acromegaly, treatment with ocreotide leads to tumour shrinkage in approximately 50% of patients. The relief of symptoms is often more marked than the changes in growth hormone concentration. The response appears to be determined by the density of somatostatin receptors on the tumour cells. It can be used concomitantly with bromocriptine. The suppressive effects can continue for many years. Ocreotide has also been used successfully in the treatment of thyrotrophin secreting adenomas and non-secretory pituitary adenomas.

Pancreatic islet cell tumours secrete a variety of hormones in excess leading to most of their clinical manifestations. They include vipomas, insulinomas, gastrinomas and glucagonomas. Ocreotide can have a marked effect, at least initially on the symptoms they produce. After several months the symptoms recur despite increases in the dose used. It is thought that tumour evolution leading to cells with fewer or no somatostatin receptors is responsible for this effect.

In carcinoid tumours therapy with ocreotide reduces symptoms, can lead to tumour shrinkage and may prolong life. Control of symptoms can be achieved in around 80% of patients with metastatic disease.

A variety of gastrointestinal tract disorders are amenable to ocreotide therapy. Some studies have suggested that it is useful in the treatment of variceal haemorrhage and may be as effective as endoscopic sclerotherapy. It has not been shown to be beneficial in the treatment of bleeding secondary to peptic ulcer disease. It is beneficial in the treatment of pancreatic pseudocysts and in the prevention of complications from pancreatic surgery when administered perioperatively. It has also been shown to be beneficial in relieving symptoms in secretory diarrhoeas.

The side-effects include nausea, abdominal cramps, diarrhoea and flatulence. These symptoms often subside with continued therapy. In the longer term the development of cholesterol gall stones occurs in 20–30% of patients though important clinical consequences are unusual.

Further development of somatostatin analogues with actions on different receptor subtypes may lead to new therapies for many of the conditions mentioned above.

Reference

Lamberts S W J, Van Der Lely A, De Herder W W et al 1996 Drug therapy. Ocreotide. New England Journal of Medicine 334: 246-254.

---

61. Fibrosing colonopathy

A. F B. T C. F D. F E. F

Between 1993 and 1994 13 children with cystic fibrosis who were receiving high-strength pancreatic enzyme supplements were reported to have developed large bowel strictures. All required surgical resection and the pathology was found to be a new disease entity. Fibrosing colonopathy was the name given to this new disease which is defined by distinct histological criteria.

A case-control study of the UK cystic fibrosis population was performed. 7600 patients were identified compiling almost all of the cystic patients treated in the UK over a 10-year period. 14 cases of fibrosing colonopathy were identified, all but one had been reported to the Committee on Safety of Medicines. Four matched patient controls were selected for each of these cases. No cases were identified prior to 1993 when the first high-strength pancreatic enzymes were introduced to the UK. There was a strong association between use of these drugs in the 2 years before surgery and development of the colonopathy, and those who developed fibrosing colonopathy were taking twice the dose of the control group.

The study showed that Nutrizym 22 and Pancrease HL were associated with the development of fibrosing colonopathy, whereas Creon 25 000 was not. The other risk factors identified were gender (boys were more at risk than girls), more severe cystic fibrosis and concomitant use of laxatives.

The high-dose preparations are not recommended for use in children under 15 years of age. The total dose of pancreatic enzyme supplements used in patients with cystic fibrosis should not usually exceed 10 000 units of lipase per kilogram of body weight per day.

Reference

Smyth R L, Van Velzen D, Smyth A R et al 1994 Strictures of ascending colon in cystic fibrosis and high-strength pancreatic enzymes. Lancet 343: 85-86

62.   Beta 2 agonists

A. F   B. T   C. F   D. F   E. F

Beta 2 adrenergic bronchodilators are used in the treatment of bronchial asthma and reversible obstructive airway disease. Beta 2 agonists exert their effect by interaction with beta 2 receptors. These receptors which are present on virtually all cells, are linked to a stimulatory guanine-nucleotide-binding protein, which when activated leads to a rise in cyclic AMP. Both beta 1 and beta 2 receptors are present in the lung but the beta 2 receptors are almost entirely responsible for the bronchodilation. Beta 2 receptors are downregulated in response to high dose or prolonged exposure to beta agonists. This is effected through receptor phosphorylation, internalization and by reduced transcription of messenger RNA. The resultant desensitization is known as tachyphylaxis. Upregulation, or increased production is stimulated by glucocorticosteroids and thyroid hormone.

Long and intermediate-acting beta agonists are not broken down by catechol O-methyltransferase. They have extended side chains which are highly lipophilic and have high affinity for the receptors.

The side chain of salmeterol binds to a specific site within the beta 2 receptor that allows prolonged activation.

As well as causing bronchodilation, beta 2 agonists inhibit the release of inflammatory mediators by mast cells and basophils, inhibit cholinergic neurotransmission and enhance mucocillary clearance. The principal side-effect of beta 2 agonists is tremor. They also frequently cause tachycardia and palpitations through a direct effect on beta 2 receptors within the heart and in response to peripheral vasodilation. The acute metabolic affects of beta 2 agonists include hyperglycaemia, hypokalaemia and hypomagnesaemia.

By using the inhaled route the systemic side-effects can be minimized. With optimal technique approximately 12% of the drug is delivered to the lungs by a metered-dose inhaler. Nebulizers require 6 to 10 times the dose to produce the same degree of bronchodilation. Some experts believe that the supervised use of a spacer is as effective as a nebulizer in the emergency setting.

Reference

Nelson H S 1995 Drug therapy: B-adrenergic bronchodilators. New England Journal of Medicine 333: 499-506.

63. Quinine sulphate and minocycline

A. T   B. F   C. F   D. F   E. T

Quinine sulphate and minocycline are commonly prescribed for benign conditions and recent reports have focused on the indications for their use.

Quinine sulphate is commonly prescribed for the treatment of nocturnal cramp. A study in Glasgow found over half the patients taking quinine for cramp were also on drugs whose recognized side-effects included cramp. Nifedipine, cimetidine, salbutamol, terbutaline, and diuretics all cause cramp. The side-effects of quinine include tinnitus, haemolytic anaemia and drug fever. Quinine in overdose may cause severe visual impairment. Although a recent meta-analysis found quinine to be an effective treatment for cramp, it should not be prescribed unless other cramp-inducing agents which can be stopped have been.

Minocycline is commonly used for the treatment of acne but may produce serious side-effects. It has been reported to cause a drug-induced chronic active hepatitis associated with polyarthralgia and positive antinuclear antibodies but negative antibodies to DNA. Other drugs causing chronic active hepatitis include nitrofurantoin, methyldopa, and diclofenac. Minocycline has also been reported in association with eosinophilic pneumonitis, where patients suffered from cough, dyspnoea and fever, with pulmonary infiltrates on chest X-ray and eosinophilia on the blood film. Reports of such immunological complications with tetracycline and oxytetracycline are extremely rare. Minocycline may also cause hyperpigmentation of skin, teeth and internal organs, and causes a dose-dependent vestibulitis. Tetracycline can aggravate pre-existing lupus, and can cause benign intracranial hypertension. All tetracyclines are contraindicated in pregnancy. Both tetracycline and oxytetracycline are cheaper and probably safer than minocycline for the treatment of acne.

References

Ferner R E, Moss C 1996 Minocycline for acne. British Medical Journal 312: 138

Gough A, Chapman S, Wagstaff K et al 1996 Minocycline induced autoimmune hepatitis and systemic lupus erythematosus-like syndrome. British Medical Journal 312: 169-172

Mackie M A, Davidson J 1995 Prescribing of quinine and cramp inducing drugs in general practice. British Medical Journal 311: 541

Man-Son-Hing M, Wells G 1995 Meta-analysis of efficacy of quinine for the treatment of nocturnal leg cramps in elderly people. British Medical Journal 310: 13-16

64.   The oral contraceptive pill

A. F   B. F   C. T   D. T   E. T

In 1995 the Committee on Safety of Medicines reported to the Government on preliminary results of studies which were showing an excess risk of venous thromboembolism (VTE) in users of the newest brands of oral contraceptive pills containing desogestral and gestodene. A press warning was released before the results had been published for peer scrutiny, and before many doctors had received any information about the changing situation.

The studies which were subsequently published in December were: a subanalysis of data from the large WHO study of women in 10 countries taking third-generation pills; a case-control study of oral contraceptive users from the British General Practice Research data base; and a re-analysis of the Leiden thrombophilia study. A further trial from the transnational research group was published in January 1996. Despite the different designs and populations all the studies showed an approximate two-fold excess risk of venous thromboembolism in takers of third generation OCPs. This increased risk could not be explained by any known or expected bias or by any confounder. This excess risk is superimposed upon the baseline risk of pill taking which confers three times the risk of VTE upon users of second generation pills. Ignoring high risk groups some studies calculated the excess risk for third generation pill users to be as high as nine.

Some researchers believed that the third-generation pill might confer hidden advantages to the user through its beneficial effects on lipid profile, such as a reduction in myocardial infarction. The transnational research group did find a three fold reduction in incidence of myocardial infarction in users of the third generation pills but this was not statistically significant and further studies are now unlikely. More importantly this group found that those most at risk from taking the pill are smokers. Smoking while taking the pill results in a ten-fold increased risk of having a myocardial infarction.

When prescribing any OCP a careful family and personal history of venous thromboembolism must be taken and where appropriate a thrombophilia screen performed. The woman should also be counselled about the dangers of smoking while taking the pill. Blood pressure should be checked before prescribing the pill, and at follow-up, as it can cause hypertension. The patient should be warned that taking rifampicin and other enzyme inducers may make the pill ineffective and an alternative form of contraception should be used.

References

Department of Health 1995 New advice on oral contraceptives. Department of Health, London

Farley T M M, Meirik O, Chang C L et al 1995 Effect of different progestagens in low oestrogen oral contraceptives on venous thromboembolic disease. Lancet; 346: 1582-1588

Jick H, Jick S S, Gurewich V et al 1995 Risk of idiopathic cardiovascular death and non-fatal venous thromboembolism in women using oral contraceptives with differing progestagen components. Lancet 346: 1589-1593

Lewis A L, Spitzer W O, Heinemann L A J et al 1996 Transnational research group on oral contraceptives and the health of young women. Third generation oral contraceptives and risk of myocardial infarction: an international case-control study. British Medical Journal 312: 88-90

McPherson K 1996 Third generation oral contraceptives and venous thromboembolism. British Medical Journal 312: 68-69

Poulter N R, Chang C L, Farley T M M et al 1995 Venous thromboembolic disease and combined oral contraceptives: results of international multicentre case-control study. Lancet 346: 1575-1582

Spitzer W O, Lewis A L, Heinemann L A J et al 1996 Transnational research group on oral contraceptives and the health of young women. Third generation oral contraceptives and risk of venous thromboembolic disorders: an international case-control study. British Medical Journal 312: 83-88.

65. Retinoic acid

A. T   B. F   C. F   D. T   E. F

The retinoids are vitamin A derivatives that play critical roles in normal development, growth and differentiation. The oxidized form of vitamin A is retinoic acid, which is important for maintaining epithelial cellular integrity. Vitamin A deficiency in vivo leads to squamous metaplasia, which is reversed by vitamin A therapy. Vitamin A is also essential for normal vision and reproduction. Retinoic acid receptors fall into a number of groups. One group binds retinoic acid in the gastrointestinal mucosa, another is found in the cytoplasm, and may act as cellular storage sites, another has homology with the steroid receptor superfamily and acts as a hormone-dependent transcription factor that activates genes by binding to DNA.

Acute pro-myelocytic leukaemia (APL) accounts for 15% of adult cases of acute myeloid leukaemia. It represents a clonal expansion of immature pro-myelocytes. In the French American British classification it is designated M3. APL is characterized clinically by a haemorrhagic diathesis with accelerated intravascular coagulation, hyperfibrinolysis and thrombocytopenia. Approximately 90% of patients with APL have a reciprocal translocation between chromosomes 15 and 17. The gene breakpoints involved in this translocation involve the retinoic acid alpha receptor on the long arm of chromosome 17 and the pro-myelocytic leukaemia gene (a transcription factor) on the long arm of chromosome 15. The fusion product acts as a retinoic acid dependent transcription factor. The protein resulting from this fusion appears to inhibit myeloid maturation.

Oral all-trans retinoic acid (ATRA) therapy induces transient complete remissions in most patients with APL. Conventional chemotherapeutic agents induce clinical remissions in APL by producing a cytotoxic effect leading to bone marrow hypoplasia and death of leukaemic cells. In contrast, ATRA alters the growth and maturation of APL cells in vivo. This maturation presumably results from interaction of ATRA with the t(15;17) gene product, but the exact mechanism remains obscure.

Therapeutic activity of retinoids has been observed in premalignant and overtly malignant settings other than APL. Retinoids inhibit the conversion of oral hairy leucoplakia to oral cavity cancer, they cause regression of squamous cell carcinoma, they reduce the incidence of secondary aerodigestive tract cancer in patients following complete resection of head and neck cancer, they induce anti-tumour responses in some cutaneous malignancies and have activity in treating cervical dysplasia.

A putative tumour suppressor gene in lung cancer has been located on chromosome 3 and the retinoic acid beta receptor maps to the same region. It may be that abnormalities of retinoic acid receptor function play a key role in the deregulation of lung cancer cells.

Reference

Early E, Dmitrovsky E 1995 Acute pro-myelocytic leukaemia: retinoic acid response and resistance. Journal of Investigative Medicine 43: 337-344

66. Metformin

A. T   B. T   C. F   D. T   E. F

Metformin is a biguanide and has been used to treat non-insulin dependent diabetes mellitus (NIDDM) for many years in Europe. It has only recently received approval from the Food and Drug Administration in the United States of America.

It lowers plasma fasting glucose levels and glycosylated haemoglobin levels in patients with NIDDM. It reduces hepatic glucose production and this is principally due to impaired hepatic gluconeogenesis but it also appears to inhibit hepatic glycogenolysis. It increases the efficiency of muscle glucose uptake. It suppresses the appetite and can lead to weight reduction. Unlike the sulphonylurea drugs metformin does not increase insulin secretion.

Metformin reduces plasma total cholesterol, low-density lipoprotein (LDL) cholesterol and triglycerides. All of these are desirable effects in helping to reduce risk profile for the development of macrovascular disease. The common side-effects of metformin are nausea and diarrhoea but these are usually mild and transient and may disappear with dose reduction. Symptoms of hypoglycaemia do occur especially when metformin is prescribed in combination with a sulphonylurea.

Another biguanide phenformin was withdrawn from the market following evidence that it caused lactic acidosis. This was reported to occur at a frequency of 0.25 to 1.0 case per 1000 patient years of treatment. Metformin also causes lactic acidosis but at an estimated incidence of 0.03 per 1000 patient years. The risk of inducing lactic acidosis with associated hypoxia, shock and renal failure is one of the major disadvantages of metformin therapy.

References

Crofford O B 1995 Metformin. New England Journal of Medicine 333: 588-589

DeFronzo R A, Goodman A M 1995 Efficacy of metformin in patients with non-insulin-dependent diabetes mellitus. New England Journal of Medicine 333: 541-549

Stumvoll M, Nurjhan N, Perriello G et al 1995 Metabolic effects of metformin in non-insulin-dependent diabetes mellitus. New England Journal of Medicine 333: 550-554

67. Low-molecular-weight heparins

A. F   B. T   C. T   D. T   E. T

Heparin is used in the treatment and prophylaxis of thromboembolic disease. Standard unfractionated heparin is a heterogeneous preparation which consists of polysaccharide chains of enormously variable length and molecular weights which range from 3000 to 30 000. Low-molecular-weight heparins with weights between 4000 and 6000 have recently been developed. These shorter chain polysaccharides are produced by enzymatic or chemical depolymerization of standard heparin molecules. Low-molecular-weight heparins confer several theoretical advantages over the older unfractionated heparins and have been shown to have clinical advantages in trials.

Heparin works by binding to and enhancing the activity of antithrombin III. The binding region consists of a unique pentasaccharide sequence which is randomly distributed throughout the chains. Standard heparin has similar activity against thrombin and factor Xa whereas the low-molecular-weight heparins have more marked inhibitory activity against factor Xa. The reason for this difference is that the inactivation of thrombin requires that a molecule of heparin binds both antithrombin III and thrombin forming a ternary, which usually requires a chain length of 18 saccharide units or more. There is a very low proportion of such molecules in the low-molecular-weight heparin preparations. The inactivation of factor Xa only requires the binding of antithrombin III to the heparin molecule and the subsequent interaction of antithrombin III with factor Xa.

There are other differences in their actions. Low-molecular-weight heparins can inactivate factor Xa when it is platelet bound. It is more resistant to inactivation by platelet factor 4, it has less pronounced effects on platelet function and vascular permeability. It has more favourable bioavailability and pharmacokinetics. Its half life is also longer.

Clinical trials have now shown that some of these preparations can be administered once or twice daily with dose adjustments for body weight only. There is no need to measure clotting. It has been found to be as effective and at least as safe as standard heparin. Meta-analyses have shown non-significant trends towards improved safety and efficacy in the initial treatment of deep vein thrombosis. The newer preparations are also less likely to induce thrombocytopenia.

Work by Koopman et al and also Levine et al has demonstrated that enoxaparin and nadroparin-Ca are safe when used for out-patient treatment of selected patients with proximal deep vein thromboses. The adverse event profiles were very similar to the standard heparin regime used as a control in both studies. The number of days spent in hospital were markedly reduced with between 36 and 49% of patients not requiring hospital admission. The use of these new agents, despite the increased drug costs may prove to be highly cost-effective over all.

References

Koopman M W, Prandoni P, Piovella F et al 1996 Treatment of venous thrombosis with intravenous unfractionated heparin administered in the hospital as compared with subcutaneous low-molecular-weight heparin administered at home. New England Journal of Medicine 334: 682-687

Leizorovicz A, Simonneau G, Decousus H et al 1994 Comparison of the efficacy and safety of low-molecular-weight heparins and unfractionated heparins in the initial treatment of deep vein thrombosis: a meta-analysis. British Medical Journal 309: 299-304

Lensing A W, Prins M H, Davidson B L et al 1995 Treatment of deep vein thrombosis with low-molecular-weight heparins: a meta-analysis. Archives of Internal Medicine 155: 601-607

Levine M, Gent M, Hirsh J et al 1996 A comparison of low-molecular-weight heparin administered primarily at home with unfractionated heparin administered in the hospital for proximal deep-vein thrombosis. New England Journal of Medicine 334: 677-681

Schafer A I 1996 Low-molecular heparin – an opportunity for home treatment of venous thrombosis. New England Journal of Medicine 334: 724-726

HAEMATOLOGY
68. Blood products
A. T   B. F   C. F   D. T   E. T

Blood product transfusion has many uses and is associated with many risks. Blood components such as red and white cells are separated from whole blood donations and have a short shelf life. Products such as immunoglobulins and factor VIII are manufactured from blood and have a shelf life of many months.

Red cell and white cell transfusions require ABO crossmatching. White cell preparations contain many erythrocytes so ABO incompatibility may cause severe transfusion reactions. With the advent of recombinant granulocyte-colony stimulating factors their use in immunosuppressed patients is declining.

Red cell transfusions are usually given as red cells resuspended in optimal additive solutions such as SAG-M (sodium chloride, adenine, glucose and mannitol). These cells lack coagulation factors and platelets and therefore large transfusions are associated with an increased risk of bleeding.

In the general population cytomegalovirus (CMV) infection is common and probably as many as one in two units of donated blood are positive for anti-CMV. Immunosuppressed patients may be given leucocyte depleted blood which reduces the risk of CMV infection. In addition, leucocyte depleted blood will reduce transfusion reactions with human leucocyte antigen (HLA) antibodies.

Platelet transfusions do not require crossmatching but HLA antibodies may develop after recurrent transfusions and HLA matched platelet transfusion is available. Platelets are given to cover high risk procedures in thrombocytopenic patients, to treat chemotherapy induced thrombocytopenia or thrombocytopenia secondary to leukaemia or aplastic anaemia. Occasionally they are used as supportive therapy in disseminated intravascular coagulation (DIC). Platelet transfusion is not beneficial in thrombotic thrombocytopenic purpura (TTP).

Fresh frozen plasma (FFP) derived from blood or plasma donation has a long shelf life when stored at -30°C. FFP contains clotting factors, anticoagulants, immunoglobulins, C1-esterase inhibitor, alpha-1-antitrypsin, albumin and fibronectin. Its use is indicated in DIC and TTP and to reverse warfarin overdose.

Standard human immunoglobulin provides temporary passive prophylaxis against hepatitis A, rubella and measles. Hyperimmune globulins are useful for the treatment of these infections and also for rabies, tetanus, diphtheria, CMV and pseudomonas infections. Intravenous immunoglobulin is used to treat immunoglobulin deficiency and a range of other disorders, such as Guillain-Barré syndrome, Wegener's granulomatosis and immune thrombocytopenic purpura. Specific immunoglobulins can be used for herpes zoster exposure in pregnancy, hepatitis B exposure following needle stick injury and rhesus incompatibility.

All blood products are screened for human immunodeficiency virus, hepatitis C, hepatitis B surface antigen and syphilis. Selected units are screened for CMV and at risk units are screened for malaria antibodies. The risk of transmission following these procedures is now very small but not absent. People who received human growth factor prior to 1985 can potentially transmit prion disease causing Creutzfeldt Jakob disease and are excluded as donors. All preparations containing cells can potentially transmit viral infections. FFP and cryoprecipitate can also transmit infections but not those which depend on cells for survival. Most manufactured products probably undergo virus destruction in their preparation and are low risk, e.g. immunoglobulin. However hepatitis C transmission has been described. Factor VIII is heat treated which seems to eliminate HIV and hepatitis C, but some viruses such as parvovirus can survive this method of preparation.

References

Power J P, Lawlor E, Davidson F et al 1995 Molecular epidemiology of an outbreak of infection with hepatitis C in recipients of anti-D immunoglobin. Lancet 345: 1211-1213

The risks and uses of donated blood 1993 Drugs and Therapeutics Bulletin 33: 89-92

69. Disseminated intravascular coagulation

A. F.   B. T   C. F   D. F   E. T

Disseminated intravascular coagulation (DIC) is a clinical diagnosis which is supported by the laboratory findings of thrombocytopenia, a prolonged prothrombin time and activated partial thromboplastin time, reduced levels of fibrinogen and increased fibrinogen degradation products. Red cell fragmentation may be seen on the blood film but is not pathonomic of the disease. Prothrombin time and activated partial thromboplastin time are prolonged in only 70% and 50% of cases respectively. High plasma concentrations of fibrinogen degradation products are present in 85% of patients but are not specific, as they are also found to be elevated in patients who have recently undergone surgery, in patients with haematomas, and in patients with liver or renal failure.

The normal response to tissue damage involves a localized production of thrombin at the site of injury resulting in coagulation and the stemming of any blood loss. If thrombin is generated next to healthy endothelium this process is rapidly halted. Thrombin is either neutralized by antithrombin or is inactivated by being bound to thrombomodulin. The thrombin-thrombomodulin complex activates the protein C system which further tips the balance towards anticoagulation. In DIC the production of thrombin is not contained and it is released into the wider circulation causing microvascular thrombosis, tissue ischaemia and organ damage. In response to the tissue ischaemia and in an attempt to maintain microvascular patency, excess plasmin is generated causing systemic fibrinogenolysis and local fibrinolysis which in turn results in the haemorrhagic manifestations of the disorder.

Tissue necrosis factor and interleukin-1 can elicit production of tissue factor by endothelial cells and monocytes and reduce the expression of thrombomodulin. Thus in inflammatory reactions there is a shift towards a hypercoagulable state.

Acute DIC is most commonly caused by infection. About 10–20% of patients with gram negative infections have evidence of DIC. Other causes include placental abruption, amniotic fluid embolism, trauma and transfusion with ABO incompatible red blood cells. Chronic DIC may result from malignancy particularly adenocarcinoma. Heparin is useful in preventing the venous thromboembolism which is a common manifestation of this condition. The other causes of chronic DIC are the retained dead fetus syndrome, liver disease and severe localized intravascular coagulation accompanying aortic aneurysms, haemangiomas or empyemas.

The haemorrhagic sequelae of DIC may be spontaneous bruising, gastrointestinal, respiratory tract and surgical wound bleeding, or an intracranial bleed. The excess thrombin generated results in thromboses which may cause renal failure, coma, liver and respiratory failure, skin necrosis, gangrene and venous thromboembolism. The patient may also have signs of the underlying condition.

Treating the underlying condition is essential when treating a patient with DIC. The best use of blood components and the absolute indications for anticoagulation are not known. Vitamin K may help reverse the coagulopathy of critically ill patients, and maintenance of blood volume and tissue perfusion is essential. The decision to start replacing blood components depends not on absolute values but on whether the patient is bleeding or is about to have a procedure. Platelet concentrates are given at a dose of 1 donor unit per 10 kg of body weight and fresh frozen plasma at a dose of 15 ml/kg body weight with an aim to maintain the fibrinogen concentration above 0.5 g/l. Fresh frozen plasma is better than cryoprecipitate as it contains more fibrinogen as well as all the anticoagulation factors and anticoagulants. The indications for using heparin have not been established in most cases of DIC and it should be used only with extreme caution. In patients with cancer and large vessel thrombosis heparin has been shown to be beneficial when given in doses which prolong the activated partial thromboplastin time to twice normal. Treatment with natural inhibitors of thrombin such as antithrombin and protein C have shown some encouraging results in initial studies.

Reference

Baglin T 1996 Disseminated intravascular coagulation: diagnosis and treatment. British Medical Journal 312: 683–687

70. Colony stimulating factors

A. **T**   B. **T**   C. **T**   D. **T**   E. **T**

Colony stimulating factors (CSF) are a group of molecules that stimulate haemopoiesis. They can now be produced in pure form by recombinant DNA technology.

Mature peripheral blood cells are produced from pluripotent stem cells through leucopoeitic, erythropoeitic or thrombopoeitic lineages of development. CSFs are able to direct development of progenitor cells down one or more lineage. Erythropoietin promotes formation of red cells and the recently discovered and produced thrombopoietin stimulates platelet production.

Granulocyte-CSF (G-CSF) is produced by endothelial cells, monocytes and fibroblasts and acts predominantly on cells in the granulocyte-monocyte lineage, increasing the number of neutrophils in peripheral blood. Granulocyte macrophage-colony stimulating factor (GM-CSF) is produced by many cell types, and promotes neutrophil, monocyte and megakaryocyte production. GM-CSF and G-CSF cause a transient leucopenia followed by a sustained rise in the peripheral leucocyte count.

Randomized controlled trials of G-CSF and GM-CSF have established that they reduce the duration of severe neutropenia following both conventional chemotherapy and high dose chemotherapy with bone marrow transplantation. They reduce the duration and incidence of infection, allowing earlier discharge from hospital and may reduce mortality. CSFs facilitate the harvesting of progenitor cells from the peripheral blood and may prove useful in the treatment of aplastic anaemia, myelodysplasia and AIDS.

In acute infections and endotoxaemia circulating levels of G-CSF, macrophage-CSF as well as interleukin-1 (IL-1), IL-6, IL-8 and tumour necrosis factor are increased. These factors are probably responsible for the leucocytosis which is associated with many infections. Clinical trials of G-CSF in community acquired pneumonia and endotoxaemia are now under way. The recent discovery of thrombopoietin holds much promise for the treatment of thrombocytopenia.

Adverse reactions such as bone pain and liver dysfunction with G-CSF, and rashes and myalgia with GM-CSF although common rarely prevent therapy. The fever associated with GM-CSF can lead to diagnostic difficulties in those at risk of sepsis. Vasculitis, deep vein thrombosis, pulmonary embolus, as well as pleural and pericardial effusions have been reported with high dose GM-CSF therapy. G-CSF and GM-CSF cost about £80 per day at standard dose.

References

Dale C D 1995 Where now for colony stimulating factors? Lancet 346: 135-136

Stewart W P 1993 Granulocyte and granulocyte-macrophage colony stimulating factors. Lancet 342: 153-157

71. Thrombophilia

A. T   B. F   C. F   D. F   E. T

Thrombophilia is said to exist when an individual possesses a discrete prothrombotic mutation. These mutations give rise to conditions known as the primary hypercoagulable states. The most important and most studied of these are the antithrombin III / heparin disorders, the protein C/protein S disorders and the fibrinolytic disorders.

Antithrombin III inhibits blood coagulation by inactivating thrombin, as well as factors XIIa, XIa, IXa and Xa. Heparin acts by binding to antithrombin III, altering its configuration and thereby enhancing its neutralizing ability. Antithrombin III deficiency is inherited in an autosomal dominant manner. There is a wide variation in the incidence of thrombosis between different kindreds, and qualitative as well as quantitative abnormalities of antithrombin III exist, requiring functional rather than immunological assays for diagnosis.

When thrombin binds to the endothelial receptor thrombomodulin, activated protein C is released from endothelium to form a complex with protein S. This complex then inactivates factors Va and VIIIa. Protein C and S deficiencies are autosomally inherited, homozygous protein C deficiency resulting in neonatal purpura fulminans. Heterozygous protein C deficiency occurs in 0.5% of the population, the majority of this group being symptom free. In families with a history of thrombosis, 50% of members heterozygous for protein C deficiency will have thrombosis. Qualitative as well as quantitative protein S and protein C abnormalities exist. These factors are vitamin-K-dependent and screening for deficiency should occur before starting warfarin therapy. Protein C has a shorter half-life than the other vitamin-K-dependent factors, resulting in a transient hypercoagulable state on the initiation of warfarin therapy in some individuals with protein C deficiency. This can lead to the rare complication of warfarin induced skin necrosis.

Various abnormalities of the fibrinolytic system exist including hypo and dysplasminoginaemia, reduced tissue plasminogen activator release, and increased levels of plasminogen activator inhibitor. All result in a reduced fibrinolytic response to fibrin formation, and a hypercoagulable state.

Secondary hypercoagulable states include immobility, obesity, heart failure, and the postoperative state. Clinical thrombosis usually only occurs when a secondary hypercoagulable state exists in an individual with one or more underlying primary hypercoagulable state. In patients with recurrent thrombosis, more than one mutation affecting the clotting system may exist.

The management of patients with a primary hypercoagulable state is controversial. Patients with recurrent thrombosis and an underlying primary hypercoagulable state will benefit from long-term anticoagulation. Patients with an abnormality detected on thrombophilia screening are unlikely to have clinical problems unless there is a strong family history or past medical history of thrombotic episodes. They should therefore only receive prophylaxis against thrombosis when a secondary state occurs.

Resistance to activated protein C due to a point mutation of the factor V gene (the Leiden mutation) has been described and is the most common primary hypercoagulation disorder detected, occurring in up to 65% of patients with venous thrombosis.

References

Greengard J S, Eichinger S, Griffin J H et al 1994 Variability of thrombosis among homozygous siblings with resistance to activated protein C due to an arg to gln mutation in the gene for factor V. New England Journal of Medicine 331: 1559-1562

Rees D C, Cox M, Clegg J B 1995 World distribution of factor V Leiden. Lancet 346: 1133-1135

Ridker P M , Hennekens C H, Lindpaintner K et al 1995 Mutation in the gene coding for coagulation factor V and the risk of myocardial infarction, stroke, and venous thrombosis in apparently healthy men. New England Journal of Medicine 332: 912-917

Schafer A I 1995 Hypercoagulable states: molecular genetics to clinical practice. Lancet 344: 1739-1742

72. The antiphospholipid syndrome

A. F.   B. T   C. T   D. F   E. T

The antiphospholipid syndrome is a hypercoagulation disorder sometimes associated with autoimmune disorders such as systemic lupus erythematosus (SLE). It may also present as a primary syndrome of recurrent thromboses, early miscarriage and thrombocytopenia in its own right.

It should be suspected in patients who present with venous or arterial thrombosis particularly when recurrent or in unusual sites. It is one of the commonest causes of Budd-Chiari syndrome, a rare condition which is otherwise usually associated with malignancy. Renal vein thrombosis and adrenal infarction are uncommon manifestations.

Associated clinical conditions not directly linked to thrombosis include livedo reticularis, heart valve lesions, haemolytic anaemia and myelopathy.

Diagnosis is made by finding the clinical features in the presence of the antiphospholipid antibody. Treatment is with warfarin aiming for an INR of 3–4. In pregnancy low dose aspirin and subcutaneous heparin are used instead of warfarin which is teratogenic. Corticosteroids may be useful and end arterial limb thrombosis has been successfully treated using prostaglandin I-2 analogues such as iloprost.

References

Hughes G R V, Khamashta M A 1994 The antiphospholipid syndrome. Journal of the Royal College of Physicians 28: 301-304

Zahavi J, Charach G, Schafer R et al 1993 Ischaemic necrotic toes associated with antiphospholipid syndrome and treated with iloprost. Lancet 342: 862

73. Deep venous thrombosis

A. T   B. F   C. F   D. F   E. T

Deep venous thrombosis is a common medical condition. In the hospital setting it is mostly associated with old age, immobilization, previous thrombosis or recent surgery. High risk surgery includes major abdominal operations, orthopaedic surgery and neurosurgery. Other risk factors include pregnancy, trauma and hypercoagulable states. They may be caused by occult malignancies and these are more common in patients under 50. Of the inherited hyper-coagulable states protein C, S and antithrombin III deficiency are the most commonly recognized.

Recently Ridker et al investigated a point mutation on the gene coding for factor V associated with resistance to activated protein C. In a large prospective study of 14 916 healthy men, 704 had venous or arterial thrombosis. The presence of the mutation was significantly higher in the venous thrombosis group.

For pre-operative prophylaxis the use of compression stockings and subcutaneous heparin has greater efficacy than the use of aspirin, although the latter will decrease the incidence by about 30%. Intravenous thrombolysis with streptokinase may produce complete lysis of thrombus and restores patency in a greater proportion of patients compared to heparin alone, but there is uncertainty as to whether this treatment reduces the incidence of the post-phlebitic syndrome and it has no advantage over heparin in the prevention of pulmonary embolus.

A recent publication by Schulman et al suggests that 6 months of anticoagulation confers a significant reduction in recurrence of thrombosis compared with 6 weeks, but whether a period of anticoagulation between these time intervals will produce a similar advantage remains to be clarified. It does however seem that initial heparinization and use of warfarin is superior to warfarin alone in preventing symptomatic extension or recurrence of venous thrombosis.

References

Ridker P M, Hennekens C H, Lindpaintner K et al 1995 Mutation in the gene coding for coagulation factor V and the risk of myocardial infarction, stroke and venous thrombosis in apparently healthy men. New England Journal of Medicine 332: 912-917

Schulman S, Rheiden A, Lindmater P et al 1995 Anticoagulant therapy after a first episode of venous thromboembolism. New England Journal of Medicine 332: 1661-1665

Weinmann E E, Salzman E W 1994 Deep-vein thrombosis. New England Journal of Medicine 311: 1630-1640

74.   Aplastic anaemia

A. F.   B. T   C. F   D. T   E. T

Aplastic anaemia is an uncommon condition with an incidence of 1 in 2 million in Europe. Males and females are affected equally. There are two incidence peaks, one in early adult life and the second in old age. It is diagnosed by finding pancytopenia in the presence of a fatty bone marrow with scattered normal haemopoietic precursors, megaloblasts and sometimes haemophagocytosis. Cytogenetic analysis is normal. These features differentiate it from other pancytopenias, notably myelodysplasia where the marrow is hypocellular with abnormal developing cells and cytogenetics, and myelofibrosis where the marrow is inaspirable and fibrotic. Severe disease is diagnosed in the presence of two of the following three criteria: neutrophils <500/ul, platelets <20 000/ul and reticulocytes <1% of the peripheral blood film.

There are many causes of acquired aplastic anaemia. Iatrogenic causes include cytotoxic chemotherapy and external gamma irradiation. Drugs such as sulphonamides, carbimazole, propylthiouracil, penicillamine and allopurinol cause aplastic anaemia as an idiosyncratic reaction. It has been linked to occupational benzene exposure. In children aplastic anaemia often follows parvovirus infection and flaviviruses have also been implicated. It is a rare complication of pregnancy, which may be cured by termination.

The pathophysiology of idiopathic aplastic anaemia is thought to be an abnormal immune response. The disease is associated with HLA DR2 and responds well to immunosuppression with anti-lymphocyte or anti-thymocyte globulins. Activated cytotoxic T cells seem to express gamma interferon and tumour necrosis factor (TNF) beta. mRNA coding for gamma interferon is expressed in aplastic bone marrow but not in normal marrow and both gamma interferon and TNF beta inhibit progenitor cells in vitro.

Both allogeneic bone marrow transplant from an HLA matched sibling and immunosuppression are effective therapeutic options. Retrospective studies show no difference in long-term survival. Bone marrow transplantation however results in cure rates of up to 65% in younger patients, and is recommended if there is a suitable donor. Secondary malignancy is a long-term complication of both therapeutic options. The rate of malignancy is reported to be as high as 18% in those treated with immunosuppression, compared to just 3% in the transplant group.

Reference

Young N S 1995 Aplastic anaemia. Lancet 346: 228-232

75.   Absent or dysfunctioning spleen
A. **T**   B. **T**   C. **T**   D. **F**   E. **T**

Splenic macrophages have an important filtering and phagocytic role in removing bacteria and parasitized red blood cells from the circulation. The liver is partially able to take over this role in patients who lack a functioning spleen, but requires an intact complement system and high levels of specific antibodies.

Congenital asplenia is rare and found in conjunction with cardiac abnormalities and biliary atresia. Functional hyposplenism is indicated by the presence of red cells containing Howell-Jolly and Heinz bodies; the blood film may also show thrombocytosis and monocytosis. Functional hyposplenism may occur secondary to sickle cell disease, thalassaemia major, essential thrombocythaemia and lymphoproliferative disorders. It also occurs in coeliac disease, inflammatory bowel disease and dermatitis herpetiformis. Patients who have had bone marrow transplants are at risk from infection because of chronic graft-versus-host disease, but in some there is also evidence of hyposplenism, and all patients should be immunized against pneumococcal infection 9–12 months after transplant. Partial splenectomy or autotransplantation of splenic tissue is increasingly practised during surgery to the spleen, but it is not known what degree of splenic function these patients retain. Splenectomy is used for the treatment of patients with hereditary spherocytosis, immune thrombocytopenic purpura, and autoimmune haemolytic anaemia.

Patients under 5 years of age have a much greater risk of infection, as do those on immunosuppressive treatment. Most serious infections in asplenic patients are due to encapsulated bacteria such as *Streptococcus pneumoniae*, *Haemophilus influenzae* type b, and *Neisseria meningitidis*. Other infections to which these patients are particularly susceptible include *Escherichia coli*, malaria, babesiosis and *Capnocytophaga canimorsus*.

The guidelines state that all patients who lack a functional spleen should receive pneumococcal immunization. The current vaccine is a polyvalent vaccine containing purified capsular polysaccharide from the 23 most prevalent serotypes. Immunization should be carried out at the earliest possible opportunity, except in patients on immunosuppressive treatment, when it should be delayed for 6 months, but prophylactic antibiotics should be given in the meantime. Patients should be vaccinated at least 2 weeks prior to elective surgery. Reimmunization is recommended every 5–10 years, but antibody levels may decline more rapidly than expected in asplenic patients. Patients not already immunized should receive *H. influenzae* type b vaccine. Meningococcal immunization is not routinely recommended as the vaccine covers group A and C infections and not group B which is the commonest type in the

UK; in addition the immunity conferred is short lived. It is, however, recommended before travelling to sub-Saharan Africa, India, or Nepal. Travellers should also be warned of the increased risk of severe *Falciparum malaria* infection. Influenza vaccine is recommended annually.

Lifelong prophylactic phenoxymethylpenicillin or erythromycin if penicillin-allergic, is recommended in all cases but especially in the first 2 years after splenectomy, in all children up to the age of 16, and in those with impaired immunity from a secondary cause. In addition patients becoming febrile or unwell should have a supply of amoxycillin or erythromycin to start taking immediately, and should be advised to seek medical attention without delay. Patients should be educated about the risk to themselves of untreated infections and should be supplied with an information leaflet and a card to alert health care workers. These are available from the Department of Health.

> **Reference**
>
> Working party of the British committee for standards in haematology clinical haematology task force 1996 Guidelines for the prevention and treatment of infection in patients with an absent or dysfunctional spleen. British Medical Journal 312: 430-433

76. Bone marrow transplantation

A. T   B. T   C. F   D. F   E. F

Bone marrow transplantation (BMT) is used in the treatment of haematological and systemic malignancies and for the treatment of haemopoietic and immunological disorders. Autologous BMT involves harvesting and freezing the patient's own haemopoietic stem cells prior to bone marrow ablative treatment. The stem cells are then reinfused into the blood and migrate to and recolonize the bone marrow. Allogeneic transplants use donor stem cells. These may be syngeneic (from an identical twin), matched-related or matched-unrelated.

BMT consists of three phases, the conditioning phase, the transplant or supportive phase and the post-transplant phase. In the conditioning phase, cycles of high dose chemotherapy with or without radiotherapy are given in an attempt to reduce the number of malignant or diseased cells below a critical level. This is the therapeutic part of the procedure. The conditioning regimen is chosen for its anti-tumour, immunosuppressive or myeloablative effects. Bone marrow toxicity would be the dose limiting factor if there were no means to rescue the bone marrow.

In patients undergoing chemotherapy prior to autologous transplantation a point is reached where the patient is said to be in complete remission. At this point just as the marrow begins to recover from the last dose of chemotherapy, and at a time when there is a high concentration of pluripotential stem cells present in the bone marrow and peripheral blood, the bone marrow or peripheral blood progenitor cells are harvested and frozen. Apheresis is used to collect and concentrate peripheral blood progenitor cells. Bone marrow is harvested by repeated aspiration, and the marrow obtained can be treated in vitro to remove red cells, T cells or tumour cells. Patients are then given high dose myeloablative chemotherapy and total body irradiation.

The transplant/supportive phase covers the time from when the cells are reinfused to the time when the full blood count recovers. During this phase the patient needs to be protected from exposure to infection, to be treated aggressively when infection does occur with intravenous antibiotics plus or minus antiviral and antifungal agents, and to have blood and platelet support as required. Frequently severe mucositis, nausea and anorexia follow the total body irradiation and the last dose of chemotherapy so nutritional support may also be needed.

Complications arise, secondary to the toxic effects of the conditioning treatment, from graft-versus-host disease (GVHD) and from severe immunosuppression.

GVHD occurs when immunocompetent lymphocytes are grafted into an immunodeficient recipient. It is most frequently seen in allogeneic transplants, but rarely a similar syndrome can occur after autologous transplantation. Acute GVHD can be reduced by depleting the donor marrow of T cells, but this increases the likelihood of graft rejection and of malignant relapse. Acute GVHD occurs in the first 2 months following transplant and mainly affects the skin, liver, gastrointestinal tract and lungs. Chronic GVHD occurs more than 100 days post-transplant and clinically resembles scleroderma.

Infection is a significant cause of morbidity and mortality in BMT patients. Infections occurring during the supportive phase result from neutropenia and mucositis and often reflect overgrowth of colonizing bacteria and fungi. The prophylactic use of antibiotics, early empirical treatment of neutropenic sepsis and the use of colony stimulating factors, all reduce the incidence of post-transplantation infection. Late infections result from continued impairment of cellular and humoral immunity long after the white cell count has recovered.

The advantages of autologous transplantion are that there are no problems with matching donors and that it rarely causes GVHD. In addition, the time to bone marrow recovery tends to be shorter, particularly when peripheral stem cells are used. The disadvantages of autologous grafts are that the patient does not benefit from the graft-versus-tumour effect, and that tumour cells present in the graft are reinfused into the patient and may result in malignant recurrence. Monoclonal antibodies, chemotherapeutic agents, and the concentration of haemopoietic stem cells by positive selection, have all been used in attempts to purge autologous grafts of malignant cells.

Other areas of development include T cell subtyping to try and select out those cells which exert useful anti-tumour effects from those causing harmful GVHD, and ex vivo gene transfer to introduce chemotherapy resistance into graft cells.

Reference

Bociek R G, Stewart D A, Armitage J O 1995 Bone marrow transplantation – current concepts. Journal of Investigative Medicine 43; 2: 127-141

77. Chronic myeloid leukaemia

A. **T**   B. **T**   C. **F**   D. **F**   E. **F**

CML is a disorder of the multipotent stem cell. The myeloid progenitor cell and granulocyte compartments become grossly expanded. In over 90% of cases the Philadelphia chromosome is found. This results from a translocation from the long arm of chromosome 22 to the long arm of chromosome 9 resulting in an abnormal c-abl gene product. Even in Philadelphia negative cases, detailed molecular analysis often shows a translocation involving the c-bcr-abl gene regions. The mechanism by which the c-abl product is associated with malignant transformation is not known.

This disease is usually progressive. It starts with a benign chronic phase and terminates in an acute transformation to blast crisis. Treatment during the chronic phase includes allopurinol, blood transfusion, and chemotherapy with hydroxyurea or busulphan to control cell counts.

Allogeneic bone marrow transplantation following supralethal chemotherapy or total body irradiation has a high initial mortality (up to 25%), but allows prolonged disease-free survival for many patients.

Alpha interferons are naturally occurring polypeptides with a variety of properties, including antiviral, immunomodulatory, and growth regulating activities. These molecules have been shown to have considerable anti-tumour activity against both solid tumours and haematological malignancies.

The Medical Research Council trial of IFNa in CML was published in 1995. Following initial induction chemotherapy, 587 patients were randomized to receive chemotherapy with busulphan or hydroxyuria or IFNa. Results were analyzed on an intention to treat basis. There was a significant survival benefit in the IFNa group. Transformation from Philadelphia positive to negative in response to treatment is considered to convey considerable survival benefit. The survival benefit seen in the IFNa group was also seen in the subgroup of patients who did not transform to Philidelphia negative. Both bone marrow transplantation and IFNa therapy offer therapeutic potential in this disease.

References

Allan N C, Richards S M, Shepherd P C A 1995 UK Medical Research Council randomized, multicentre trial of interferon-alpha n1 for chronic myeloid leukaemia: improved survival irrespective of cytogenetic response. Lancet 345: 1392-1397

Wetzler M, Kantarjian H, Kurzrock R et al 1995 Interferon-alpha therapy for chronic myelogenous leukemia. American Journal of Medicine 99: 402-411

78. Chronic lymphocytic leukaemia (CLL)

A. F   B. T   C. F   D. F   E. T

CLL is a disease of late middle age and the elderly. The disease is characterized by mature B-lymphocytes in the peripheral blood with monoclonal immunoglobulins on the cell surface. The T cell marker CD5 is expressed on these B cells and is the hallmark of CLL.

Symptoms include lethargy, fever, weight loss and infections. Signs may include lymph gland, liver and splenic enlargement. There is often a normochromic normocytic anaemia which may become aggravated by Coombs' positive haemolysis. Thrombocytopenia is a late feature, as is gammaglobulinaemia. Prognosis can be assessed using the Rai system of clasification. Stage 0 indicates the presence of a raised lymphocyte count, stage I also includes lymphadenopathy, stage II includes splenomegaly or hepatomegaly, in stage III the haemoglobin is less than 11 g/dl and stage IV includes thrombocytopenia with a platelet count of less than 100. Other poor prognostic features include rapid lymphocyte doubling time, diffuse lymphocyte infiltration of the marrow and trisomy 12 in the karyotype.

Patients with early disease have an excellent prognosis and do not need drug treatment. A meta-analysis of trials of drug treatment in early CLL revealed a worse prognosis in the treated group. In patients with more advanced disease chlorambucil is the agent of choice. The role of combination therapy such as CHOP remains controversial. The nucleoside derivatives such as fludarabine show promise as second line agents. Trials of interferon alpha and bone marrow transplantation are under way for more advanced disease, but their use is not yet established.

Reference

Hamblin T J 1995 The CME lecture. Chronic lymphocytic leukaemia – new drugs and management. Journal of the Royal College of Physicians, London 29; 5: 419-421

INFECTIOUS DISEASES

79.   Human plague

A. F   B. T   C. F   D. F   E. F

Reports of an outbreak of human plague in India in 1994 led to a wave of media coverage. Most of the 6300 suspected cases reported by October 1994 were probably not caused by *Yersinia pestis*, the gram negative bacillus which is the causative organism of human plague. The bacillus is usually caught following a bite from fleas living on wild rodents. Person to person spread can rarely occur in the pneumonic form, particularly in overcrowded conditions. The incubation period is 1–7 days and the illness takes one of four forms. If infection follows a flea bite, swollen painful regional lymphadenopathy (buboes) occurs in the area draining the inoculation site. This is accompanied by fever, chills, malaise, myalgia and prostration. The pneumonic form is characterized by a productive cough, often with haemoptosis and pulmonary infiltrates on chest X-ray. Septicaemic plague may result in endotoxic shock and disseminated intravascular coagulation without localizing signs of infection. Plague meningitis is less common.

Laboratory diagnosis depends on culture from body tissues or fluids, detection of rising antibody titres by haemaglutination or the more recent technique of fluorescent antibody staining of antigens in tissues.

Management includes isolation, supportive measures and antibiotic treatment with streptomycin or tetracycline in adults and sulphonamides or chloramphenicol in children. Prophylactic tetracycline or sulphonamide is recommended for those in close personal contact with a case of pneumonic plague. Inactivated plague vaccine can be given to those visiting a plague focus, but its effectiveness is unknown.

Reference

Campbell G L, Hughes J M 1995 Plague in India: A new warning from an old nemesis. Annals of Internal Medicine 122; 2: 151-153

80.   Ebola virus

A. T   B. T   C. F   D. F   E. T

In April and May 1995 an outbreak of Ebola virus haemorrhagic fever in Zaire resulted in more than 100 cases and nearly 100 deaths. Ebola and Marburg are filoviruses having a long filamentous appearance on electron microscopy. Marburg was first described, after an outbreak was traced to contact with green monkeys which had been trapped in Uganda. The natural reservoirs of these viruses are not known. Both lead to a virtually indistinguishable illness which starts with severe frontal headache and high fever followed by generalized pains particularly in the back. Stabbing chest pains are well described. Bloody diarrhoea often leads to dehydration and the disease may mimic typhoid in its early stages. Dry throat and cough are often prominent. Between days 5 and 7 a maculopapular rash occurs which is most prominent on white skin. Severe haemorrhage may then ensue and death is frequent between days 7 and 16. Treatment involves supportive care and case isolation. The outbreak's high profile in both the general and medical press make the infection a likely MRCP subject.

References

Outbreak of Ebola viral haemorrhagic fever – Zaire 1995 Morbidity Mortality Weekly Report 44: 381

Simpson D I H 1995 The filovirus enigma. Lancet 345: 1252-1253

81. Malaria

A. **T**   B. **F**   C. **F**   D. **F**   E. **F**

The guidelines for travellers from Britain to areas of malaria risk were updated in March 1995. The new guidelines stress the importance of seeking expert and up-to-date advice regarding malaria prophylaxis because of increasing drug resistance. Mosquito bites should be avoided by using insect repellent, repellent-impregnated bednets and by wearing long-sleeved clothes at night. Malaria should be suspected in anyone with a relevant travel history for up to 1 year after returning home, regardless of whether or not they have taken prophylaxis. It should also be suspected in travellers whose aeroplane has touched down in a malaria area regardless of whether the patient left the 'plane ('airport malaria'). The diagnosis may require repeated thick and thin films especially in people who have taken prophylaxis. For travellers who may be isolated from medical services standby therapy is recommended which they can start themselves on if they develop a fever.

The principles of treatment are the administration of appropriate anti-paracytic agents (usually quinine in *F. malaria*), supportive therapy and monitoring for complications. Features of severe *F. malaria* include coma, convulsions, renal failure, the acute respiratory distress syndrome, severe anaemia, shock, haemoglobinuria, hypoglycaemia, and DIC. Thrombocytopenia is almost universal in patients with *F. malaria*, and does not usually mean that DIC is present. Patients with features of severe malaria should be transferred to an intensive care unit, as they can deteriorate rapidly.

The side-effects of anti-malarial medication have received recent media attention in the UK. Mefloquine is a very effective agent both in prophylaxis and treatment. Its side-effects include psychiatric disturbances in a proportion of users. Patients should be warned about possible side-effects before starting therapy. Mefloquine should be avoided in the first trimester of pregnancy, and patients should be advised not to get pregnant for 3 months after stopping therapy.

References

Brabley D J, Warhurst D C 1995 Malaria prophylaxis: guidelines for travellers from Britain. British Medical Journal 319: 709-714

Molyneux M, Fox R 1993 Diagnosis and treatment of malaria in Britain. British Medical Journal 306: 1175-1180

82. Meliodosis

A. T   B. F   C. F   D. T   E. F

Meliodosis is the name given to infection by *Pseudomonas pseudomallei*, a gram negative bacillus endemic in tropical areas in South East Asia especially Thailand, Central and South America, southern China and northern Australia. In these areas infection poses a significant public health problem. Sporadic cases, usually of chronic disease, occur in temperate climates where a history of residence in or travel to an endemic area is usually found. Infection is caused by direct contact with contaminated soil or water.

The disease can present in four different ways, acute, subacute, chronic or subclinical. Virtually any organ can be affected but pulmonary involvement is the most common. Chest X-ray appearances include consolidation, lung abscess, nodules, cavitation or pleural effusion. The acute disease presents with fulminant septicaemia, or less frequently with pneumonia. Subacute illness may be clinically indistinguishable from pulmonary tuberculosis presenting with a low grade fever and weight loss over a period of months. Meliodosis may be chronic with suppurative abscesses often at more than one site. 5% of patients have hepatosplenomegaly. Reactivation many years after primary infection may be secondary to the development of an immunocompromised state. Subclinical meliodosis results in an asymptomatic chronic carrier state which rarely converts to clinical illness.

Blood culture or pus culture is the most effective way of diagnosing meliodosis. Serology is also helpful. A feature of the bacillus is its resistance to aminoglycosides. It may also develop resistance during treatment. Single agent therapy is therefore often disappointing. Polytherapy with long courses of antibiotics is required.

Reference

Ip M, Osterberg L G, Chau P Y et al 1995 Pulmonary meliodosis. Chest 108:1420-1424

83. Brucellosis

A. **T**   B. **T**   C. **F**   D. **F**   E. **T**

Brucellosis is an uncommon bacterial infection usually acquired in Mediterranean and Middle Eastern countries. It is usually related to the ingestion of unpasteurized dairy products. In the UK infection is most commonly seen in workers in high risk occupations, such as farm workers, abattoir workers and butchers. Person to person transmission is rare.

The infective organism is a gram negative, non-spore forming aerobic coccobacillus. Four species cause disease in humans: *Brucella melitensis* is the most common world-wide and causes the most severe acute infections. The others are *Brucella suis, Brucella canis* and *Brucella abortus*. *B. abortus* causes abortion in sheep and cattle. In an acute illness blood cultures are positive in 50–80% of patients but these may take up to 6 weeks to grow. Bone marrow culture may also be positive. Serological tests are available to facilitate diagnosis.

Symptoms of infection are usually non-specific with fever, malaise, weight loss, anorexia and depression being common presenting features. A granulomatous reaction can set up in any organ, the commonest manifestations of localized infection being osteomyelitis, splenic abscesses, genito-urinary tract infection including epididymo-orchitis, pulmonary disease and endocarditis. Altered bowel habit is common. Neurological complications are uncommon but include meningitis and peripheral neuropathy. The most common cause of death is endocarditis, usually of the aortic valve and this is more common in men. Clinical examination is often unhelpful in making the diagnosis. Splenomegaly, hepatomegaly or lymphadenopathy may be present, but one of these signs is found in only 50% of patients. Brucellosis can also be asymptomatic or subclinical, and can develop into a chronic illness lasting for more than a year after initial infection.

Treatment is with antibiotics. WHO guidelines recommend polytherapy including a tetracycline, such as doxycycline. Streptomycin, gentamicin and rifampicin are useful adjuncts. A Jarisch-Herxheimer reaction can complicate treatment.

Reference

Friedland J S 1993 Uncommon infections: brucellosis. Prescribers Journal 33: 24-28.

84. Tick-borne diseases

A. **T** B. **T** C. **F** D. **T** E. **T**

Our knowledge of tick-borne diseases has increased dramatically over the last 3 decades. Rocky Mountain spotted fever is a ricketsial infection transmitted by the wood tick *Dermacentor andersoni* and the dog tick *Dermacentor variabilis*. Before the advent of antibiotics, approximately 70% of patients developing the infection died. In the 1970s more than 1000 cases were reported per year.

Lyme disease is the most commonly reported vector-borne disease in the USA. In 1994 more than 13 000 cases were reported. *Ixodes* ticks transmit both Lyme disease and babesiosis.

Human ehrlichiosis is caused by *Ehrlichia chafeensis* and is transmitted by *Amblyomma americanum* ticks. It was discovered in the 1980s and a recent report has revealed that up to 12.5% of members of some communities based near wildlife reserves in the USA are seropositive. The disease typically occurs in spring and summer and there is generally a history of a tick bite. In serious infections patients present with headache, fever, leucopenia, thrombocytopenia and abnormalities of liver function tests. The disease may be fatal. A similar disease called human granulocytic ehrlichiosis has been recognized and is thought to be transmitted by *Ixodes scapularis* or *D. variabilis*.

Primary prevention by reducing exposed skin and by using insect repellents has been shown to be effective in reducing the incidence in endemic areas. Doxycycline is the treatment of choice for Rocky Mountain spotted fever and human ehrlichiosis. These diseases usually respond to treatment in 24–48 hours.

References

Fishbein D B, Dennis D T 1995 Tick-borne diseases: a growing risk. New England Journal of Medicine 333: 452-453

Strandaert S M, Dawson J E, Schaffner W et al 1995 Ehrlichiosis in a golf-orientated retirement community. New England Journal of Medicine 333: 420-425

85. Lyme disease

A. **F** B. **F** C. **F** D. **F** E. **F**

Lyme disease is caused by the spirochaete *Borrelia burgdoferi*. The mode of transmission is by a tick vector, particularly *Ixodes ricinus* in Europe and *Ixodes scapularis* in the USA. Lyme disease has early and late features. Early disease has two stages. Stage I presents with 'flu-like symptoms and a characteristic rash known as erythema migrans. This is a macular rash which spreads away from the site of the infection. Patients may not recall the tick bite as the rash can take up to 16 weeks to appear. In most cases stage I disease is self limiting. However, a proportion of patients progress to more serious disease with potentially debilitating long-term sequelae and therefore antibiotic treatment is recommended. Despite treatment approximately 1% of patients will progress to stage II or III disease. Tetracyclines, penicillin and cephalosporins have all been shown to be effective. Erythromycin is less effective.

Stage II disease occurs weeks to months later and many organs may be affected by an inflammatory response to invading spirochaetes. The most common manifestation is an intermittent oligoarthritis. More serious complications are neurological and cardiac. Bannwarth's syndrome comprises painful meningoradiculoneuritis associated with a cerebrospinal fluid lymphocytosis. Lyme carditis can be life threatening.

Late disease (Stage III), with chronic arthritis, acrodermatitis chronica atrophicans, encephalopathy and cardiomyopathy, occurs months to years after infection. The most common site for the development of acrodermatitis chronica atrophicans is the lower leg. Epidermal atrophy develops following a bluish-red discoloration of the skin. Myalgia and sensory neuropathy are frequently seen in association with this manifestation of late Lyme disease.

The diagnosis is usually serological, however the polymerase chain reaction looks promising for future use. Serology may be negative in 50% of cases with Stage I disease. Low titres of IgG antibodies may be present in the absence of active disease indicating past exposure rather than active disease.

References

O'Connell S 1995 Lyme disease in the United Kingdom. British Medical Journal 310: 303-309

Pfister H, Wilske B, Weber K 1994 Lyme borreliosis: basic science and clinical aspects. Lancet 343: 1013-1020

86.   Anti-retroviral therapy (HIV)

A. **T**   B. **T**   C. **T**   D. **T**   E. **T**

Human immunodeficiency virus (HIV) is a retrovirus. It binds to cells through the interaction of virus-envelope glycoproteins (gp 120) and CD4 molecules on the surface of some human cell types. The virus then internalizes and disassembles, and its RNA genetic code is transcribed by the viral enzyme reverse-transcriptase into DNA, which can integrate into the host cell genome. Viral genetic material can then be expressed, processed and reassembled as progeny virus that can be released to continue infection.

Anti-retroviral drugs include the nucleoside analogue reverse-transcriptase inhibitors like zidovudine, zalcitabine, didanosine and stavudine, non-nucleoside reverse-transcriptase inhibitors and protease inhibitors. This last class of drugs inhibit the HIV-protease enzyme which cleaves viral glycoproteins to yield gp120 and gp 41.

Early trials of zidovudine versus placebo suggested a slowing of disease progression and a survival benefit from starting the drug early during the disease free period, compared to delaying treatment to the development of AIDS. These trials were terminated early, after initial promising results, in order to allow all patients the perceived benefits of zidovudine therapy. The benefits of early therapy were shown to be short lived in the Concorde study. 1749 asymptomatic HIV positive patients were randomized to immediate or delayed treatment with zidovudine. Patients were analysed at 1 and 3 years in terms of disease progression, death and drug side-effects. The results showed that, after a mean follow-up of 3.3 years, survival was not significantly different between the two groups. The 3 year estimated survival probabilities were 92% in the immediate group ,and 94% in the deferred group. Similarly, there was no significant difference in progression of HIV disease. In the separate analysis of data from the first year, there was a slight advantage to being in the immediate group. This advantage was lost by 18 months. Although there was a consistent difference in CD4 counts, there was no relation between this and a delay in the progression of disease. Analysis of drug side-effects showed an increase in adverse effects in the group treated with zidovudine early.

The Concorde study does not support the use of zidovudine as monotherapy in early asymptomatic HIV infection, and reminds us of the dangers of interpreting the findings of short-term studies and of stopping studies early, rather than allowing them to continue to their predetermined end-points.

The preliminary results of the Delta and ACTG175 trials comparing zidovudine combined with didanosine or zalcitabine against zidovudine alone in patients with HIV infection have been announced. Delta divided patients naive to zidovudine from those with previous exposure (Delta 1 and 2). 12% of patients in Delta 1 and 17% of patients in Delta 2 had AIDS. Delta 1 showed a significant reduction in mortality and progression of disease with combination therapy, whereas Delta 2 did not. The results of ACTG175 were similar. Trials of protease inhibitors and various combinations of anti-retroviral drugs are currently under way.

Another area receiving considerable interest is immunotherapy to augment the host immune response to HIV infection. By manipulating the cytokines which orchestrate the immune response, it may be possible to kill more effectively virally infected cells.

References

Bridges S H, Saryer N 1995 Gene therapy and immune restoration for HIV disease. Lancet 345: 427-432

Choo V 1995 Combination superior to zidovudine in Delta trial. Lancet 1995; 346: 895

Concorde Coordinating Committee 1994 Concorde: MRC/ANRS randomized double blind controlled trial of immediate and deferred zidovudine in symptom-free HIV infection. Lancet 343: 871-881

Emery S, Cooper D A 1995 Anti-retroviral therapy of human immunodeficiency virus type-1 infection. Australian and New Zealand Journal of Medicine 25: 344-349

Lipsky J J 1994 Concorde lands. Lancet 343: 866-867

Pinching A J 1996 Managing HIV disease after Delta. British Medical Journal 312: 521-522

87.   Vertical transmission of HIV

A. **T**   B. **T**   C. **F**   D. **F**   E. **F**

In the USA 7000 HIV infected women give birth to 1000 to 2000 HIV infected infants each year. The prevalence of HIV infection is as high as 30% amongst child-bearing women in some parts of Africa. Clearly strategies to reduce vertical HIV transmission are urgently needed. There is growing evidence that in 50–70% of case transmission occurs late in gestation or during delivery. Strategies that are currently under study to reduce vertical transmission include elective caesarean delivery, the use of vaginal antiseptics during labour and anti-viral therapy given to mother and infant.

A trial of zidovudine therapy in pregnancy and in the new born has been published. In a group of 477 HIV infected pregnant women with CD4 counts above 200 who had not had anti-retroviral therapy during the current pregnancy, a double-blind placebo controlled trial of zidovudine was conducted. Mothers were given zidovudine orally during pregnancy and intravenously during labour. Infants were given oral zidovudine for the first 6 weeks of their life. The proportion of infants infected at 18 months was 8.3% in the zidovudine group and 25.5% in the placebo group, corresponding to a 67.5% relative risk reduction. Minimal short-term toxic effects were observed.

The possibility that zidovudine may increase birth defects or may have long-term adverse effects in exposed children has not been excluded. By inducing resistance, the treatment of women with zidovudine during pregnancy may deny them effective therapy later in their infection. Whether the results of this study can be extrapolated to women with more advanced disease and how zidovudine or other anti-retroviral agents can be used to maximal effect, have yet to be established. In order to be able to offer strategies to reduce vertical HIV infection, women have to know their HIV status, necessitating testing of all pregnant women. This has obvious ethical implications. Expensive anti-retroviral agents are unlikely to be affordable in those countries where the problem of vertical transmission is greatest.

References

Peckham C, Gibb D 1995 Current concepts: mother-to-child transmission of the human immunodeficiency virus. New England Journal of Medicine 333: 298-302

Rogers F M, Jaffe H W 1995 Reducing the risk of maternal- infant transmission of HIV: a door is opened. New England Journal of Medicine 331; 18: 1222-1223

The Paediatric AIDS Clinical Trials Group Protocol 076 Study Group 1995 Reduction of maternal-infant transmission of human immunodeficiency virus type 1 with zidovudine treatment. New England Journal of Medicine 331; 18: 1173-1180

88. HIV neurology
A. F   B. F   C. T   D. T   E. F

89. HIV neurology
A. T   B. T   C. T   D. F   E. F

Human immunodeficiency virus (HIV) is associated with a wide range of neurological abnormalities. These can be broadly divided into degenerative, neoplastic and infective.

HIV dementia is thought to be a direct consequence of HIV infection. HIV infected cells are seen within the central nervous system (CNS). HIV gp41 antigen has also been identified in the brain at postmortem in 60–70% of patients with HIV dementia. The mechanism of infection is uncertain. HIV may enter the brain through infected monocytes or through a possible cytokine mediated disruption of the blood brain barrier. Typically, HIV dementia is a feature of advanced disease with CD4 lymphocyte counts of <200 cells/mm3. Neuropsychiatric impairment is rare in early HIV infection and is difficult to detect without formal cognitive testing. As the dementia progresses cognitive, motor and behavioural abnormalities become more pronounced. Psychomotor retardation is a feature of severe dementia. Overt psychoses such as mania are recognized. The diagnosis of HIV dementia is one of exclusion. Cerebrospinal fluid (CSF) abnormalities include elevated beta 2 microglobulin, elevated immunoglobulins, the presence of oligoclonal bands and a leucocytosis. Computed tomography (CT) or magnetic resonance imaging (MRI) reveal cerebral atrophy, ventricular enlargement and white matter abnormalities. Zidovudine is not thought to be helpful in preventing HIV dementia but it does reduce progression once the diagnosis has been made.

Progressive multifocal leucoencephalopathy (PML) is a demyelinating condition associated with HIV infection. It is caused by infection with a human papillomavirus (or papovavirus) called the JC virus. Focal lesions which do not enhance with contrast are seen on CT scan. MRI reveals multiple characteristic lesions in the parieto-occipital white matter. The definitive diagnosis requires biopsy. Histology reveals pronounced demyelination and enlarged oligodendrocytes containing multiple virions. The prognosis is poor. No therapy has been shown to be consistently successful, but there is some evidence that anti-viral therapy delays progression in these patients. There have been several reports on the successful use of cytarabine in affected individuals.

Other important causes of space occupying cerebral lesions in HIV disease are cerebral toxoplasmosis and primary cerebral lymphoma. Both cause ring enhancing lesions on CT. Toxoplasmosis, a protozoal infection, is the commonest cerebral mass lesion in acquired immunodeficiency syndrome (AIDS). Focal signs are present in 70% of patients. Headache, fever, lethargy and seizures are all common. The diagnosis is favoured if there are multiple cerebral lesions in conjunction with detectable toxoplasma antibodies. An empirical trial of treatment with pyrimethamine and sulphadiazine or clindamycin is usually commenced. If there is no improvement after 7 to 10 days then an alternative diagnosis should be considered. Toxoplasmosis usually presents when the CD4 count is <200 cells/mm³. It is thought that toxoplasmosis in HIV patients is due to reactivation of quiescent disease rather than primary infection.

The main alternative diagnosis is lymphoma. This usually occurs when the CD4 count is <100 cells/mm³. The lymphoma is invariably of B cell origin. A single lesion on CT scan favours the diagnosis of lymphoma, as does the absence of anti-toxoplasma antibodies. Definitive diagnosis is by biopsy or detection of lymphoma cells in the CSF. Treatment with radiotherapy or chemotherapy may improve survival in some cases. Without treatment the prognosis is grave.

CNS infections may be focal or diffuse. Tuberculosis, histoplasmosis and aspergillus may all cause focal disease. TB meningitis may also occur. Syphilitic gummata are also seen. Treponemal infection may be concurrent with HIV infection. Syphilis may reactivate after previous treatment for primary infection, or be acquired subsequent to HIV infection. A positive serum VDRL may help with diagnosis in those patients in whom neurosyphilis is suspected but is not diagnostic. A positive CSF VDRL is diagnostic but false negative tests occur.

Cytomegalovirus (CMV), as well as causing retinitis, may target the brain stem and spinal cord causing a diffuse encephalitis or myelitis. CMV encephalitis is associated with very low CD4 counts and has a poor prognosis. The blood brain barrier is poorly penetrated by standard anti-CMV therapy such as gancyclovir and foscarnet.

Cryptococcus is a common fungal infection in AIDS. It causes a meningitis with relatively little inflammation and hence the typical features of photophobia and neck stiffness are often absent. The diagnosis is made by India ink staining of the CSF, positive CSF culture or a positive CSF cryptococcal antigen. Treatment with amphotericin B, flucytosine or fluconazole may be effective.

Other CNS infections include *Candida albicans*, coccidiomycosis, herpes zoster, herpes simplex, *Trypanosomiasis cruzi* and nocardia. Myelopathy may be caused by vacuolar myelopathy, lymphoma, toxoplasmosis, varicella zoster granulomatous myelitis, herpetic necrotizing myelitis, CMV and vitamin B12 deficiency.

References

Levine A M 1990 Lymphoma in acquired immunodeficiency syndrome. Seminars in Oncology 17: 104-112

Lipton S A, Gendelman H E 1995 Dementia associated with the acquired immunodeficiency syndrome. New England Journal of Medicine 332: 934-939

Simpson D M, Tagliati M 1994 Neurologic manifestations of HIV infection. Annals of International Medicine 121: 769-785

Sweeney B J, Miller R F, Harrison M J G 1993 Progressive multifocal leucoencephalopathy. British Journal of Hospital Medicine 50: 187-192

90. Streptococcal throat infections

A. **T**   B. **F**   C. **F**   D. **T**   E. **T**

Streptococcal sore throat is a common clinical condition which is usually self limiting but can have serious sequelae. Symptom-free carriers tend to carry relatively few organisms and are much less likely to develop complications. They are not an important reservoir of infection. Overall *Streptococcus pyogenes* can be isolated in only about 30% of cases of sore throat although in children of school age the figure is nearer 50%.

The typical features of streptococcal sore throat include fever and pain of sudden onset, dysphagia, pharyngeal or tonsillar exudate, and enlarged anterior cervical lymph nodes. These features are present in only 15% of patients making a definite diagnosis difficult on clinical grounds alone. Infection with *Arcanobacterium haemolyticum* can produce a similar picture including a scarlet fever type rash. It usually affects 10–20 year-olds and responds well to erythromycin.

Streptococcal infections can lead to a variety of complications including bacteraemia, rheumatic fever, glomerulonephritis, arthritis, erythema nodosum and erythema multiforme. Some of these complications can be severe; the mortality from streptococcal bacteraemia is 50%. Invasive streptococcal infection is more common than meningococcal septicaemia and there is often no obvious portal of entry.

The decline in the incidence of rheumatic fever in industrialized communities earlier this century started before the introduction of antibiotics. It is thought to have been a result of improvements in environmental and social conditions as well as a decline in the number of strains with the potential to cause rheumatic fever. Rheumatic fever is now on the increase again with several clusters of disease in relatively affluent communities. This increase coincides with an increase in more virulent and invasive strains, leading to more cases of necrotizing fasciitis, toxic shock syndrome and bacteraemia.

In order best to manage streptococcal sore throat, early diagnosis is necessary. This allows the appropriate use of antibiotics in patients with bacterial infection and avoids their inappropriate use in viral sore throat. A variety of tests have been developed to help speed up the diagnosis. Rapid antigen tests have been used in some specialist centres with up to 90% diagnostic sensitivity.

Delaying treatment of streptococcal sore throat for 48 hours seems to reduce early and late recurrence. This may be because type specific antibody production is impaired with early antibiotic therapy. Treatment should be continued for 10 days because shorter courses are less successful and recurrence is more common. The clinical failure rate for a 10-day course of penicillin is about 11%. Eradication occurs in about 95% of cases with various cephalosporins, but at a greater financial cost than with penicillins.

Reference

Diagnosis and treatment of streptococcal sore throat Feb 1995 Drugs and Therapeutic Bulletin 33; 2: 9-12

---

91. Group A streptococcal infections

A. **T**   B. **T**   C. **T**   D. **F**   E. **F**

Lancefield Group A streptococcal infections encompass a number of clinical syndromes either through direct local infection or through nonsuppurative sequelae of infection such as rheumatic fever and glomerulonephritis. Skin and soft-tissue infections include streptococcal pyoderma or impetigo, erysipelas and acute cellulitis. More dangerous are necrotizing fasciitis and the streptococcal toxic shock like syndrome.

Media attention has followed a number of outbreaks of necrotizing fasciitis. Several factors predispose to infection including penetrating injuries, cuts, burns, varicella infection, childbirth and even muscle strain. An outbreak in the early 1990s in Gloucestershire was in some cases related to surgery. Initial presentation is with pain and swelling usually of a limb, which then develops clear fluid-filled bullae which rapidly become purple. Gangrene, muscle necrosis and compartment syndromes follow and are fatal if not promptly treated with surgical debridement, fasciotomy and high dose penicillin. Penicillin is less efficacious in the presence of large numbers of organisms and in overwhelming infection clindamycin is often useful. Often the infection is polymicrobial and more than one antibiotic is required.

Streptococcal toxic shock like syndrome is caused by group A streptococcus and is characterized by early onset shock and multiorgan failure. In 50% of cases necrotizing fasciitis is present. Laboratory investigations may show a left shift in neutrophil count, uraemia, hypocalcaemia, elevated creatinine kinase, haematuria and hypoalbuminaemia. The mortality is high.

Pneumococcus is a group D alpha haemolytic streptococcus and gas gangrene is usually caused by clostridia species.

References

Bisno A L, Stevens D L 1996 Streptococcal infections of skin and soft tissues. New England Journal of Medicine 334: 240-245

Burge T S, Watson J D 1994 Necrotizing fasciitis. British Medical Journal 308: 1453-1454

Thomson H, Cartwright K 1995 Streptococcal necrotizing fasciitis in Gloucestershire: 1994. British Journal of Surgery 82: 1444-1445

92. Human parvovirus B19

A. F   B. F   C. T   D. T   E. T

Parvovirus B19 is best known as the cause of fifth disease (slapped cheek syndrome or erythema infectiosum). However the infection, most common in children aged 4 to 11 is usually asymptomatic or causes a nonspecific respiratory tract infection. Fifth disease often occurs in outbreaks, but unless the characteristic red cheeks are prominent it may be misdiagnosed as rubella or allergy.

Arthropathy occurs in 80% of adult women infected. Most commonly it is a symmetrical small joint arthritis although wrists, knees and ankles may be involved. Symptoms of arthralgia or arthritis usually subside after 2 weeks, but in a small minority may persist for years. Rarer presentations associated with parvovirus B19 infection include vasculitis, peripheral neuropathy, nephritis and myocarditis.

Aplastic crisis following infection in patients with sickle cell anaemia is well recognized, however this complication may also occur in other haemolytic states such as hereditary spherocytosis. The crisis usually lasts 5–7 days before the virus is cleared. In immunocompromized patients such as those with AIDS, parvovirus can cause a chronic anaemia. This has been successfully treated by administration of human immunoglobulin.

Maternal infection during pregnancy results in a spontaneous abortion rate in the second trimester of 10 times that expected. Infection in the second or third trimester sometimes results in hydrops fetalis, with anaemia and occasionally myocarditis in the fetus. There is some suggestion that parvovirus B19 infection of the fetus may result in congenital red cell aplasias. With no convincing evidence of an increase in congenital abnormalities, infection is not considered an indication for therapeutic abortion.

Diagnostic tests are commercially available in kit form, but as yet are only used in a few laboratories. The interpretation of a positive result requires consideration of past exposure. The development of an effective vaccine is awaited particularly by those caring for patients at risk of aplastic crisis.

References

Cohen B 1995 Parvovirus B19: an expanding spectrum of disease. British Medical Journal 311: 1549-1552

Pattison J R 1994 Human parvovirus B19 British Medical Journal 308: 149-150

93. Meningococcal infection

A. **T**   B. **F**   C. **F**   D. **F**   E. **F**

Meningococcal infection is caused by the gram negative coccus *Neisseria meningitidis*. In the UK it is more common in the winter months and has two peaks of incidence, in infancy and teenage years. The carriage rate of meningococcus in the general population may be as high as 25%. Transmission is via the respiratory route. Influenza infection and smoking are recognized predisposing factors. Patients with complement C5 and C9 deficiencies are at increased risk of infection. World-wide, groups A and C meningococcus are the commonest cause of meningitis. In the UK, group B meningococcus is most common.

Most patients present with meningitis. They have fever, headache, photophobia, neck stiffness and vomiting. There may be a characteristic purpuric rash and lumbar puncture and blood cultures are needed to confirm the diagnosis. Rarely, the cerebrospinal fluid fails to reveal the organism. In these cases meningococcal infection can be confirmed by antigen detection using the polymerase chain reaction. The overall mortality from meningitis is 3–5%. If there is no shock and central nervous system involvement is not severe, then the prognosis is good as long as treatment is initiated promptly. This is not true for meningococcal septicaemia. The rash is more common in cases with septicaemia and rapid hypovolaemic shock is a common finding. Disseminated intravascular coagulation frequently occurs. Multiorgan failure is common and intensive therapy is needed. Mortality in septicaemia may be as high as 20%.

In the UK meningococcus is sensitive to benzylpenicillin and this remains the treatment of choice. World-wide, penicillin resistance is increasing. Other common causes of meningitis, *Haemophilus influenzae* and *Streptocccus pneumoniae*, may be clinically indistinguishable and are not as sensitive to penicillin. If the causative organism is not known then a third generation cephalosporin is a better choice of antibiotic.

Close contacts should be treated prophylactically with rifampicin or ciprofloxacin. An effective vaccine against meningococcus group B is not available. There are polysaccharide vaccines available for groups A and C. In Britain outbreaks of group C disease are occasionally seen and vaccination is given to contacts at risk of exposure. This vaccine is also available to travellers to endemic areas.

A randomized controlled trial of the use of dexamethasone in bacterial meningitis in children concluded that dexamethasone did not affect the rate at which the cerebrospinal fluid becomes free of infection. Long-term follow-up up to 15 months suggested, however, that neurological sequelae of infection were significantly less frequent in the dexamethasone treated group compared to the placebo group. The use of dexamethasone for adults with meningococcal meningitis varies between units.

References

Klein N J, Heyderman R S, Levin M 1993 Management of meningococcal infections. British Journal of Hospital Medicine 50: 42-49

Letter from the Chief Medical Officer Feb 1994 Meningococcal infection: meningitis and septicaemia.

Nathavitharana K A, Tarlow M J 1995. Advances in treating bacterial meningitis. Update 51: 69-76

Schaad U B, Lips U, Gnehm H E et al 1993 Dexamethasone therapy for bacterial meningitis in children. Lancet 342: 457-461

Tunkel A R, Scheld W M 1995 Acute bacterial meningitis. Lancet 346: 1675-1680

94. Influenza

A. F   B. F   C. T   D. F   E. T

Influenza A is a single stranded RNA orthomyxovirus. It is a common virus causing a non-specific febrile illness associated with myalgia, headache and cough. It is transmitted by the nasopharyngeal route and is clinically indistinguishable from many other viral respiratory illnesses. The influenza A virus coat has haemagglutinins and neuraminidase peptides. The appearance of novel subtypes of these resulting from an epidemiological phenomenon called antigenic shift causes pandemic or worldwide outbreaks of influenza. Minor changes or antigenic shifts cause influenza epidemics. Pandemics are uncommon, there have been four this century, and they usually arise in Asia.

Laboratory diagnosis is facilitated by serological tests, virus isolation, antigen detection by immunofluorescence or ELISA and gene amplification using the polymerase chain reaction (PCR). Serological tests, which depend on the demonstration of a rise in antibody titre over time, are useful to confirm a diagnosis but are unhelpful for acute diagnosis, unlike immunofluorescence or PCR. Most cases are diagnosed clinically. Laboratory techniques are used for epidemiological surveillance and for identifying symptomatic at-risk patients during an epidemic. An epidemic is defined as more than 100 new cases per week per 100 000 population. At-risk patients in such outbreaks may be suitable for either amantidine prophylaxis or treatment. These include patients with chronic respiratory or cardiovascular illnesses who have not been vaccinated. Health workers and nursing home residents should also be considered for prophylaxis. Vaccination is contraindicated in egg, polymyxin or neomycin sensitivity.

Amantidine is the only effective anti-influenza drug available for use in the UK. It is ineffective against influenza B and C, but highly effective at reducing virus shedding in influenza A. If started within 48 hours of symptom onset, the duration of symptoms may be reduced by about one third. There are few serious side-effects but its use should be restricted in pregnancy. High doses are teratogenic in rats. Ribavirin, interferon alpha and a neuraminidase inhibitor are all potential alternatives currently undergoing evaluation.

Vaccination is recommended annually for all age groups at risk of severe influenza infection. Such groups include those with diabetes, renal failure and the immunosuppressed. The current vaccine is a non-live, subunit trivalent preparation with two A and one B subunit. Studies have shown a greatly reduced incidence of complications and mortality following its use, particularly in the elderly.

Complications of influenza include otitis media, pneumonitis and secondary bacterial pneumonia especially *Staphylococcus aureus* and meningococcal infection. Other complications are probably related to immune mechanisms rather than a direct consequence of infection and include Guillain-Barré syndrome, toxic shock syndrome, myocarditis and Reye's syndrome.

Reference

Wiselka M 1994 Influenza: diagnosis, management and prophylaxis. British Medical Journal 308: 1341-1345.

---

95. *Clostridium difficile*

A. T   B. F   C. F   D. F   E. T

Clostridium difficile is a spore forming, anaerobic, gram positive bacillus. It is the commonest enteric pathogen in patients in hospital, and nosocomial infection, usually associated with broad spectrum antibiotic use causes considerable morbidity and mortality. The use of broad spectrum antibiotics is thought to change the normal intestinal flora, allowing *C. difficile* to become established and to proliferate. The source of infection may be endogenous, exogenous from the environment or directly from a carrier. Almost all antibiotics have been implicated, however broad spectrum antibiotics, particularly orally administered penicillins, cephalosporins and clindamycin are most commonly involved. Even antibiotics with in vitro activity against *C. difficile* can precipitate disease.

Toxigenic strains of *C. difficile* produce two exotoxins, A and B. Toxin A is an enterotoxin, thought to bind to mucosal receptors, which enters the cell and causes fluid secretion and mucosal damage. Toxin B is a cytotoxin, which also binds to specific membrane receptors but is 1000 times more potent in tissue cultures than toxin A. Non-toxigenic strains are usually not pathogenic.

Carriage rates in healthy volunteers vary from 0 to15% depending on detection methods used and populations studied. If healthy volunteers are given antibiotics, their carriage rate increases to about 45%. Carriage rates are high in neonates but rarely cause disease, possibly due to immaturity of the mucosa and lack of toxin receptors. Colonization is thought to result from the ingestion of spores, which can survive for years. Spores can be found on patients and healthcare workers' hands, as well as on beds and floors. Once in the colon spores convert to the vegetative organism.

C. difficile causes a spectrum of illness, from mild watery foul smelling diarrhoea to life-threatening pseudomembranous colitis with toxic megacolon and perforation. The white cell count is often raised and sigmoidoscopy reveals a patchy non-specific colitis.

Pseudomembranous colitis produces more systemic symptoms, and sigmoidoscopy reveals pathognomonic raised yellow plaques.

Diagnosis depends on stool tests, endoscopic appearance and response to antibiotic withdrawal and specific antibiotic therapy. Culture is the most sensitive method of *C. difficile* detection and allows study of outbreak epidemiology. Detection of the cytopathic effect of toxin B in tissue culture has high sensitivity and specificity, but takes 48–72 hours. ELISA for detection of toxin A is now available and although expensive allows rapid diagnosis. PCR techniques are being developed to allow rapid detection of pathogenic strains.

Management of a patient with *C. difficile* associated disease includes withdrawal of the offending antibiotic, rehydration, isolation and drug treatment. Isolation with full enteric precautions should only be stopped when diarrhoea resolves and toxin can no longer be detected in the stool. Oral metronidazole or vancomycin for 7–10 days are probably equally effective. Relapse is rarely due to antibiotic resistance but is usually caused by re-infection or germination of residual spores. A vaccine designed to produce IgA against toxin A is being investigated.

Reference

Tabaqchali S, Jumaa P 1995 Diagnosis and management of *Clostridium difficile* infection. British Medical Journal 310: 1375-1381.

RHEUMATOLOGY

96.   Paget's disease of bone

A. T   B. F   C. F   D. F   E. F

97.   Paget's disease of bone

A. F   B. T   C. F   D. F   E. T

Paget's disease is a progressive bone disease of unknown cause. There is some evidence to suggest that it may result from a slow virus infection. It is common, affecting up to 10% of elderly people, although many of these will be asymptomatic. The condition is three times more common in men than women. It is characterized by a localized disorganization of bone remodelling due to a primary abnormality of osteoclasts.

Patients most commonly present with bone pain, commonly around the major joints. Deformity is also common, including bowing of weight bearing bones which may be associated with pathological stress fractures. Complete transverse fractures may also occur. Skull deformity with frontal bossing and maxillary enlargement is characteristic. Basilar invagination may cause brain stem compression with long tract signs or internal hydrocephalus. Cranial nerves may be compressed as they exit the skull, auditory and ocular nerves being most commonly affected.

Diagnosis is based on the combination of symptoms, X-ray signs and raised levels of bone turnover markers. Radiographs of painful or deformed bones are usually diagnostic, showing areas of mixed lysis and sclerosis. Long bones may have an increased diameter. Scintigraphy is useful in revealing the extent and distribution of disease but is non-specific. Serum calcium, phosphate, parathyroid hormone and vitamin D are usually normal. The concentration of alkaline phosphatase (AP) reflects the rate of bone formation. When disease is very localized and total serum AP is normal, bone specific AP may be raised, allowing the diagnosis to be made. Bone specific AP is also very useful in patients with abnormal liver function, where the interpretation of total serum AP is difficult. Osteocalcin is a vitamin D and K dependent protein which binds calcium and has a strong affinity for hydroxyapatite. It is a reliable index of osteoblast activity but is not a useful index of disease activity in Paget's disease.

Among markers of resorption, excretion of pyrodinoline and urinary hydroxyproline have the best diagnostic accuracy. Where a single sclerotic vertebra is found, the differential diagnosis includes malignancy and osteomyelitis, and bone biopsy may be necessary to make a definitive diagnosis.

The aims of treatment are to reduce pain and the risk of long-term complications. This requires analgesia, surgical management of fractures and joint disease and measures to reduce bone turnover. Bisphosphonates are potent anti-resorptive agents that have led to a dramatic improvement in the treatment of Paget's disease. Etidronate, pamidronate and tiludronate are currently licensed in the UK.

Reference

Hosking D, Meunier P J, Ringe J D et al 1996 Paget's disease of bone: diagnosis and management. British Medical Journal 312: 491-494

98.   Osteoporosis

A. **T**   B. **F**   C. **F**   D. **T**   E. **T**

Osteoporosis is a condition of low bone mass or osteopaenia associated with low-trauma fractures particularly of vertebral bodies, the distal forearm and the proximal femur. There are two commonly recognized types of primary osteoporosis. Type 1, or post-menopausal bone mass loss, is an acceleration of the normal rate of bone loss and principally affects trabecular bone. This can continue for up to 10 years after the menopause. Type II is age related bone loss and affects men and women equally, being non-specific for trabecular and cortical bone. Risk factors for primary osteoporosis are female sex, older age, low body-mass index, smoking, heavy alcohol intake, hypogonadism and early menopause. Secondary causes should be sought. Drugs, endocrinological, rheumatological or malignant conditions may all predispose to osteoporosis.

Peak bone mass is usually reached by 30 years and declines steadily thereafter at a rate of 1% per annum. Bone densitometry will help identify high risk groups and should be offered to women with early menopause, those with vertebral deformity or X-ray evidence of osteopaenia, and long-term corticosteroid users. In post-menopausal women with a lumbar spine bone density one standard deviation below the mean for age-related density, HRT is indicated. Treatment involves symptom control, treatment of predisposing diseases, manipulation of potentially hazardous environments to minimize the risk of falls, and preventative and therapeutic pharmacological manipulation of the process of bone remodelling. A lot of recent work has focused on the use of bisphosphonates. These inhibit both bone resorption (the basis for their therapeutic use) and bone remineralization (giving rise to concern about osteomalacia with long-term use). They vary in potency and their efficacy in inhibiting resorption is independent of their inhibition of mineralization. Currently, cyclical regimens of etidronate and calcium regimes are being evaluated. Trials have confirmed a transient increase in bone mass in lumbar vertebrae and femurs, and claims have been made for a preventative role in fracture incidence. These claims need further substantiation with larger trials.

References

Compston J E 1994 The therapeutic use of bisphosphonates. British Medical Journal 309: 711-715

Doherty M, Deighton C, Compston J 1994 Osteoporosis. Medicine International. 22: 209-212

Francis R M 1995 Oral bisphosphonates in the treatment of osteoporosis: a review. Current Therapeutic Research 56: 831-851

Peel N, Eastell R 1995 ABC of Rheumatology osteoporosis. British Medical Journal 310: 989-992

99.   Rheumatoid arthritis

A. F   B. F   C. T   D. F   E. T

A number of autoimmune diseases have been shown to be linked to different major histocompatibility class (MHC) antigens. Rheumatoid arthritis is associated with MHC class II DR4/DR1 molecules and ankylosing spondilitis with the MHC class 1 antigen HLA-B27.

The increased susceptibility of patients with MHC class II DR4/ DR1 for rheumatoid arthritis (RA) is important but other genes and environmental factors are known to play a major role in the development of the disease. The importance of non MHC genes has been clearly demonstrated in various family studies, but the concordance rate in monozygotic twins is only 12–30% and thus the disease must be under environmental as well as genetic control. The environmental factors implicated in the pathogenesis of rheumatoid arthritis have included exposure to silica dust and a variety of infectious agents. Some case-control studies and a recent meta-analysis have argued that administration of oestrogen may protect against severe forms of the disease.

The finding of large numbers of activated CD4 positive T cells in close proximity to antigen presenting cells in inflamed synovial fluid suggested a possible pivotal role for MHC class II dependent T cell activation in the pathogenesis of the inflammatory process. More recently the idea that synovial T cells are the primary players in the pathogenesis of rheumatoid joint disease has been challenged by two observations: there appears to be a high concentration of monokines in the synovial fluid but relatively little in the way of T cell derived cytokines, and secondly anti-CD4 antibody treatment has been shown to be ineffective in treating the disease in the first placebo controlled trial of the drug. The failure of this treatment was in sharp contrast with the impressive results gained using neutralizing antibodies to tumour necrosis factor-alpha (TNF-alpha).

None of the current drugs used for treating rheumatoid arthritis is curative. They are designed to reduce pain and inflammation but some do manage to slow the progression of the underlying disease process. New immune modulating therapies are being studied and a better understanding of the underlying disease process may shed light on the mechanisms of action of some of the currently available drugs, and provide the rationales for new drug combination therapies. Little is known of the mechanisms by which so-called disease-modifying anti-rheumatic drugs (DMARDs) work. In vitro studies have shown that chloroquine interferes with antigen processing and presentation, that sulphasalazine inhibits lymphocyte activation, and D-penicillamine inhibits T cell proliferation. The action of corticosteroids is better understood. Steroids suppress phagocytosis and inhibit the production of pro-inflammatory cytokines by monocytes, macrophages and T cells. It is thought that these actions may be mediated through the production of transforming growth factor-beta (TGF-beta). Cyclosporin A is used in severe rheumatoid arthritis (RA) and is known to inhibit T cell dependent immune reactions by inhibiting the production of cytokines, such as interferon gamma (IFN-gamma) and interleukin-2 (IL-2). The fact that cyclosporin A is an effective treatment lends support to the role of T cells in the disease process, but the improvement in symptoms is both slow and incomplete so IL-2 and IFN-gamma are unlikely to be the only factors driving the disease.

Recent studies suggest that very early treatment with DMARDs may improve prognosis as evaluated by clinical symptoms and inflammatory activity. In addition, a recent controlled trial has shown beneficial effects from treatment with a combination of DMARDs, as opposed to treatment with a single agent. New trials are needed to evaluate the efficacy of different treatment combinations.

New immune therapies may be directed at blocking stages in the immune cascade such as blocking the action of monokines, or at redirecting the underlying immune process by using, for example, vaccines. Blockade of the pro-inflammatory cytokine TNF-alpha with neutralizing monoclonal antibodies was shown to improve dramatically clinical symptoms and reduce C-reactive protein concentrations and other signs of inflammation in a double-blind placebo controlled study of human RA. The long-term consequences of TNF blockade on anti-tumour defence and antimicrobial action is unclear, but preliminary results from phase II trials have shown an increase in infection rate. Desensitization to the presumed antigen through immunization or oral tolerization is also under investigation.

Reference

Klareskog L, Ronnelid J, Holm G 1995 Immunopathogenesis and immunotherapy in rheumatoid arthritis: an area of transition. Journal of Investigative Medicine 238: 191-206

100. Gout

A. **F**   B. **F**   C. **F**   D. **T**   E. **T**

The commonest manifestation of gout is an acute inflammatory arthritis, most often affecting the first metatarsophalangeal joint in middle-aged men. The pathophysiology is of urate crystal deposition in the synovial fluid, usually associated with a raised serum uric acid concentration. Uric acid is the breakdown product of the purines adenine and guanine degraded by xanthine oxidase and it is excreted by the kidneys. Following glomerular filtration and proximal tubular reabsorption, the distal tubules secrete uric acid into the urine. Uncommonly a urate crystal nephropathy can be a consequence of gout. Several factors predispose to hyperuricaemia. These include impaired renal function, alcoholism, myeloproliferative disease, drugs such as low dose aspirin, thiazides, pyrizinamide and cytotoxics and congenital abnormalities such as in the Lesch-Nyhan syndrome. Hyperlipidaemia does not predispose to hyperuricaemia.

Non-steroidal anti-inflammatory drugs (NSAIDS) are the most effective treatment for acute gout. An alternative agent is colchicine which inhibits intracellular microtubule formation. Gastrointestinal side-effects are common, especially diarrhoea, and these limit the dose which can be given. Allopurinol is used to prevent chronic tophaceous arthritis in recurrent attacks of gout. It competitively inhibits xanthine oxidase thereby increasing the concentration of xanthine, which is more soluble. If used during an acute episode it will prolong the attack and may itself precipitate acute gout. The reason for this is thought to be related to large shifts in intra- and extra-cellular urate gradients. It is therefore initiated when the condition is quiescent and combined initially with a NSAID or colchicine.

Hyperuricaemia per se does not need treatment in an otherwise healthy individual. Cytotoxic agents can cause massive cellular breakdown and allopurinol is indicated as preventative treatment in patients undergoing chemotherapy. Other drugs used in chronic gout include sulphinpyrazone and probenecid. These are uricosuric agents, increasing renal urate excretion and are contraindicated in patients with urate stones. They need to be used cautiously in renal failure.

References

Emmerson B T 1996 The management of gout. New England Journal of Medicine 334: 445-451

Goodacre J A, Carson Dick W 1995 Treatment of gout. Prescribers Journal 35: 105-110

Snaith M C 1995 ABC of rheumatology: gout, hyperuricaemia and crystal arthritis. British Medical Journal 310: 521-524

101. Raynaud's phenomenon

A. F   B. T   C. F   D. T   E. T

Raynaud's phenomenon is the name given to the characteristic colour changes seen in the digits of up to 5% of the population in response to cold. The white, blue, red sequence was first recognized to be a local effect of cold when its induction was demonstrated in otherwise warm patients on immersion of their hands into cold water. A mainstay of treatment is to avoid cold exposure to the extremities. However, in some cases, especially those associated with autoimmune diseases, vasodilator drugs are needed. The most useful are the calcium channel antagonists. Severe disease with prolonged vasoconstriction may cause digital ulceration and necrosis, and intensive vasodilatory treatment with prostacyclins is then indicated.

The majority of affected patients are women. 5% of new patients will go on to develop an underlying autoimmune disease, the commonest of which is systemic sclerosis but rheumatoid arthritis, Sjögren's syndrome, systemic lupus erythematosus and myositis are all recognized associations. Abnormal nailfold capillaries and a positive anti-nuclear factor help to predict the likelihood of these conditions developing.

Recent work to try and elucidate the cause of Raynaud's phenomenon has centred on the skin microvasculature and perivascular innervation. Increased amounts of endothelin-1 have been detected in patients with Raynaud's but this is not thought to be the primary pathological abnormality. Patients with Raynaud's phenomenon have decreased numbers of nerve endings releasing calcitonin gene related peptide (CGRP) and there is evidence for a central role of CGRP in the pathogenesis of Raynaud's phenomenon. CGRP is the most potent endogenous vasodilator so far discovered and early trials of its intravenous therapeutic use have been promising.

References

Isenberg D A, Black C 1995 ABC of rheumatology. Raynaud's phenomenon, scleroderma and overlap syndromes. British Medical Journal 310: 795-798

Report of a meeting of physicians and scientists 1995. Raynaud's phenomenon. University College Medical School, London. Lancet 346: 283-290

RENAL MEDICINE

102. Adult polycystic kidney disease

A. F.   B. F   C. T   D. T   E. T

Adult polycystic kidney disease (APKD) shows autosomal dominant inheritance. It is a major cause of chronic renal failure accounting for 10% of all patients requiring long-term haemodialysis. The formation of multiple thin-walled cysts causes progressive renal enlargement and eventual renal failure due to a combination of nephron compression and outflow obstruction. Few nephrons remain within the renal tissue between cysts on microscopic examination. Instead this area is usually replaced by fibrotic tissue. It has been proposed that apoptosis (programmed cell death) may be a contributory mechanism in the inevitable loss of renal function in these patients.

Three different forms of APKD have been identified. The most common, APKD-1, accounts for 85% of cases and the gene has been localized to chromosome 16 near the alpha haemoglobin gene. This gene has now been cloned. A variety of mutations may occur within its structure and this may account for the inter-family variability in disease severity and progression. The gene for APKD-2 has been localized to chromosome 4. The locus for APKD-3 is currently unknown. Different kindreds show variable rates of progression suggesting a degree of polymorphism.

Flank pain, haematuria, nocturia and hypertension may be presenting features of APKD. 10% of patients have renal stones and renal colic may be a consequence of stone or blood clot passage. 75% will develop hypertension. End stage renal failure may occur at any age necessitating renal replacement therapy. Despite this, only 50% of adults with APKD-1 develop end stage renal failure. Haematuria may cause anaemia but polycythaemia is also recognized secondary to increased erythropoietin production. Malignant transformation of renal cysts may occur. Associated abnormalities include mitral valve prolapse in 25% and Berry aneurysms causing intracranial haemorrhage in 10% of patients. Cysts may also form in the liver, spleen, ovaries and pancreas. Proteinuria is common but does not usually reach nephrotic levels.

Management involves early detection of the disease necessitating screening of family members with ultrasound. Identification of the gene loci for APKD may soon allow genetic screening. Once a diagnosis of APKD has been established, blood pressure control should be meticulous as this has been shown to delay any deterioration in renal function. Urinary tract infection should be treated early and patients should be regularly screened for complications of the disease.

References

Grantham J J 1995 Polycystic kidney disease – there goes the neighbourhood. New England Journal of Medicine 333: 56-57

Saggar-Malik A K, Jeffrey S, Patton M A 1994 Autosomal dominant polycystic kidney disease. British Medical Journal 308: 1183-1184

Woo D 1995 Apoptosis and loss of renal tissue in polycystic kidney diseases. New England Journal of Medicine 333: 18-25

103. Haemodialysis related amyloidosis

A. F   B. T   C. T   D. F   E. F

Haemodialysis associated amyloidosis is a complication of long-term renal replacement therapy. It is seen most commonly in haemodialysis patients after 10–15 years but is also well described in patients on peritoneal dialysis. It does not occur in patients with a functioning renal transplant.

Carpal tunnel syndrome is a characteristic presentation. Another common manifestation is osteoarthropathy. Symptoms are recurrent arthralgia, joint effusions, synovitis, tendinitis and stiffness of large and medium sized joints. The differential diagnosis is extensive and complicated by hyperparathyroidism and renal osteodystrophy. Because visceral involvement is very rare in this type of amyloidosis, diagnosis depends on the histopathology of the joints and synovium. Rectal biopsy is unhelpful.

Symptoms are due to the deposition of A-beta-2-microglobulin-amyloid of which beta-2-microglobulin is the precursor. Beta-2-microglobulin has long stretches of beta-pleated sheets and is a prerequisite for amyloid formation. 95% of excretion is renal and so, for this type of amyloidosis to occur, uraemia is a necessary precondition. However, other mechanisms must be involved as not all uraemic patients exhibit clinical symptoms.

A common constituent of all types of amyloid is serum amyloid P (SAP) protein. An isotope scan using radiolabelled SAP to aid the diagnosis of amyloidoses has been developed and is available at specialist centres. The specificity and sensitivity of this scan has yet to be evaluated.

Reference

Floege J, Ehlerding G 1996 Beta-2-microglobulin-associated amyloidosis. Nephron 72: 9-26.

---

104. *Escherichia coli* O157:H7

A. **T**   B. **T**   C. **F**   D. **T**   E. **F**

Escherichia coli O157: H7 was first described in 1983. It can cause asymptomatic infection, non-bloody diarrhoea, bloody diarrhoea, haemolytic-uraemic syndrome (HUS) or thrombotic thrombocytopenic purpura (TTP). Its serotype is designated by its somatic (O) and flagellar (H) antigens. The incidence is not known but it is estimated to cause 21 000 infections in the USA each year. It can affect all ages but it tends to cause more serious illness in the very young and the elderly. Clinical infection tends to occur most commonly in the warmer months.

Major outbreaks have occurred through the consumption of contaminated ground beef but transmission can also occur from raw milk and from contaminated water. Person to person transmission has been described.

The organism produces a shigella-like toxin and this acts locally producing a histological appearance similar to *Clostridium difficile* colitis. It is thought that vascular damage may lead to the leakage of toxins such as lipopolysaccharide into the circulation which then initiate the extra-gastrointestinal complications such as HUS and TTP.

During an outbreak about 6% of cases develop HUS and about 1% of cases die. The illness in symptomatic individuals typically starts with non-bloody diarrhoea and severe abdominal cramps. The stools may become bloody by the second or third day. Fever is not a prominent feature. The disease can mimic an acute surgical abdomen. Barium enema examination may reveal thumbprinting and sigmoidoscopy may reveal oedema, hyperaemia, ulceration or even a pseudomembrane.

Antibiotic therapy for the acute diarrhoeal illness has not been shown to be beneficial and some studies suggest it may be harmful. Anti-motility drugs are contraindicated as they have been shown to increase the incidence of major complications.

References

Boyce T G, Swerdlow D L, Griffin P M 1995 *Escherichia coli* O157: H7 and the haemolytic-uraemic syndrome. New England Journal of Medicine 333: 364-368

Riley L W 1983 Haemorrhagic colitis associated with a rare *Escherichia* serotype. New England Journal of Medicine 308: 681-685

---

105. Haemolytic uraemic syndrome
A. T   B. T   C. F   D. T   E. F

The haemolytic uraemic syndrome (HUS) is characterized by the triad of acute renal failure, thrombocytopenia and micro-angiopathic haemolytic anaemia. It is commonest in children and while some cases are drug related or idiopathic, most follow an episode of infectious diarrhoea. The most common causative agent is *Escherichia coli* serotype O157: H7 followed by *Shigella dysenteriae* serotype 1. Both are thought to produce shigella-like endotoxins which have an affinity for a glomerular transmembrane protein. Binding to this protein mediates endothelial cell damage and initiates intravascular platelet activation and thrombus formation. Similar affinity for an erythrocyte membrane protein may participate in haemolysis but this is not fully established.

HUS is one of a group of microangiopathic haemolytic disorders which includes thrombotic thrombocytopenic purpura (TTP). HUS affects the kidney preferentially and unlike TTP and septicaemia associated disseminated intravascular coagulation (DIC), rarely presents with disturbance of the coagulation pathways. Moderate proteinuria in the region of 1–2g/24hrs is usual as is microscopic haematuria. Frank haematuria is occasionally seen.

Renal biopsy reveals intraluminal platelet aggregates in renal arterioles. The exact site depends on whether the HUS is related to diarrhoea or not. Complete obstruction of renal microvasculature may produce glomerular and tubular necrosis. This may result in hypertension and dialysis-dependent renal failure.

Treatment is supportive, and haemodialysis may be required. Fresh frozen plasma (FFP) improves outcome and is the mainstay of active treatment. If oliguria is marked then plasmapharesis may be needed to allow space in the intravascular compartment for FFP. Platelets should be avoided as, paradoxically, they can exacerbate the thrombocytopenia. Aspirin may be of some benefit. The prognosis is usually good, reflecting the self-limiting natural history of the disease.

References

Boyce T G, Swerdlow D L, Griffin P M 1995 *Escherichia coli* O157: H7 and the haemolytic-uraemic syndrome. New England Journal of Medicine 333: 364-368

Moake J L 1994 Haemolytic-uraemic syndrome: basic science. Lancet 343: 393-397

Nield G H 1994 Haemolytic-uraemic syndrome in practice. Lancet 343: 398-401

---

106   Renal disease in diabetes mellitus

A. **T**   B. **T**   C. **F**   D. **F**   E. **F**

The pattern of renal disease in diabetes is changing. The number of young diabetics reaching end stage renal failure is falling and this probably reflects improved diabetic care, particularly tighter glycaemic control. Diabetic renal disease still poses a formidable problem, with up to 30% of insulin-dependent diabetics under the age of 30 showing evidence of nephropathy. Onset of nephropathy usually occurs 15–25 years after the diagnosis of insulin-dependent diabetes mellitus (IDDM). Patients with NIDDM also develop nephropathy but the proportion is smaller.

Three main processes damage the kidney in DM: infection, ischaemia and glomerular damage. Women with bladder stasis from autonomic neuropathy are particularly prone to recurrent ascending urinary infections with secondary chronic interstitial damage. Acute pyelonephritis with papillary necrosis can also occur. Ischaemic renal damage can occur due to hypertrophy and hyalinization of the afferent and efferent vessels or secondary to large vessel atherosclerosis causing renal artery stenosis.

Glomerular damage is probably caused by a combination of hyperglycaemia (with protein glycosylation) and microvascular changes. The earliest changes are renal hypertrophy with an increased glomerular filtration rate. Histologically there is thickening of the basement membrane associated with leakage of albumin. In more advanced nephropathy, renal biopsy reveals diffuse or nodular glomerularsclerosis, the latter also being known as the Kimmelstiel-Wilson lesion. Not all renal disease in diabetics is due to diabetic glomerulosclerosis. Other possible intrinsic renal pathology as well as vascular disease should be considered, especially if evidence of other tissue damage, for example, retinopathy is absent. Once end stage renal failure is reached vascular disease makes peritoneal dialysis and transplantation preferable methods of renal replacement, although in practice haemodialysis is often required. Some transplant centres are adding pancreatic grafts at the time of surgery, although pancreatic graft life has been limited by fibrosis and subsequent failure.

References

Clark C M, Lee D A 1995 Prevention and treatment of the complications of diabetes mellitus. New England Journal of Medicine 332: 1210-1217

The Diabetes Control and Complication Trial Research Group 1993 The effect of intensive treatment of diabetes on the development and progression of long-term complications in insulin-dependent diabetes mellitus. New England Journal of Medicine 329; (14): 977-986

107. Diabetic nephropathy
A. T   B. T   C. F   D. F   E. F

Studies in the early eighties showed strong correlation between the presence of microalbuminuria and the progression to frank proteinuria and eventual end stage renal failure. A more recent study following a larger cohort of patients (155) with microalbuminuria showed that the predictive value of this test is weaker than was thought. Of those with a single raised urinary albumin excretion measurement, 19% developed clinical nephropathy at 5 years follow up and only 31% showed a progressive rise in albumin excretion. These results suggest that although microalbuminuria remains a useful risk marker for the subsequent development of nephropathy, a single abnormal value should be interpreted with caution. Microalbuminuria is not detectable on routine dipstick testing. New dipsticks which detect albumin levels of 40-200mg are now available and are used by some practitioners for screening. Qualitative assays on early morning or overnight urine are preferable for analysis.

In patients with microalbuminuria who have normal serum creatinine, ACE inhibitors will reduce the rate of progression to overt proteinuria. Part of this effect is due to a reduction in blood pressure, but studies have revealed that some of this renoprotective effect is independent of blood pressure control. The mechanism of protection is not clear but in animal studies the reduction in glomerular hypertension seen with ACE inhibitors has been associated with reduction in the development of histological lesions.

ACE inhibitors have also been shown to reduce by almost 50% the rate of progression of established nephropathy in IDDM. This is also partly independent of their anti-hypertensive effect. Thiazides should not be used in diabetics as their metabolic side-effects of hyperglycaemia and hyperlipidaemia interfere with good glycaemic control and add to the risk factors already present for cardiovascular disease.

Although ACE inhibitors can precipitate acute renal failure when given to patients with renal artery stenosis (especially if bilateral), their use is not absolutely contraindicated. In diabetics where an ACE inhibitor is indicated (for hypertension, heart failure or nephropathy) they can be introduced with careful monitoring of blood pressure and renal function. If a diabetic has evidence of extensive atherosclerosis or has asymmetrical kidneys suggesting renal artery stenosis, further investigation with renogram, doppler flow ultrasound or arteriography should be considered prior to initiating therapy.

References

Almdal T, Norgaard K, Feldt-Rasmussen B et al 1994 The predictive value of microalbuminuria in IDDM: a 5-year follow-up study. Diabetes Care 17: 20-25

Krolewski A S, Lattel L M B, Krolewski M et al 1995 Glycosylated haemoglobin and the risk of microalbuminuria in patients with insulin-dependent diabetes mellitus. New England Journal of Medicine 332: 1251-1255

Lewis E J, Hunsicker L G, Bain R P et al 1993 The effects of ACE inhibition on diabetic nephropathy. New England Journal of Medicine 329: 1456-1462

Microalbuminuria Collaborative Study Group 1995 Intensive therapy and progression to clinical albuminuria in patients with insulin-dependent diabetes mellitus and microalbuminuria. British Medical Journal 311: 973-977

Viberti G, Mogensen C E, Groop L C et al 1994 Effect of captopril on progression to clinical proteinuria in patients with insulin-dependent diabetes mellitus and microalbuminuria. Journal of the American Medical Association 271: 275-279

108. Membranous glomerulonephritis

A. **F**   B. **T**   C. **F**   D. **F**   E. **T**.

Membranous glomerulonephritis is the commonest cause of nephrotic syndrome in adults. Other causes include focal segmental glomerulosclerosis (FSGS) occurring in 15%, and minimal change glomerulonephritis, occurring in 20%. Minimal change glomerulonephritis is the commonest cause of nephrotic syndrome in children, accounting for 90% of cases. The commonest cause of glomerulonephritis in adults is IgA nephropathy. The histological lesion in membranous glomerulonephritis is a thickened glomerular basement membrane with subepithelial deposition of IgG and C3, seen on immunofluorescence.

Nephrotic syndrome or proteinuria are the most common presentations of membranous glomerulonephritis. It is usually idiopathic but it can complicate illnesses such as systemic lupus erythematosus and sickle cell disease. It is a recognized idiosyncratic effect of drugs such as gold and penicillamine and can be caused by infections such as hepatitis B and malaria. In the elderly it is commonly associated with malignancy, especially carcinoma. Minimal change glomerulonephritis has an association with lymphoma, particularly Hodgkin's disease.

The natural history of membranous glomerulonephritis is varied. 20–30% will undergo spontaneous remission. 15–20% will progress to end stage renal failure(ESRF). The remainder have a partial remission or remain stable. Treatment is controversial. A regime of alternating steroids and chlorambucil known as the Ponticelli regime has been shown to preserve renal function and induce remission in some patients. Chlorambucil is carcinogenic and asymptomatic disease with normal renal function may not warrant intensive therapy. Cyclophosphamide is an alternative agent. Nephrotic syndrome associated with membranous glomerulonephritis is usually actively treated because of the risk of secondary complications associated with the syndrome, such as venous thrombosis (due to functional anti-thrombin III deficiency). Poor prognostic indicators include increasing age, male sex and heavy proteinuria.

References

Mason P D, Pusey C D 1994 Glomerulonephritis: diagnosis and treatment. British Medical Journal 309: 1557-1563

Ponticelli C, Zucchelli P, Imbusciati E et al 1984 A controlled trial of methylprednisolone and chlorambucil in idiopathic membranous nephropathy. New England Journal of Medicine 310: 946-950

Robertson S, Isles C, More I 1995 Glomerular disease made easier: 2. British Journal of Hospital Medicine 53: 323-326

ENDOCRINOLOGY
109. Insulin-dependent diabetes mellitus
A. F.   B. F   C. T   D. T   E. T

Insulin-dependent diabetes mellitus (IDDM) presents with symptoms of polyuria, polydipsia and weight loss associated with hyperglycaemia and ketosis. Both genetic and environmental factors are implicated in its pathogenesis. It is more common in HLA DR3 and DR4 individuals and at least 95% of patients have one or both of these antigens. HLA DR1, 8 and 16 are also associated and there is an even stronger association with the DQ antigens. Certain HLA antigens are protective, for example, HLA DR11 and HLA DR15. A risk factor for developing IDDM is having a first-degree relative with the condition, the highest risk being with identical twins or HLA identical siblings. 33% of identical twins show concordance for IDDM, compared to nearly 100% for non-insulin-dependent diabetes mellitus (NIDDM). People whose fathers have IDDM are three times more likely to develop the disease than those whose mothers have it.

Viral infection is postulated to be the triggering environmental factor for disease development in susceptible individuals. At least 80% of beta islet cells have to be lost before symptomatic IDDM develops. Rubella virus is associated with congenital IDDM and several autoantibodies are described in patients with IDDM, including those to the enzyme glutamate decarboxylase which shares a common amino acid sequence with a coxsackie virus protein (genetic mimicry). Other autoantibodies include anti-islet cell antibodies and anti-insulin antibodies. These are present in 0.5% of normal individuals, about 4% of people with diabetic relatives and 70–80% of newly diagnosed diabetics.

Reference

Atkinson M A, Maclaren N K 1994 The pathogenesis of insulin-dependent diabetes mellitus. New England Journal of Medicine 331: 1428-1435.

110. Human insulin

A. T   B. F   C. T   D. T   E. F

Human insulin is a polypeptide hormone which is encoded by a gene on the short arm of chromosome 11. It is stored in pancreatic islet beta cells as proinsulin, which consists of two polypeptide chains A and B which are linked to each other by three bridging disulphide bonds and C-peptide. Proinsulin is cleaved prior to release within the cells to insulin and C-peptide. C-peptide and insulin are therefore released in equimolar amounts, although after an overnight fast the plasma concentration may differ by a factor of 10 because of the different rates of renal C-peptide excretion and hepatic insulin metabolism. The human insulin molecule consists of 51 amino acids and is highly conserved across species, differing from porcine insulin by only one amino acid and from bovine insulin by three. The C-peptide is not as closely conserved. Insulin release is stimulated by many factors including arginine, glucose, glucagon, gastrin and secretin. Inhibitors of release include somatostatin, interleukin-1 and alpha adrenergic stimulation.

Reference

Hall R, Besser M 1989 Fundamentals of clinical endocrinology, 4th edn. Churchill Livingstone, Edinburgh

111. Tight diabetic control

A. F   B. T   C. F   D. T   E. F

In 1993 a landmark paper was published which showed for the first time that tight diabetic control can reduce the development and progression of the microvascular complications of diabetes. The Diabetes Control and Complication Trial Research Group studied 1441 patients with insulin-dependent diabetes, 726 with no retinopathy at base line and 715 with mild retinopathy. These groups formed the primary and secondary prevention groups respectively. Patients were assigned to either tight diabetic control, attempting to achieve near normoglycaemia, or conventional therapy. After a mean follow-up of 6.5 years, it was shown that the tight control group suffered fewer complications. There was a 76% reduction in the development of retinopathy in the primary prevention group and a 54% reduction in the progression of retinopathy in the secondary prevention group. Intensive therapy reduced the development of microalbuminuria by 39%, of albuminuria by 54% and of neuropathy by 60%. In the intensive therapy group there was a two to three-fold increase in the incidence of hypoglycaemia. The study was not able to establish a reduction in macrovascular complications. Earlier studies had shown a worsening of diabetic retinopathy with tight control, but this appears to be a temporary phenomenon with abnormalities disappearing after 18 months, and longer term follow-up showing a clear reduction in progression with tight control.

It is thought to be hyperglycaemia and the glycosylation of proteins that leads to the microvascular complications of the disease. The ideal level of glycaemia to strike a balance between microvascular complications and hypoglycaemia, was not established by the trial. The relevance of the trial to patients outside a trial setting has been questioned, particularly whether such close patient surveillance would be possible.

Whether tight diabetic control reduces complications in non-insulin-dependent diabetics is currently under scrutiny in the United Kingdom Prospective Diabetes Study (UKPDS) and in the Veterans Affairs Cooperative Study on Glycaemic Control and Complications in NIDDM (VACSDM).

References

Clark C M, Vinicor F 1996 Risks and benefits of intensive management in non-insulin-dependent diabetes mellitus. Annals of Internal Medicine 124; 1 pt 2: 81-85

The Diabetes Control and Complication Trial Research Group 1993 The effect of intensive treatment of diabetes on the development and progression of long-term complications in insulin-dependent diabetes mellitus. New England Journal of Medicine 329 (14): 977-986

112. Diabetes and pregnancy

A. T   B. F   C. F   D. T   E. T

Patients with diabetes need additional surveillance during pregnancy. Pre-conception care will improve the outcome of the pregnancy. There is an increased incidence of spontaneous abortion in patients who have poorly controlled diabetes (reflected by a glycosylated haemoglobin of >12%) in the first trimester of pregnancy, even if the control is improved thereafter. Overall, women with IDDM have a fetal mortality rate of 3%. With good glycaemic control diabetics have no greater risk of spontaneous abortion than non-diabetic women.

All diabetic pregnancies are associated with higher rates of infection compared to non-diabetic pregnancies. 80% of insulin-dependent diabetic women will have at least one episode of infection. 4% will have pyelonephritis, a rate four times higher than for non-diabetic women. There are significantly higher rates of urogenital, wound, respiratory, endometrial and candida infections.

Pre-eclampsia is much more common in diabetic pregnancies than non-diabetic pregnancies and is associated with a far greater perinatal mortality rate (60 deaths per 1000 live births compared with 3.3 per 1000 live births for non-diabetic women). Pre-existing hypertension and nephropathy further increase the risk of pre-eclampsia and in these diabetics the diagnosis may be difficult.

Some pre-existing complications of diabetes may improve in pregnancy. In normal, non-diabetic pregnancies, creatinine clearance increases. This occurs in about one third of diabetic women with nephropathy. An equivalent proportion will, however, show declining renal function and may progress to require dialysis during the pregnancy. Premature delivery is common in patients needing renal replacement therapy. The management of retinopathy during pregnancy is difficult. Pregnancy itself can aggravate retinopathy considerably. There is also a worsening of retinopathy as diabetic control is improved, as is often the case during pregnancy. Frequent fundoscopy and early ophthalmic referral is advisable. Peripheral neuropathies are not usually problematical but autonomic neuropathy may cause difficulties by exacerbating postural hypotension and impairing the recognition of hypoglycaemia. Diabetic gastroparesis will contribute to emesis and nutritional control may then become difficult.

Ketoacidosis may develop as a result of hyperemesis, beta sympathomimetic agents and infections. Pregnancy induces relative insulin resistance. Ketoacidosis now affects only a small proportion of diabetic pregnancies in the UK due to improved antenatal care, but it is serious and it is associated with a high rate of fetal loss (up to 20%). The management of ketoacidosis in pregnancy is the same as in non-pregnant diabetic patients.

References

Garner P 1995 Type 1 diabetes mellitus and pregnancy. Lancet 346: 157-161

Kanz N K, Herman W H, Becker M P et al 1995 Diabetes and pregnancy: factors associated with seeking pre-conception care. Diabetes Care 18: 157-165

113. Aldosterone

A. **F.**   B . **F** C. **T**   D. **T**   E. **T**

Aldosterone is a potent mineralocorticoid differing characteristically from other steroids by an aldehyde group at C18. It is synthesized in the zona glomerulosa in normal adults where the enzyme aldosterone synthetase is expressed. Only in the autosomal dominant disorder 'glucocorticoid suppressible hyperaldosteronism' is aldosterone inappropriately regulated by adrenocorticotrophic hormone (ACTH) with synthesis in the zona fasciculata. Renin, angiotensin and potassium are all implicated in the normal regulation of aldosterone synthesis. Aldosterone excess leads to salt and water retention with resulting hypertension and potassium depletion. Conversely, hypoaldosteronism leads to hyponatraemia and hyperkalaemia. Primary hypoaldosteronism is characterized by an elevated plasma renin to aldosterone ratio, in contrast to secondary hypoaldosteronism where renin concentrations are low. The converse is true in hyperaldosterone states.

There are several inherited defects of aldosterone synthesis. The most common is congenital adrenal hyperplasia due to 21-hydroxylase deficiency. This is inherited in an autosomal recessive manner and two thirds of cases exhibit mineralocorticoid deficiency. Excess androgen secretion makes this disorder clinically separate from cholesterol desmolase and 3-beta-hydroxysteroid hydrogenase deficiencies which may also be salt wasting but where the genitalia are ambiguous. Aldosterone synthase deficiency is autosomal recessive in inheritance. It may present in neonates or in childhood where it is associated with growth retardation. These children are usually asymptomatic in adulthood concurring with observations in congenital adrenal hyperplasia that salt wasting often improves with age. Adrenoleucodystrophy and congenital adrenal hypoplasia are both X-linked conditions. The latter is closely linked to the Duchenne gene locus and occasionally the two conditions are seen together in combination with glycerol kinase deficiency. Acquired adrenal insufficiency is most commonly autoimmune in nature. It may be part of a polyglandular deficiency syndrome. Type I is associated with hypoparathyroidism and mucocutaneous candidiasis and is rare. Type II occurs mostly in young women and is associated with autoimmune thryoiditis and insulin-dependent diabetes mellitus.

Hypoadrenalism may also be secondary to infections such as tuberculosis or human immunodeficiency virus or to drugs such as ketoconazole.

Reference

White P C 1994 Disorders of aldosterone biosynthesis and action. New England Journal of Medicine 331: 250-258

114. Cushing's syndrome
A. **T**   B. **T**   C. **T**   D. **F**   E. **F**

Cushing's syndrome results from the pathological manifestations of glucocorticoid excess. It may be caused by excessive oral or parenteral administration of glucocorticosteroids, by steroid secreting adrenal tumours or by ectopic production of adrenocorticotrophic hormone (ACTH) (most commonly from a small cell carcinoma of the lung). Cushing's disease shares the same symptoms and signs as Cushing's syndrome but specifically results from excess production of ACTH by corticotroph tumours in the anterior pituitary.

The diagnosis of Cushing's disease can be difficult. Corticotrophin releasing hormone (CRH) produces an exaggerated response in those with Cushing's disease. Enhanced high resolution nuclear magnetic resonance imaging can locate the site of a corticotroph tumour in only 50% of cases but is more sensitive than CT scanning or petrosal venous sampling.

High dose dexamethasone tests (2mg qds for 2 days or an overnight test with 8mg given at 11pm) have a specificity of 100% in the diagnosis of Cushing's disease. In Cushing's disease the 24-hour urinary cortisol excretion is reduced by more than 90% but this test is only 65% sensitive. Greater sensitivity of up to 90% can be achieved with a high dose overnight test and when 17-hydroxycorticosteroids are also measured. Metyrapone stimulation tests can further improve accuracy. Petrosal venous sampling combined with peripheral venous sampling and CRH stimulation is 100% sensitive and specific in distinguishing Cushing's disease from ectopic corticotrophin excess. It is however an expensive procedure with a complication rate of 0.2–23% which includes permanent brain stem damage.

Reference

Orth D N 1995 Medical progress: Cushing's syndrome. New England Journal of Medicine 332: 791-803

115. Thyrotoxicosis
A. F.   B. T   C. F   D. F   E. T

Thyrotoxicosis should be suspected in any patient with unexplained weight loss, heat intolerance, excessive sweating, increased appetite, tachycardia or fatigue. Less common presentations include pruritus, muscle weakness and thirst. Other recognized presentations include oligomenorrhoea in young women and heart failure in the elderly.

The serum thyroid stimulating hormone (TSH) level is the most useful confirmatory test. It is characteristically low. Very rarely, when secondary causes such as TSH secreting tumours are the cause, it will be elevated. Usually the free thyroxine (T4) level is elevated, but if normal then T3 thyrotoxicosis may be present and T3 levels should be checked. High T4 levels will be seen in patients where deiodination of T4 to T3 is inhibited. This occurs in patients taking drugs such as dexamethasone, propanolol and amiodarone. In severe systemic illness a high T4 but normal TSH or a low T4 with normal TSH, are both compatible with a diagnosis of the sick euthyroid syndrome.

Grave's disease and toxic multinodular goitre are the commonest causes of thyrotoxicosis. Other causes include Hashimoto's disease, post partum and viral thyroiditis, factitious thyrotoxicosis associated with excess thyroxine ingestion, pregnancy when hyperemesis gravidarum is a presenting feature and ectopic thyroid hormone secretion from metastatic follicular cell carcinoma or struma ovarii. It is extemely rare for primary thyroid malignancy to present with thyrotoxicosis.

History and examination are essential parts of the investigation of thyrotoxicosis. Autoimmune diseases are often familial. Recent pregnancy or pain over the thyroid area may suggest a diagnosis of thyroiditis, while the drug history may reveal amiodarone as the cause. Grave's disease is associated with ophthalmopathy, dermopathy and acropachy. The goitre of Grave's disease is usually smooth and diffusely enlarged as opposed to the bulky irregular goitre of multinodular disease.

In Grave's disease autoantibodies to thyroid peroxidase (thyroid microsomal antibodies) are present in 90% of patients compared to 10% of the normal population. Anti-TSH receptor antibodies are more specific to autoimmune disease. Thyroglobulin antibodies are uncommon in Grave's disease but common in Hashimoto's disease which can cause either hyper- or hypothyroidism.

Radioisotope scans are useful in the diagnosis of thyrotoxicosis. In thyroiditis radioisotope uptake is decreased. As thyrotoxicosis is transient in this condition an accurate diagnosis alters the management. Decreased uptake is also seen in thyroxine excess and iodide induced thyrotoxicosis. Increased uptake is characteristic of Grave's disease and of multinodular goitre. A toxic adenoma will show increased uptake but if the scan is equivocal the patient should have a fine needle aspirate to exclude malignancy.

Reference

Kendall-Taylor P 1995 Investigation of thyrotoxicosis. Clinical Endocrinology 42: 309-313.

---

116. Hyperprolactinaemia

A. F   B. T   C. F   D. F   E. F

Hyperprolactinaemia has many causes. Prolactin is produced by the anterior pituitary gland and is the only anterior pituitary hormone predominantly under the inhibitory control of dopamine acting on D2 receptors. Dopamine antagonists will therefore cause hyperprolactinaemia and this accounts for many of the iatrogenic cases. Drugs such as metaclopramide, domperidone, phenothiazines and sulpiride are all dopamine antagonists. Other drugs which can cause a raised prolactin include oestrogen, methyldopa, opiates and danazol. Prolactin levels are physiologically high during pregnancy and lactation.

After drugs the next most common cause of hyperprolactinaemia is pituitary adenomata. These can be either micro (<1cm) or macro (>1cm) prolactinomas or mixed tumours where prolactin is secreted along with growth hormone or adrenocorticotrophin. Other causes of hyperprolactinaemia need to be excluded such as pituitary stalk compression, polycystic ovaries, renal failure, cirrhosis, hypothyroidism and porphyria. Much rarer causes are histiocytosis X and ectopic secretion of prolactin from bronchial or renal tumours.

Dopamine agonists are the mainstay of medical treatment for prolactinomas. A gradual reduction in size of the tumour is usual but occasionally they induce rapid tumour shrinkage and cerebrospinal fluid leaks. Bromocriptine has common side-effects such as nausea, postural hypotension, headache and dizziness which can limit its use. Less commonly it can cause retroperitoneal fibrosis, pleural effusions and dyskinesia. More selective D2 agonists are cabergoline and quinagoline which are useful alternatives to bromocriptine.

Reduction of prolactin levels is more successfully achieved with medical treatment than with surgery. There is, however, a chance of cure with surgery although there is also a high recurrence rate. Surgery is usually offered in resistant cases, when there is drug intolerance or when large tumours are causing chiasmal compression and threatening sight.

The main risk of prolactinomas in pregnancy is that high oestrogen levels can stimulate rapid tumour growth particularly in patients with macroprolactinomas. Bromocriptine is thought to be safe in pregnancy but vigilance must be increased with formal visual field monitoring and computed tomography or magnetic resonance imaging if necessary. Serum prolactin levels are altered in normal pregnancy and levels do not therefore correlate well with tumour enlargement.

References

New drugs for hyperprolactinaemia 1995 Drugs and Therapeutics Bulletin 33: 65-67

Jones T H 1995 The management of hyperprolactinaemia. British Journal of Hospital Medicine 53: 374-378

117. Human chorionic gonadotrophin

A. **T**   B. **F**   C. **T**   D. **T**   E. **T**

Human chorionic gonadotrophin (HCG) is a glycoprotein consisting of an alpha and beta subunit. The alpha subunit is common to other glycoproteins like luteinizing hormone, follicle stimulating hormone and thyroid stimulating hormone (TSH), but its beta subunit is distinct. Beta HCG is normally raised in pregnancy when it is secreted by the syncytioblast of the placenta. Levels rise within the first few days of pregnancy and peak towards the end of the first trimester.

Another clinical use of beta HCG is as a tumour marker. Choriocarcinoma is nearly always associated with grossly elevated levels and mild clinical hyperthyroidism and a goitre may develop due to its weak TSH activity. Other tumours commonly associated with raised beta HCG levels are germ cell tumours, teratomas and seminomas. 21% of breast cancers have an associated high beta HCG level and with metastatic disease this may rise to 50%. Carcinoma of the pancreas, ovary and bladder are less commonly associated with high levels.

Measurement of beta HCG is helpful in the management of germ cell tumours and trophoblastic disease. Elevated levels indicate the presence of active disease and may precede clinical recurrence. The converse, however, is not true and the absence of detectable beta HCG should not be taken as evidence of cure.

HCG can also be used diagnostically. A stimulation test is useful for assessing the hypothalamic-pituitary-testicular axis in patients with suspected hypogonadotrophic hypogonadism, and in detecting the presence of functional testicular tissue when the testes are impalpable. Because it stimulates Leydig cells to produce testosterone an HCG stimulation test will differentiate between disorders of testosterone synthesis and androgen insensitivity.

Reference

Pandha H S, Waxman J 1995 Tumour markers. Quarterly Journal of
    Medicine 88: 233-241

118. Gynaecomastia

A. T   B. F   C. F   D. T   E. T

Gynaecomastia is the name given to benign hypertrophy of male
breast tissue. It is very common, particularly in neonates, during
early puberty and with advancing age. 25% of cases will be
idiopathic and a further 25% will be related to puberty. Of the
remainder most are related to drugs.

A large number of drugs cause gynaecomastia. The strongest
associations are with anabolic steroids, chorionic gonadotrophin
and its analogues, oestrogens and oestrogen agonists.
Associations with spironolactone, cyproterone, flutamide,
ketoconazole, cimetidine and digoxin treatment are well
recognized. Illicit drugs such as heroin and marijuana have been
reported to cause gynaecomastia and epidemiological studies or
challenge-rechallenge studies on small groups of patients have
described roles for captopril, enalapril, nifedipine, diazepam,
penicillamine and phenytoin as aetiological agents in
gynaecomastia.

Of the remainder of cases cirrhosis, primary and secondary
hypogonadism, testicular tumours, hyperthyroidism and renal
disease will account for the majority. In most instances a careful
history and examination accompanied by renal, liver and thyroid
function tests will reveal the cause. Very occasionally non-
trophoblastic cancers such as lung, kidney, stomach and liver
cancer can cause gynaecomastia. This is probably due to ectopic
chorionic gonadotrophin secretion stimulating testicular aromatase
production. This increases aromatization of testosterone to
oestrogen leading to a state of relative androgen deficiency. The
glycogen storage disorder Pompe's disease and
hypoparathyroidism are not associated with gynaecomastia.

Several mechanisms for the development of gynaecomastia have
been proposed. These include increased oestrogen concentration,
decreased androgen concentration, androgen receptor
insensitivity and hypersensitivity of breast tissue.

In men oestrogens are produced by the testes and by
aromatization of androgens in extragonadal sites, particularly
adipose tissue, liver and muscle. Increased oestrogen synthesis
occurs in Leydig cell tumours. Increased aromatization occurs in
sex cord tumours and germ cell tumours. It is also seen in
hyperthyroidism, testicular feminization and obesity. Sex hormone
binding globulin binds oestrogens and androgens. Androgens are
more tightly bound and therefore drugs displacing steroids will

cause a relative increase in free oestrogens, such as ketoconazole and spironolactone. Such hyperoestrogenic states also cause a relative decrease in androgens. Androgen deficiency is commonly seen in ageing and in primary and secondary hypogonadism. Hermaphroditism is a consequence of androgen receptor inactivity or deficiency.

The treatment of gynaecomastia may be medical or surgical, if no underlying cause is found. Medical treatment is most effective whilst there is continuing breast tissue proliferation. Options include non-aromatizable dihydrotestosterone or anti-oestrogenic clomiphene and tamoxifen. Aromatase inhibitors may prove useful in the future.

Reference

Braunstein G D 1993 Gynaecomastia. New England Journal of
Medicine 328: 490-495

NEUROLOGY
119. Atrial fibrillation and stroke
A. **F.**   B. **T**   C. **F**   D. **F**   E. **T**

Atrial fibrillation (AF) is a common arrhythmia. It is associated with rheumatic and non-rheumatic heart disease. In rheumatic heart disease the risk of thromboembolism is about 18% per year and anticoagulation with warfarin is recommended provided there are no contraindications. Non-rheumatic AF is also associated with an increased incidence of stroke which increases with age. The issue of whether aspirin or warfarin should be used as primary prevention in these patients is the subject of much current debate.

Several trials have examined the use of anticoagulants and aspirin in non-rheumatic AF. Patient selection for these trials was carefully specified and in patients receiving warfarin the INR carefully monitored and adjusted within pre-specified margins. Translating these conditions to clinical practice is not always easy.

Chronic AF and paroxysmal AF carry a similar risk of stroke. The risk of stroke is highest during the first few months after diagnosis or during the transition of paroxysmal AF to chronic AF. Other important risk factors for stroke in AF are previous thromboembolism, hypertension, congestive heart failure and diabetes. Several trials have confirmed that in the absence of additional risk factors patients with AF under the age of 60 have no greater risk of stroke than the general age-matched population. There is no indication to anticoagulate patients under 60 with lone AF.

Meta-analysis of the trials addressing stroke prevention in non-rheumatic AF show that compared to placebo, there is an overall reduction in relative risk of stroke of about 22% using aspirin and of 69% using warfarin. These benefits are seen in patients over the age of 60 and reach significance in the over 65s. However, there is some disagreement about the exact benefits of warfarin over aspirin. The large Second Stroke Prevention in Atrial Fibrillation (SPAF-2) showed low rates of primary thromboembolic disease in patients under 75 years of age treated with aspirin who had no other risk factors, and suggested that warfarin would not confer sufficient additional risk reduction to justify its use in this group. The substantial annual risk of thromboembolism in the over 75s was reduced from 4.8% in the aspirin treated group to 3.6% in the warfarin treated group. This did not reach statistical significance. The results from this trial are at odds with the main body of evidence which advocates the use of warfarin over aspirin in patients with AF over 65 years of age. Generally it is recommended that older patients with AF should receive warfarin if there are no contraindications.

References

Boston area anticoagulation trial for atrial fibrillation investigators 1990 The effect of low dose warfarin on the risk of stroke in patients with non-rheumatic atrial fibrillation. New England Journal of Medicine 323: 1505-1511

European Atrial Fibrillation Trial Study Group 1993 Secondary prevention in non-rheumatic atrial fibrillation after transient ischaemic attack or minor stroke. Lancet 342: 1255-1262

Ezekowitz M D, Bridgers S L, James K E et al 1992 Warfarin in the prevention of stroke associated with non-rheumatic atrial fibrillation. New England Journal of Medicine 327: 1406-1412

Petersen P, Boysen G, Godtfredsen J et al 1989 Placebo controlled, randomized trial of warfarin and aspirin for prevention of thromboembolic complications in chronic atrial fibrillation. (AFASAK). Lancet i: 175-179

Stroke Prevention in Atrial Fibrillation (SPAF) Investigators 1991 Stroke prevention in atrial fibrillation study: final results. Circulation 84: 527-539

SPAF Investigators 1994 Warfarin versus aspirin for prevention of thromboembolism in atrial fibrillation: SPAF II study. Lancet 343: 687-691

120. Acute stroke

A. T   B. T   C. F   D. F   E. F

121. The treatment of acute stroke

A. T   B. T   C. T   D. T   E. F

In recent years the treatment of acute stroke with antiplatelet drugs and thrombolysis has been evaluated in a number of large prospective studies including the Multicentre Acute Stroke Trial (MAST), the International Stroke Trial (IST) and the Chinese Acute Stroke Trial.

In acute stroke as in myocardial infarction, thrombolytic drugs have been shown to result in early recanalization of arteries. In acute myocardial infarction, thrombolysis given within 6 hours reduces mortality by 30 in 1000 patients treated, and aspirin alone reduces mortality rates from 13 to 10%. So far the results from the large muliticentre stroke trials are less encouraging.

MAST-I, a two-by-two study comparing aspirin, streptokinase, both aspirin and streptokinase, or neither drug, in the treatment of acute stroke, showed an excess in 10-day mortality in patients treated with thrombolysis, with an insignificant reduction in disability at 6 months. The trial was stopped and analysed early in the Italian study because of concern that there might be excess mortality in the thrombolysis group. The risk of haemorrhagic transformation increased with the length of time between symptom onset and administration of streptokinase.

A systematic review of eight completed trials of thrombolysis in stroke was published in the Cochrane Database of Systematic Reviews showing a significant excess of deaths from all causes in the patients treated with thrombolysis.

The possible benefits of heparin are being assessed in IST, a study of 20 000 patients treated with aspirin, heparin, both drugs or neither within 48 hours of the onset of symptoms of stroke.

In recent years there has been much debate over the value of acute stroke units. A recent overview of all the trials has shown that patients treated in stroke units do better than those treated on the general wards but the reason for this was not clear. One year after a stroke 33% of patients will have died, 22% will be dependent, and 45% independent. Most recovery takes place in the first few weeks but still useful recovery can occur at 6–12 months. The risk of having a second stroke within 5 years is 30%.

The lateral medullary syndrome is caused by posterior inferior cerebellar artery (PICA) or vertebral artery thromboembolism. It presents with sudden vertigo, vomiting, ipsilateral ataxia and contralateral loss of pain and temperature sensation.

Weber's syndrome is a second distinct set of brain stem symptoms and signs, consisting of a third nerve palsy with contralateral hemiplegia. Paralysis of upward gaze may also be present.

Loss of consciousness is not a feature of a simple anterior circulation stroke, but may occur with a posterior circulation stroke or transient ischaemic attack (TIA). Amaurosis fugax and aphasia are both features of anterior circulation disease.

References

Humphrey P R D 1995 Management of transient ischaemic attacks and stroke. Postgraduate Medical Journal 71: 577-584

Multicentre Acute Stroke Trial–Italy Group 1995 Randomized controlled trial of streptokinase, aspirin, and combination of both in treatment of acute ischaemic stroke. Lancet 346: 1509-1514

Oxfordshire Community Stroke Project 1983 Incidence of stroke in Oxfordshire: first year's experience of a community stroke project. British Medical Journal 287: 713-716

122. Carotid endarterectomy

A. T   B. F   C. F   D. T   E. F

500 000 new strokes occur each year in the USA. Of these 20–30% are due to carotid artery disease. The role of carotid endarterectomy in symptomatic patients with a severe (greater than 70%) stenosis has now been established. The Medical Research Council European Carotid Surgery Trial recruited 2518 patients who had had a non-disabling stroke, a transient ischaemic attack (TIA) or a retinal infarct, and had stenosis of the appropriate carotid artery. They were randomized to surgery plus best medical management or best medical management alone. The results from the moderate stenosis (30–68%) group have yet to be published. In the severe stenosis group, surgery in addition to best medical management reduced the risk of ipsilateral stroke from 16.8 to 2.8% and reduced the risk of disabling stroke, stroke death or surgical death from 11 to 6%. These findings have been supported by the results of the North American Symptomatic Endarterectomy Trial.

In the general population 0.5% of 50–60-year-olds have carotid artery stenosis and this rises to 10% of the over 80-year-olds. Prospective epidemiological studies of these populations have found that of those with severe stenosis, 2% per year will have an ipsilateral stroke. The Asymptomatic Carotid Artery Stenosis (ACAS) study followed 1659 patients with no previous symptoms of cerebrovascular disease for a mean of 2.7 years. Patients with a greater than 60% stenosis were randomized to receive best medical care with or without carotid endarterectomy. The aggregate risk over 5 years of ipsilateral stroke or any perioperative stroke or death was 5.9% in the surgical group, and 11% in the medical group.

Although there is now general agreement about the benefits of carotid artery surgery for symptomatic patients with severe stenosis, the benefits of surgery in asymptomatic patients are less clear cut. It may be that asymptomatic patients at highest risk can be identified and targeted for surgical intervention.

A recent Italian study has looked at both the prevalence and the natural history of carotid lesions in young patients (15–44 years) with a history of TIA or stroke. Of the 240 patients studied there was a low prevalence of high grade symptomatic carotid artery stenosis and occlusion. The 5-year prognosis was benign in patients with internal carotid artery occlusion but poor in patients with high grade carotid stenosis.

References

Carolei A, Marini C, Nencini P et al 1995 Prevalence and outcome of symptomatic carotid lesions in young adults. British Medical Journal 310: 1363-1366

European Carotid Surgery Trialists Collaborative Group 1991 MRC European carotid surgery trial. Lancet 337: 1235-1243

Executive Committee for the Asymptomatic Carotid Atherosclerosis Study 1995 Endarterectomy for asymptomatic carotid artery stenosis. Journal of the American Medical Association 273: 1421-1428

Humphrey P R D 1995 Management of transient ischaemic attacks and stroke. Postgraduate Medical Journal 71: 577-584

North American Symptomatic Endarterectomy Trial Collaborators 1991 Beneficial effect of carotid endarterectomy in symptomatic patients with high-grade carotid stenosis. New England Journal of Medicine 325: 445-453

123. Vascular dementia

A. F   B. T   C. F   D. F   E. T

Vascular dementia is one of the three most common causes of dementia and may be the commonest in the over 85-year-olds. Symptomatic stroke increases the risk of developing dementia nine fold. Vascular dementia and multi-infarct dementia are not synonymous. Although multiple cerebral infarcts can cause dementia, white matter ischaemia from other vascular events and a single strategically placed infarct can also result in dementia. In multi-infarct disease the site of the lesions has been shown to be more important than their size in the development of dementia. The dementia which results from multiple cortical infarcts usually has features of cortical dysfunction such as amnesia, aphasia, apraxia and agnosia. In contrast patients with evidence of lacunar infarct dementia may exhibit the classical signs of hemiparesis, small stepping gait, dysarthria, dysphagia, with cognitive impairment of a subcortical nature, typically psychomotor slowing, poor concentration, indecision, and mental apathy. Lacunar infarcts are often associated with white matter disease and both conditions are commonly associated with hypertension. Dementia resulting from a single infarct is recognized to occur in patients with the angular gyrus syndrome. This presents with fluent dysphasia, visuospatial disorientation, agraphia and memory loss. Single infarcts in the thalamus, caudate and globus pallidus, and hippocampus are also recognized as causes of dementia.

White matter is particularly vulnerable to ischaemia because its blood supply consists of long penetrating end arterioles. Pathologically low attenuation of the white matter represents demyelination, reactive gliosis and arteriosclerotic changes in the blood vessels. White matter lesions are associated with hypertension, heart disease and diabetes, and they are thought to result in dementia by disrupting the connections between cortical and subcortical areas. White matter lesions are found in 70–90% of patients with vascular dementia, and between 10 and 20%; and 70 and 80% of patients with Alzheimer's disease, depending on the age group. Magnetic resonance imaging shows that 100% of normal adults over the age of 85 have white matter disease; new evidence shows that these subjects may have subtle changes in cognitive function on neuropsychological testing. The role of white matter disease in vascular dementia is still unclear.

Vascular dementia typically presents with a sudden onset and subsequent stepwise decline in cognitive function, and with a history of stroke and transient ischaemic attacks. Evidence of focal neurological deficit supports the diagnosis as does the presence of a source of thromboembolism such as atrial fibrillation, valvular heart disease or carotid artery disease. Computerized tomography usually shows evidence of cerebrovascular disease. It is important to address vascular risk factors as the disease is preventable, and there is evidence that controlling blood pressure and diabetes and prescribing aspirin can improve cognitive function. Investigations should include a search for other treatable causes of dementia, such as hypothyroidism, neurosyphilis, vitamin B12 deficiency, cerebral vasculitis, normal pressure hydrocephalus and frontal lobe tumours, and a search for any risk factors for thromboembolic disease.

Reference

Amar K, Wilcock G 1996 Vascular dementia. British Medical Journal 312: 227-231

124. Dementia

A. F   B. F   C. T   D. T   E. T

600 000 people in England and Wales suffer from dementia. Dementia is defined as an acquired global impairment of intellect, memory and personality without impairment of consciousness. In the early stages there is usually loss of short-term memory with relative preservation of long-term memory. Depression, anxiety and irritability commonly accompany the intellectual deterioration and in the latter stages paranoid delusions and even auditory and visual hallucinations may occur.

Pseudodementia is a term used to describe a patient who appears withdrawn and apathetic as a result of depression and it is especially important to think of this diagnosis in elderly patients. About 25% of the elderly suffer from a psychiatric disability, mainly anxiety and depression. 10% of people over 65 years of age and 20% of those who are over 80 have dementia. The three most common causes of dementia are Alzheimer's disease, vascular dementia and Lewy body type dementia; the first two are reviewed elsewhere in this book.

Parkinson's disease is complicated by dementia in 10–20% of cases. The dementia is typically subcortical presenting with apathy and poor concentration. The parkinsonian features usually respond to dopaminergic drugs which can be helpful if there is doubt about the diagnosis.

A number of other neurodegenerative disorders have prominent extrapyramidal signs and differentiating them from Parkinson's disease can be difficult. Lewy body type dementia is characterized by marked fluctuations in symptoms, prominent extrapyramidal signs, florid early visual hallucinations and delusions, and poor tolerance to neuroleptics. Progressive supranuclear palsy has similar features to Parkinson's disease but the rigidity and bradykinesia are not improved by dopaminergic drugs. Additional characteristic features are truncal ataxia and vertical gaze palsy. Multisystem atrophy presents with a slowly progressive dementia with any combination of pyramidal tract signs, extrapyramidal features, autonomic dysfunction and cerebellar ataxia. The accurate diagnosis of these conditions often relies on post-mortem examination.

Potentially reversible causes of dementia should be excluded with blood tests and a CT scan. Patients with frontal lobe tumours may present with disinhibition and mental apathy. Other intracranial mass lesions including subdural haematomas and hydrocephalus can also be diagnosed by a CT scan and blood tests for hypothyroidism, B12 deficiency, pellagra, hypoparathyroidism, and neurosyphilis should be taken. Other causes of dementia include Wernicke-Korsakoff syndrome, Huntington's disease, multiple sclerosis, spongiform encephalopathy, heavy metal poisoning, chronic hepatic and AIDS encephalopathies, chronic hypoxia or hypoglycaemia, uraemia, dialysis and rare metabolic disorders such as Wilson's disease.

Reference

Amar K, Wilcock G 1996 Vascular dementia. British Medical Journal 312: 227-231

---

125. Prion diseases

A. **T**   B. **T**   C. **F**   D. **T**   E. **F**

Prion diseases (transmissible spongiform encephalopathies) are rare, but recent media attention about the possible transmission of 'mad cow disease' (bovine spongiform encephalopathy) to humans has focused scientific attention on these unusual diseases. They classically present with rapidly progressive neuro-degeneration with cognitive impairment, ataxia, myoclonus and motor dysfunction.

The prion diseases may be genetic, sporadic or infectious. The pathogenic prion related protein PrP is encoded by the PRNP gene on chromosome 20. This protein which is protease-resistant and insoluble accumulates in the brain. In the familial diseases, mutations of the PRNP gene are found. In the infectious forms polymorphism at codon 129 of this gene has been shown to alter susceptibility to infection. Gerstmann-Sträussler-Scheinker disease and fatal familial insomnia are examples of rare familial prion disorders.

The transmissible spongiform encephalopathies are amyloidoses in which the host-encoded protein acquires a beta-sheet conformation producing amyloid which accumulates and causes vacuolar degeneration of neurones and thus the histological features of the diseases. Renal amyloid does not occur.

Kuru, the first of the prion diseases to be identified, affected the peoples of the highlands of New Guinea. It was found to be transmitted by eating human brains as part of the local custom of cannibalism. Education about the health risks from cannibalism has resulted in the virtual eradication of the disease.

Creutzfeldt-Jakob disease (CJD) may take an infectious, genetic or sporadic form. Iatrogenic transmission has been well documented following human growth hormone therapy and corneal transplantion. It has also been transmitted to neurosurgeons peroperatively and to technicians removing pituitaries from cadavers for the extraction of growth hormone. Transmission has not been shown to occur following treatment with infected blood products.

Whether human prion disease can be transmitted from animals (i.e. cattle with bovine spongiform encephalopathy and sheep with scrapie) to humans remains controversial. The occurrence of 10 cases in young people in the UK in 1994 and 1995 has led to grave concerns that consumption of infected beef products before the introduction of tighter meat-handling regulations in 1989 may lead to an epidemic of CJD.

Reference

Almond J W, Brown P, Gore S M 1995 Creutzfeldt-Jakob disease and bovine spongiform encephalopathy: any connection? British Medical Journal 311: 1415-1421

Goldfarb L G, Brown P 1995 The transmissible spongiform encephalopathies. Annual Review of Medicine 46: 57-65

Gore S M 1996 Bovine Creutzfeldt-Jakob disease? British Medical Journal 312: 791-793

---

126. Huntington's disease
A. F   B. T   C. F   D. T   E. F

127. Trinucleotide repeats
A. T   B. F   C. T   D. F   E. T

Huntington's disease is an inherited degenerative disorder characterized by the development of progressive chorea, bradykinesia, rigidity and cognitive impairment. There is selective neuronal loss from the caudate and putamen, and neurochemical studies have shown loss of gamma-aminobutyric acid (GABA) and its synthesizing enzyme glutamic acid decarboxylase.

Chromosome 4 was identified in 1983 as the site of the defective gene. Ten years later a stretch of expanded DNA of repeating CAG trinucleotides was identified.

The Huntington's disease gene is expressed in neurones, glia and non-nervous tissues and is believed to code for a protein, Huntington, whose function remains unclear. The presence of the excess number of CAG repeats does not seem to alter the production of mRNA or the translocation into normal amounts of the protein. Deletion of the short arm of chromosome 4 is not associated with the development of Huntington's disease. The pathogenesis of Huntington's disease thus remains elusive. A number of other neurodegenerative disorders have been associated with an expanded length of trinucleotide repeats including myotonic dystrophy, spinocerebellar ataxia, spinomuscular atrophy and the fragile X syndrome.

In Huntington's disease the expanded stretch of DNA is found to be unstable when transmitted to the next generation. This explains how sporadic cases may come about and how the disease tends to present earlier and be more severe in the next generation, a feature described as anticipation.

Measurements of the length of CAG repeats have now replaced the cumbersome genetic-linkage tests to confirm the clinical diagnosis and provide an assessment of risk for relatives. Pre-test counselling is important because of the consequences of a positive diagnosis of this untreatable progressive disease for the patient and for his or her offspring, who will have a 50% chance of having the abnormal gene.

References

Gusella J F, Wexler N S, Coneally P M et al 1983 A polymorphic DNA marker genetically linked to Huntington's disease. Nature 306: 234-238

Gusella J F, MacDonald M E 1994 Huntington's disease and repeating trinucleotides. New England Journal of Medicine 330: 1450-1451

The Huntington's Disease Collaborative Research Group 1993 A novel gene containing a trinucleotide repeat that is expanded and unstable on Huntington's disease chromosomes. Cell 72: 971-983

Kremer B, Goldberg P, Andrew S E et al 1994 A world-wide study of Huntington's disease mutation: the sensitivity and specificity of measuring CAG repeats. New England Journal of Medicine 330: 1401-1406

128. Motor neurone disease

A. **T**   B. **F**   C. **T**   D. **T**   E. **T**

Motor neurone disease (MND) is a progressive neurodegenerative disorder of upper and lower motor neurones, resulting in weakness of bulbar and skeletal muscles with relative sparing of the extraocular muscles and of sphincter function. Orthopnoea is a common and early feature of the disease. Emotional lability may complicate upper motor neurone, but not lower motor neurone bulbar disease. Death results from respiratory failure about 5 years after the onset of symptoms. 5–10% of cases are familial, mostly autosomal dominant, the rest are sporadic. The term motor neurone disease covers a spectrum of conditions including amyotrophic lateral sclerosis, progressive muscular atrophy with only lower motor neurone involvement and progressive bulbar palsy. Classically there are mixed upper and lower motor neurone signs with spasticity, hyperreflexia, wasting and fasciculation. Fasciculations are the visible resting contractions of abnormally large motor units. Extensor plantars are present in up to 50% of patients and there should be no objective sensory signs. Electromyography shows a reduction in the number, but an increase in the amplitude and duration of the motor action potential.

The cause or causes of sporadic motor neurone disease remain elusive. It has an incidence of 1–2 per 100 000 population. It affects men 1.5 times more commonly than women, and trauma, heavy manual labour and exposure to a variety of toxins have been implicated in its aetiology. Bulbar onset, female sex and older age are poor prognostic features. 10–15% of kindreds with the inherited form of the disease have been found to have mutations in the Cu/Zn superoxide dismutase (SOD 1) gene on the long arm of chromosome 21.

Attempts to treat MND as an autoimmune disorder, possibly caused by antibodies to the calcium channel, with aggressive immunomodulation have been unsuccessful. The three most promising treatment strategies currently under investigation are glutamate antagonists, agents which combat free-radical damage such as N-acetylcysteine, and neurotrophic factors. Riluzole modulates glutaminergic transmission and may block voltage-dependent sodium channels and the guanylate cyclase linked second messenger. In initial studies riluzole has been shown to prolong survival and delay deterioration in muscle strength. A large multi-centre trial is now under way. Ciliary neurotrophic factor is produced by Schwann cells of peripheral nerves and has been shown to promote survival of rat and human motor neurones in culture, and slow progression of MND in murine models. Recombinant human ciliary neurotrophic factor is now being tested in patients with motor neurone disease. Insulin-like growth factor which causes motor neurone sprouting in vivo and increases the size of rat motor-end-plates and brain derived neurotrophic factor which can increase survival of motor neurones after axotomy and during development are also being investigated in clinical trials.

References

Leigh P N, Ray-Chaudhuri K 1994 Motor neurone disease. Journal of Neurology, Neurosurgery, and Psychiatry 57: 886-896

Smith R G, Appel S H 1995 Molecular approaches to amyotrophic lateral sclerosis. Annual Review of Medicine 46: 133-145

129. Muscular dystrophies

A. F   B. T   C. T   D. F   E. T

Duchenne muscular dystrophy occurs in 1 in 3000 male infants. Gower's sign describes the characteristic way patients get up by climbing up their legs with their hands. There is initially a proximal limb weakness with pseudohypertrophy of the calves. The myocardium is also affected. Creatinine phosphokinase is grossly elevated and there are characteristic changes on muscle biopsy and EMG. Carrier females also have these changes, but accurate carrier status and prenatal diagnosis can now be determined using DNA probes.

The gene defect responsible for the severe X-linked Duchenne muscular dystrophy was identified in 1986. The normal gene produces a protein dystrophin which is a large rod shaped cytoskeletal protein found at the inner surface of muscle fibres. It is completely absent in Duchenne muscular dystrophy but present in reduced amounts in the milder Becker form. The dystrophin gene is located at Xp21. One third of cases of Duchenne muscular dystrophy are due to spontaneous mutations. Other types of muscular dystrophy are autosomally inherited and do not have the defective dystrophin gene. They vary phenotypically from a Duchenne-like picture to later onset limb-girdle disease.

It is now thought that dystrophin forms part of a more complex molecule, the dystrophin-glycoprotein complex, which bridges the inner cytoskeleton and the extracellular matrix. It is defects in the other proteins in this molecule which cause the autosomal recessive disorders. Dystroglycan has an extracellular subunit which binds to merosin in the basement membrane, and a transmembrane portion which binds to dystrophin within the cell. Sarcoglycan has three subunits all of which are transmembrane glycoproteins. Defects in these three subunits have been linked with different autosomal recessive muscular dystrophies and their genes have been located. It seems that loss of function deletion mutations of these genes results in severe forms of the disease, while partial loss of function causes the milder limb girdle dystrophy. Proteins of both the dystrogycan and sarcoglycan complex are deficient in Duchenne muscular dystrophy even though the only genetic abnormality is in the dystrophin gene. This suggests that dystrophin is necessary for the correct formation of the complex. Whether the function of this complex protein is solely structural is still unknown.

Reference

Worton R 1995 Muscular dystrophies: diseases of the dystrophin-glycoprotein complex. Science 270: 755-756

130. Clinical features of multiple sclerosis

A. T   B. T   C. T   D. F   E. T

131. Interferon beta-1B as treatment for multiple sclerosis

A. T   B. F   C. F   D. F   E. T

Multiple sclerosis (MS) affects about 80 000 people in the UK. The clinical signs and symptoms are thought to be due to acute episodes of demyelination of white matter in the central nervous system. Median nerve palsy is a lower motor neurone lesion and is not caused by MS. Internuclear opthalmoplegia and vertigo may both complicate brain stem demyelination. Myokymia is a rare, continuous movement of the lower face that is seen in association with brain stem lesions. Patients often say that their symptoms are worse in hot weather.

The clinical picture is variable. 80% of patients present with relapsing/remitting disease, characterized by recurrent acute attacks followed by a partial or complete recovery from disability and a period of quiescence. Over many years this may lead into a progressive phase with increasing disability. 5% of patients have primary progressive disease, and the rest have a benign form. It is thought that the disease has polygenic inheritance but the relatively low concordance rates from twin studies show that environmental triggers also play a role in its pathoaetiology. The diagnosis requires evidence of episodes of central nervous system demyelination separated in time and place. Magnetic resonance imaging (MRI) demonstrates plaques in the white matter of the brain and spinal cord. Clinically evident neurological deficits usually correlate well with the site of lesions on MRI, but many of the lesions seen are asymptomatic.

Cerebrospinal fluid analysis usually reveals oligoclonal bands which are absent from the serum. Evidence of delayed visual evoked or somatosensory evoked potentials also support the diagnosis.

Interferons are a group of naturally occurring proteins that modify immune processes. Interferon gamma stimulates immune responses and in early trials appeared to increase the relapse rate in patients with MS. Interferons alpha and beta suppress the immune response and both have been reported to be beneficial in trials using recombinant interferon to treat MS. Interferon beta-1B is produced by a strain of *Escherichia coli*, it contains 165 amino-acids and differs from human interferon beta by having serine in place of cysteine in position 17 and no methionine at position 1.

One randomized controlled trial of interferon beta-1B has been reported. It enrolled 372 patients with relapsing/remitting MS and randomized them to placebo or interferon at low (1.6MIU) or high dose (8MIU). Patients had to have some clinical signs but be able to walk 100 m without assistance, and had to have had two relapses in the preceding 2 years. 164 patients remained in the trial at the time of the 5-year report. The trial was not analyzed on an intention to treat basis, and was probably not truly double blind as the side-effects of interferon were prominent, and up to 20% of the episodes of relapse recorded relied on self-reporting, without examination by a physician.

The higher dose was reported to reduce the frequency (the primary end point) and severity of relapses by a third, at the lower dose there was no significant difference from placebo. A secondary outcome was a reduction in the number of lesions seen on MRI in the group on high dose treatment and fewer new lesions seen in the low dose group as compared to those taking placebo. Despite this there was no evidence of any effect on disability rating as measured by the Kurtzke expanded disability status scale. This may be explained by the relapsing and remitting nature of the disease and brevity of the study, or perhaps because the processes that result in disability are not being altered by the drug. Neutralizing antibodies to interferon were detected in over 40% of the treated patients and only 11% of the placebo group. Their occurrence was related to an increase in relapse rate.

Over half the patients in the high dose group developed side-effects of flu-like symptoms compared to 18% and 19% in the other two groups. These symptoms were improved by taking NSAIDs and taking the drug at night. Other side-effects included anxiety, confusion and depression which was twice as common in the treatment group, with one suicide and four attempted suicides, compared to none in the placebo arm. A skin reaction at the site of the injection occurred in up to 80% of the high dose group. Mild lymphopenia, neutropenia and mild to moderate derangement of liver function tests were also noted.

The drug has been given marketing authorization subject to annual review in Europe, because it was felt that comprehensive information on quality, safety and efficacy had not been provided.

References

Interferon beta-1B – hope or hype? 1996 Drug and Therapeutics Bulletin 34: 9-11

The IFNB Multiple Sclerosis Study Group, the University of British Columbia MS/MRI Analysis Group 1995 Interferon beta-1b in the treatment of multiple sclerosis: final outcome of the randomized controlled trial. Neurology 45: 1277-1285

132. Guillain-Barré syndrome

A. F   B. T   C. F   D. F   E. F

Guillain-Barré syndrome (GBS) is now the commonest cause of acute areflexic paraparesis. It has an incidence mortality of 5%, and 10% of patients are left with severe disability. GBS is a syndrome characterized by acute weakness, with reduced or absent tendon reflexes, with or without sensory signs. The commonest type is an acute demyelinating polyradiculopathy with mostly motor sequelae and a good prognosis. More rarely patients have an acute purely motor axonal neuropathy (AMAN), which presents with severe weakness and has a poor prognosis. Axonal degeneration without primary inflammation is distinguished from demyelination by biopsy and EMG findings. Other forms consist of a mixed motor and sensory axonal neuropathy, and subacute and chronic inflammatory demyelinating polyradiculopathies. The Miller Fisher syndrome of ophthalmoplegia, loss of tendon reflexes, and ataxia is an axonopathy with characteristic anti-ganglioside GQ1b antibodies.

The differential diagnosis is from acute muscle disease, myasthenia and from metabolic disturbances such as hypokalaemia. It has been mistaken for hysteria and brain stem strokes. Other causes of acute motor neuropathies include toxins, vasculitis, porphyria, lymphoma and leukaemia.

GBS is a post infectious immune-mediated disease. Diseases as diverse as dengue fever, hepatitis C, and measles have been implicated in its aetiology and there have been reports of GBS following jellyfish stings and immunization with the MMR (measles/ mumps/rubella) vaccine. Great interest has recently focused on the association between *Campylobacter jejuni* infection and the AMAN-type disease. In certain parts of China there are seasonal childhood epidemics of AMAN. Serological evidence shows that 90% of these children have had recent *C. jejuni* infection. In contrast to most AMAN-type disease these children tend to make a good recovery. Sequence homology between part of a lipopolysaccharide moiety on certain forms of *C. jejuni* and the terminal carbohydrate residue of ganglioside GM1 has supported the hypothesis of cross reactivity of autoantibodies whose production is triggered by foreign antigen.

In all the forms of GBS the mainstay of treatment is supportive management of the life-threatening complications of respiratory failure, autonomic disturbance, and venous thromboembolism. Plasma exchange is widely used in an attempt to treat the underlying disease process. Other attempts at immune modulation have had mixed results. A large trial using high dose methylprednisolone failed to show any beneficial effect, but reports of a prompt sustained improvement in patients treated with intravenous immunoglobulin are encouraging, not least because of the technical difficulties, complications and limited availability of plasma exchange. The provision of good rehabilitation is vital.

Reference

Hughes R A C, Rees J H 1994 Guillain-Barré syndrome. Current opinion in neurology 7: 386-392

133. Myasthenia gravis

A. **F**   B. **F**   C. **F**   D. **T**   E. **T**

Myasthenia gravis has a prevalence of 50–125 cases per million population, with peaks in incidence in the second and third decade affecting mostly women, and a second peak in the sixth and seventh decades affecting mostly men. The cardinal symptom is fatiguable weakness of skeletal muscles. Classically the extrao- cular muscles are affected early in the disease and in 15% of patients the weakness is confined to this muscle group. In a percentage of patients the generalized weakness becomes so severe that the patient is at risk of respiratory failure. Respiratory function should be monitored with regular measurement of the patient's vital capacity.

Pathologically there is a reduction in the number of acetylcholine receptors and loss of the normal folding pattern at the post-synaptic junctions of extremity skeletal muscle. These changes are also seen in the extremity muscles when only extra-ocular symptoms are present. At myasthenic junctions the decreased number of acetylcholine receptors results in end plate potentials of diminished amplitude, which fall below the safety threshold and fail to trigger action potentials in some of the muscle fibres. In normal muscle the amount of acetylcholine released with repetitive firing declines as the nerve terminal is not able to sustain its initial rate of release. At the myasthenic junction this normal rundown results in progressively weaker muscle power as more and more fibres fail to reach threshold potential. This is illustrated by the electromyogram which shows a decremental response in the amplitude of the evoked motor action potential with repetitive stimulation. The neuromuscular abnormalities in myasthenia gravis are caused by the presence of acetylcholine receptor antibodies. These are found to be present in 80–90% of patients and are specific to the condition. Patients who are 'antibody negative' are shown by passive transfer to have antibodies present in their serum, but these are not detected by the assay. Either the antibodies are directed at epitopes not present in the soluble receptor extract, or they have too low an affinity for detection.

There is enormous heterogenicity in the antibodies which cause the disease and in the B cells which produce them. Although the production of acetylcholine-receptor antibodies is directly attributable to B cells, there is extensive evidence that T cells play a key role. One of the unsolved questions is the origin of the autoimmune response. The thymus has long been implicated. Abnormalities of thymic histology are present in 75% of patients, of these 85% have thymic hyperplasia and 15% have thymomas (associated with the presence of anti-striated muscle antibodies). A role for the thymus is also supported by the fact that thymectomy results in clinical improvement in most patients. A wide variety of other autoimmune diseases have been reported in patients with myasthenia gravis and their relatives, supporting a possible inheritable defect in immune regulation.

The mainstays of treatment have been: anti-cholinesterase drugs which form part of the diagnosis of the disease and improve symptoms; immunosuppressive treatment with corticosteroids and azathioprine which alter the underlying disease process, and plasma exchange which can provide a window of clinical improvement in which the patient may undergo thymectomy. Thymectomy offers long-term benefit with 60% of non-thymoma cases showing improvement. Paradoxically, if a thymoma is present, surgery, although necessary to remove a potentially malignant tumour, seldom results in improvement of symptoms. Intravenous immunoglobulin treatment has also been shown to produce a rapid improvement in the condition of some patients.

The cellular immunology of the disease is now the subject of intensive study, to determine precisely how T cells and B cells specific for acetylcholine receptors interact to produce pathogenic immunity. With this knowledge it should be possible to devise more specific methods of immunotherapy.

References

Drachman D B 1994 Myasthenia gravis. New England Journal of Medicine 330: 1797-1807

Havard C W H, Fonseca V 1990 New treatment approaches to myasthenia gravis. Drugs 39(1): 66-73

Kaminski H J, Mass E, Spiegel P et al 1990 Why are eye muscles frequently involved in myasthenia gravis? Neurology 40: 1663-1669

134. Functional neuroimaging

A. **T**   B. **T**   C. **T**   D. **F**   E. **F**

Traditionally, neuroimaging has been involved with determining brain structure, but in recent years techniques designed to derive information about brain function have been developed. Whilst in the main these have found application as research tools, they are also of potential clinical use in the diagnosing and monitoring of certain conditions.

Positron emission tomography (PET) uses short lived isotopes to label molecules of biological interest, which are inhaled or injected and then decay by positron emission. Each positron is annihilated within 1–2 mm of its parent nucleus by collision with an electron. This generates two gamma rays or photons which are emitted at an angle of 180° to each other. These gamma rays are then simultaneously detected by the ring detector, thus allowing a spatial image of isotope density to be created. After positron emission from deep within the structure of the brain, a percentage of the emitted photons will be attenuated by the brain structure thus limiting spatial resolution. This can be corrected for using data from a second set of images taken before the isotope is given, called a transmission scan. The spatial resolution of PET is now 3–5 mm. Commonly used isotopes are oxygen-15 with its half-life of just 2 minutes, carbon-11, and fluorine-18 with its half-life of 110 minutes.

Single photon emission computed tomography (SPECT) uses isotopes such as technetium-99 or iodine-123. These have much longer half-lives than the isotopes used in PET. This means that the isotopes do not have to be produced 'on site', so reducing cost and problems with timing, but they emit only a single photon and this limits the spatial resolution.

Functional magnetic resonance imaging (fMRI) relies on the generation of images where a change in the signal over time is thought to reflect a change in neuronal function. Two of the techniques, echo-planar imaging (EPI) and fast low angle shot (FLASH) look at change in small vessel blood flow. Reported data from EPI at high field strength include images obtained over 0.1 s with a spatial resolution of 0.75 mm. A major advantage over PET and SPECT is the avoidance of exposure to ionising radiation.

There are a few specific circumstances where functional neuroimaging techniques can provide information not available from MRI or CT which alters the clinical management of the patient. In neuro-oncology PET (18F) fluorodeoxyglucose (FDG) has been used to differentiate between tumour recurrence and radiation induced focal necrosis in patients with recurrent brain lesions post radiotherapy. Tumour recurrence shows up as high FDG uptake indicating increased metabolism, in contrast to lesions due to radionecrosis which have low uptake. In patients with refractory epilepsy in whom surgical ablation of the epileptic focus is being considered, interictal and ictal functional imaging may show areas of hypo or hypermetabolism. These images are compared with the findings on structural MRI and EEG, and are used to locate the epileptic focus. Other possible current clinical uses of functional imaging are the identification of critical gyri or sulci prior to neurosurgical or neuroradiological procedures, and the neurochemical monitoring of patients undergoing neurotransplantation for Parkinson's disease. For the moment, though, functional neuroimaging's main application is as a research tool.

Reference

Sawle G V 1995 Imaging the head: functional imaging. Journal of Neurology, Neurosurgery, and Psychiatry 58: 132-144

135. Epilepsy and driving

A. T   B. T   C. F   D. F   E. T

Approximately 4.7% of men and 3.7% of women will have at least one epileptic seizure in their life-time. Recent research from the University Department of Neurological Science at Liverpool has shown that people with epilepsy who drive have the same rates of accidents as the average driver, but they have a higher rate of accidents involving injury. In 1995 the rules about epilepsy and driving were changed. People who have epilepsy must now be fit-free for just 1 year before they can drive. Seizures not associated with loss of consciousness and myoclonic jerks are regarded as epilepsy by the DVLA, and the same driving rules apply. A person who has seizures which occur only in sleep for at least 3 years may drive. The holder of a group II licence, should be seizure-free and off medication for 10 years. Many conditions associated with brain damage have an increased risk of epilepsy. Even if no seizure has occurred, these conditions must be notified by the licence holder to the DVLA. It is the doctor's responsibility to tell the patient of their duty to inform the DVLA of his or her condition.

Reference

Chief Medical Officer's Update 5 March 1995

---

136. The persistent vegetative state

A. F   B. F   C. F   D. T   E. F

The vegetative state is defined as a clinical condition of unawareness of self and environment in which the patient breathes spontaneously, has a stable cardiovascular system, and has cycles of eye opening which may simulate sleep and waking. This can occur as part of the recovery stage from coma and only becomes 'persistent' when the diagnosis of irreversibility can be established with a high degree of clinical certainty.

Three preconditions are cited. Firstly, that there should be an established cause for the condition, such as acute cerebral injury, degenerative conditions, metabolic disorders or developmental abnormalities. Secondly, that the continued effects of sedative anaesthetic or neuromuscular blocking drugs should be excluded and thirdly, that reversible metabolic causes should be corrected or excluded. The clinical criteria state that there should be no evidence of awareness of self or environment at any time, no evidence of language comprehension, and no volitional response to external stimuli. There should be evidence of cycles of eye opening and closing, and adequate brain stem and hypothalamic function to maintain respiration and circulation. In addition there may be spontaneous blinking with retained pupillary responses. In response to ice water caloric testing, the patient will exhibit a tonic eye movement which can be conjugate or dysconjugate. The patient should not have visual fixation but there may be roving eye movements. There may be occasional movements of the head to a peripheral sound or movement, and movement of the body but in a purposeless reflex way.

The vegetative state must be distinguished from brain stem death, coma and the locked-in syndrome. This is made on clinical grounds. The diagnosis that the vegetative state is persistent cannot be made for 6 months following non-head injury brain damage or 12 months following head injury. These time intervals are based on prior experience of very late recovery from continuing (more than 4 weeks) vegetative states. The diagnosis must be made by two medical practitioners experienced in disorders of consciousness. In addition to clinical assessment they should take into account reports from carers of the reactions and responses of the patient, as these are the people who spend most time with the patient.

When the diagnosis of the persistent vegetative state has been established with identification of the cause, and a sufficient time elapsed to know that recovery will not occur, the decision to withdraw nutrition or medication resides with the medical team responsible for the patient's care. At present the courts require that this decision is referred to them before any action is taken. By contrast decisions not to intervene with new treatments do not need to be referred to the courts. This is the distinction between acts of omission and commission. The relatives should be counselled as to the decision of the medical team and their views sought but the final decision (with the court's agreement) is the doctor's responsibility.

Reference

Working Group of the Royal College of Physicians 1996 The permanent vegetative state. Journal of the Royal College of Physicians, London. 30: 119-121

---

137. Brain stem death

A. **F**   B. **T**   C. **T**   D. **F**   E. **F**

A working group of the Royal College of Physicians has updated the recommendations for the diagnosis of brain stem death. The following criteria must be fulfilled: deep coma with no respiratory effort, the absence of drug intoxication (including sedatives and neuromuscular blocking agents), the absence of hypothermia, hypoglycaemia, acidosis or electrolyte imbalance. All brain stem reflexes should be absent. The patient should have fixed pupils, absent vestibular ocular reflexes, absent corneal reflexes, no motor response in the cranial nerve distribution, no gag reflex or response to bronchial stimulation and no respiratory effort on allowing the pCO_2 to rise to 6.7 kPa. No EEG is required. Spinal reflexes are not relevant to the diagnosis and this may need to be explained to the relatives. The diagnosis must be made by a consultant or his deputy (registered for more than 5 years). The examination should be carried out on two occasions and should be confirmed by a second doctor.

The updated guidelines acknowledge that some metabolic disturbances such as hyponatraemia and diabetes insipidus are the effect rather than the cause of brain stem death, and do not preclude the diagnosis.

References

Conference of the medical royal colleges and their faculties in the United Kingdom 1979 Diagnosis of death. British Medical Journal i: 332.

Working Group of the Royal College of Physicians 1995 Criteria for the diagnosis of brain stem death. Journal of the Royal College of Physicians London 29 (5): 281-282

CARDIOLOGY

138. Hypertension in the elderly

A. T   B. F   C. F   D. T   E. T

139. Hypertension

A. F.   B. F   C. T   D. F   E. F

A progressive rise in systolic blood pressure usually accompanies ageing. It is estimated that 40% of over 65-year-olds in the USA have either borderline systolic or true hypertension. The World Health Organization defines hypertension as a blood pressure of 160/95 mmHg or greater, and in the Framingham Study a blood pressure of 140/90 mmHg was deemed borderline with 160/95 mmHg abnormal. Data from the Framingham Heart Study showed increased cardiovascular morbidity with increasing systolic blood pressure in over 65-year-olds, and elderly hypertensive patients to have double the morbidity rates of the 35–64 year olds. The complications of hypertension are due to the increased risk of developing atheroma resulting in cerebral vascular disease, coronary artery disease and peripheral vascular disease. Raised blood pressure per se results in heart failure, cerebral haemorrhage, renal disease and aortic dissection.

The rise in blood pressure with age is largely caused by loss of distensibility in the large capacitance vessels. Patients with isolated systolic hypertension have increased aortic stiffness and high peripheral vascular resistance. The arterial stiffness makes the diastolic pressures less than would be expected with the high peripheral vascular resistance. Combined systolic and diastolic hypertension is either essential hypertension of old age or secondary hypertension. If the hypertension has an abrupt onset or is accelerated, atherosclerotic renal disease should be excluded with a Mag 3 renogram after captopril or with arteriography.

The elderly have increased cardiac and vascular stiffness, reduced cardiac output and intravascular volumes, and defective cerebral autoregulation. These features typically accompany systolic hypertension. In addition the baroreflex and sympathetic nervous systems become less sensitive with age and are unable to counter the sudden fall in blood pressure which accompanies standing up and eating. Up to 20% of the elderly suffer from post prandial or postural hypotension. When assessing blood pressure in the elderly it is essential to check for postural hypotension, particularly if anti-hypertensive treatment is being considered.

Before initiating anti-hypertensive treatment other risk factors for cardiac and cerebral vascular disease should be sought and addressed, including diabetes, smoking, hyperlipidaemia and obesity. A review of the patient's lifestyle and diet is also important in order to maximize non-pharmacological blood pressure reduction. This should include weight reduction and reduced alcohol consumption where appropriate and the encouragement of gentle exercise and moderate dietary sodium restriction.

Recently published large clinical trials include the MRC Working Party 1992 report and STOP-Hypertension. These have shown that lowering elevated blood pressure in the elderly reduces the incidence of stroke and cardiovascular morbidity and mortality. The results of these trials show the major potential that blood pressure control has for reducing mortality and cardiovascular morbidity, which is the leading cause of debility in the elderly. Thiazide diuretics were the primary drug prescribed in all the recent trials, and should be first line unless there are specific contraindications or reasons for using a different class of drug. ACE inhibitors would be the drug of choice in heart failure, calcium channel blockers for sufferers of angina, and alpha-blockers for patients with prostatism. Alpha-blockers also have a beneficial effect on lipid profile and improve insulin sensitivity. Longer acting once-daily formulas may be preferred as they improve compliance, and may provide smoother blood pressure control. The initial doses should be low with gradual dose titration and blood pressure monitoring.

References

Dahlof B, Lindholm L H et al 1991 Morbidity and mortality in the Swedish trial in old patients with hypertension (STOP-Hypertension) Lancet 338: 1281-1285

Kaplan N M 1995 Hypertension in the elderly. Annual Review of Medicine 46: 27-35

MRC Working Party 1992 Medical Research Council trial of treatment of hypertension in older adults: principal results. British Medical Journal 304: 405-412

Systolic Hypertension in the Elderly Program (SHEP). Cooperative Research Group 1991 Prevention of stroke by anti-hypertensive drug treatment in older persons with isolated systolic hypertension in the elderly. Journal of the American Medical Association 265: 3255-3264

140. Hyperlipidaemia

A. **F**   B. **T**   C. **T**   D. **T**   E. **F**

Hyperlipidaemia is classified into types I to V. Type I is an excess of chylomicrons alone and is rare. Type II has two subdivisions and both are predominantly hypercholesterolaemias. Type IIa is associated with raised low density lipoproteins (LDL) and type IIb is associated with raised LDL and raised very low-density lipoproteins (VLDL). Type III has an excess of chylomicron remnants, is rare, and is associated with familial dyslipoproteinaemias. Type IV is common and consists mainly of raised triglyceride levels, while type V is uncommon and all lipid classes, including chylomicrons, are raised.

Hyperlipidaemias are therefore predominantly hypercholesterolaemias, predominantly hypertriglyceridaemias or mixed hyperlipidaemias. The disorders can be primary or secondary. Common causes of secondary hyperlipidaemia include diabetes (type II and IV), hypothyroidism (type II) and alcoholism (type IV). Mixed hyperlipidaemias are often associated with obesity and are amenable to dietary intervention. Chronic liver disease, chronic renal disease, nephrotic syndrome and oral contraceptives are also associated with mixed hyperlipidaemia or with hypercholesterolaemia. Hypertriglyceridaemia can cause acute pancreatitis.

Reference

Winder T 1994 Lipid profiles. British Journal of Hospital Medicine 51: 102-104

141. Hyperlipidaemia

A **F**   B. **F**   C. **F**   D. **F**   E. **F**

In the Scandinavian Simvastatin Survival Study, a 35% reduction in low-density lipoprotein (LDL) cholesterol resulted in a 42% reduction in mortality from coronary heart disease and a 32% reduction in coronary events, supporting the theory that lowering cholesterol in patients with coronary heart disease reduces mortality. Evidence from the West of Scotland Coronary Prevention Study has now shown that the treatment of moderate hypercholesterolaemia in people who do not have a history of heart disease can be as beneficial as the treatment of mild to moderate hypertension in reducing coronary events. Earlier trials of lipid lowering drugs in the primary prevention of coronary heart disease in men with hypercholesterolaemia had shown a reduction in the incidence of myocardial infarction, but were unable to show a survival benefit. Previous reports that deaths from non-cardiac events and particularly violent deaths and suicides, were increased in patients on lipid lowering agents, further questioned whether lipid lowering drugs reduced all cause mortality when used as primary prevention for coronary heart disease.

Pravastatin is a 3-hydroxy-3-methylglutaryl coenzyme A (HMG-CoA) reductase inhibitor which blocks endogenous synthesis of cholesterol and reduces the levels of LDL cholesterol. This class of drug has been shown to be effective in the secondary prevention of coronary heart disease. In the West of Scotland Coronary Prevention Study 6595 middle-aged men with LDL cholesterol levels in the range 4.0–6.0 mmol/l were assigned in a double-blind randomly controlled trial to 40 mg of pravastatin or placebo. 5% had a history of angina, 8% had ST and T changes on ECG, 1% had self-reported diabetes mellitus, 16% were known hypertensives and 44% were smokers. They were followed up over an average of 5 years, to determine whether the treatment of hypercholesterolaemia in a group with no history of myocardial infarction would reduce the incidence of non-fatal myocardial infarction and death from coronary heart disease. Pravastatin lowered LDL cholesterol levels by 26% and increased levels of high density lipoprotein (HDL) cholesterol by 5%. It reduced the risk of fatal and non-fatal coronary events by 30%. The relative reduction in risk attributable to pravastatin was not affected by age or smoking, and a significant effect was found in the sub-groups without multiple risk factors or pre-existing vascular disease. There was no increase in deaths from non-cardiac causes in the treatment group. It was estimated that if 1000 middle-aged men with hypercholesterolaemia were treated for the primary prevention of coronary heart disease with pravastatin for 5 years, there would be 14 fewer coronary angiograms, eight fewer revascularizations, 20 fewer non-fatal myocardial infarctions, seven fewer deaths from cardiovascular disease and two fewer deaths from other causes.

The benefits of reducing cholesterol levels in individuals with moderate hypercholesterolaemia are now well established, but for the effective prevention of coronary heart disease efforts must be made to reduce the content of saturated fat and cholesterol in the diet of the population as a whole.

References

Pedersen T R 1995 Lowering cholesterol with drugs and diet. New England Journal of Medicine 333: 1350-1351

Scandinavian Simvastatin Survival Study 1994 Randomized trial of cholesterol lowering in 4444 patients with coronary heart disease. Lancet 344: 1383-1389

Shepherd J, Cobbe S M, Ford I et al (for the West of Scotland Coronary Prevention Study) 1995 Prevention of coronary heart disease with pravastatin in men with hypercholesterolaemia. New England Journal of Medicine 333: 1301-1307

142. Peroxidation of low-density lipoprotein

A. T   B. T   C. T   D. T   E. T

Recent reports in the lay press have raised public awareness of the possibility that anti-oxidants may reduce the incidence of coronary heart disease. Free radicals are by-products of many oxidative reactions in the body, and there is growing evidence that these cause cellular damage, contributing to chronic diseases such as atherosclerosis. Oxidative modification of low-density lipoprotein (LDL) is a critical factor in atherogenesis; free radicals oxidize LDL making it more atherogenic. These free radicals are formed by lipooxygenases in smooth muscle, endothelial cells and macrophages. Whether anti-oxidant micronutrients (beta-carotene, retinyl stearate, alpha-tocopherol and gamma-tocopherol), can inhibit LDL oxidation and atheroma formation by neutralizing free radicals, has profound therapeutic and public health implications.

The fatty streak is the precursor for atheroma formation. It forms when arterial wall macrophages take up oxidized LDL (which cannot be recognized by the LDL receptor). This macrophage uptake can be regarded as a scavenger pathway, leading to the formation of 'foam cells'. In addition to the formation of lipid laden macrophages, oxidized LDL is chemotactic to monocytes, is cytotoxic to endothelial cells leading to platelet aggregation and is highly immunogenic, forming immune complexes in the arterial wall. In support of the involvement of lipid peroxidation in atheroma formation are the findings of lipid peroxides in atheromatous aorta, and raised circulating peroxide levels in diabetics, smokers and patients with coronary heart disease.

Of the fat soluble anti-oxidants the most active isomer of the vitamin E family is alpha-tocopherol. Beta-carotene is important as a singlet oxygen scavenger, and ascorbic acid is the first line of defence against oxygen radicals in the water soluble compartment. Theoretically anti-oxidants should prevent oxidation of LDL and reduce atheroma formation at the early fatty streak stage.

There is epidemiological evidence that dietary anti-oxidants reduce atherosclerosis. Fresh fruit and green vegetable consumption is inversely related to cerebrovascular mortality and vitamin C and E intake is inversely related to cardiovascular mortality. These epidemiological studies do not however, establish a causal link.

Case-control studies have yielded contradictory results. A Scottish study established a link between vitamin E deficiency and angina, and a Maryland study a protective effect for high serum beta-carotene against MI. However a Finnish study could reveal no association between anti-oxidant levels and coronary artery disease, and a Dutch study no link between anti-oxidants and cardiovascular mortality.

Further evidence for a protective effect of anti-oxidants comes from prospective cohort studies. One such study found significantly reduced rates of coronary heart disease amongst women taking vitamin E, and another amongst men. In both studies, reduced rates were only observed after more than 2 years' vitamin E supplementation. Weaker evidence exists for a protective effect from beta-carotene, and there is little cohort evidence for a protective effect from vitamin C ingestion. This type of study suggests a protective effect but cannot prove a causal relationship as many confounding factors exist.

The Cambridge Heart Anti-oxidant Study (CHAOS) compared vitamin E with placebo given for 500 days in a group of patients with known coronary heart disease. There was a significant reduction in the two primary end points of cardiovascular death plus non-fatal MI and non-fatal MI alone. There was, however, a non-significant increase in cardiovascular deaths alone in the vitamin E group. Few other randomized placebo controlled studies of anti-oxidants in the prevention of coronary heart disease have been completed, although a number of well designed large trials are currently under way. These should be able to establish whether or not we should be recommending anti-oxidant therapy as primary or secondary prevention against heart disease, but as yet enough trial evidence does not exist to draw firm conclusions. Clearly anti-oxidant therapy should not substitute for advice to avoid tobacco, lose weight and take regular exercise.

References

Hoffman R M, Garewal H S 1995 Anti-oxidants and the prevention of coronary heart disease. Archives of Internal Medicine 155: 241-246

Riemersma R A 1996 Coronary heart disease and vitamin E. Lancet 347: 776

Stephens N G, Parsons A, Schofield P M et al 1996 Randomized controlled trial of vitamin E in patients with coronary disease: Cambridge Heart Anti-oxidant Study (CHAOS). Lancet 347:781-786

143. Acute myocardial infarction

A. **F**   B. **F**   C. **F**   D. **F**   E. **T**

To date there have been four published ISIS (International Study of Infarct Survival) trials. This question addresses the first three and the next question deals with ISIS 2 in greater detail. They are all multi-centre, randomized prospective studies. Large numbers of patients were recruited to achieve the statistical power needed to detect small but significant benefits from trial treatments.

ISIS-1 evaluated the use of intravenous atenolol in 16 027 cases of suspected acute myocardial infarction (MI), following reports of benefit from beta-blockers in late mortality and late reinfarction. There were two trial arms: atenolol or placebo. In the treatment group 5–10 mg of atenolol was given intravenously followed by 7 days of 100 mg orally. The mean time after onset of symptoms was 5 hours. There were no restrictions placed on physician management of their patients. Conduction defects, cardiogenic shock, cardiac failure and bronchospasm were included as contraindications to beta-blockade and therefore entry into the trial. There was no significant increase in conduction defects in the atenolol treated group. Vascular mortality was significantly lower in the atenolol group (3.89%) compared to the placebo group (4.57%) in the first 7 days, a rate reduction of 15%. There was an overall increase in the use of inotropic agents in the first 24 hours in the atenolol group, but this coincided with the period of greatest benefit from atenolol. An improved survival rate after 1 year was also seen in the atenolol group. However, more of this group were discharged home on a beta-blocker and the longer term figures may have been reflecting the already recognized effects of these drugs on late mortality. 200 patients with suspected MI would have to be treated with atenolol for 7 days following presentation to prevent one death, one cardiac arrest and one reinfarction.

ISIS-2 evaluated the use of aspirin, streptokinase, both or neither, in 17 187 patients with suspected acute MI. A dose of 160mg of aspirin was used to achieve immediate antiplatelet effect by inhibition of cyclo-oxygenase dependent platelet aggregation. Smaller doses take several days to achieve this action. Hypotension and bradycardia were reported more often in the streptokinase groups (10% cf 2% placebo), usually whilst the infusion was in progress. Overall incidence of stroke was unchanged by thrombolysis although the proportion of haemorrhagic strokes was increased.

Aspirin alone reduced overall mortality at 35 days to 9.4%, streptokinase alone reduced overall mortality to 9.2% and the combination of both reduced overall mortality to 8%. Compared to the mortality of patients receiving neither active treatment which was 13.2%, the reduction in risk of death by combination treatment was 42%. ISIS-2 confirmed findings from previous large trials suggesting a role for thrombolysis in the treatment of acute MI and was the first large randomized trial to show a role for antiplatelet therapy in the active treatment of acute MI. Aspirin use had been established in the treatment of patients with a past history of MI to reduce vascular mortality and in unstable angina. The effect of aspirin and thrombolytic therapy appeared independent of anticoagulant use, confirming findings by Italian investigators in the second GISSI trial, and this was then further investigated in the ISIS-3 study. It is estimated that for every 1000 patients presenting with acute MI about 50 deaths will be prevented by treatment with streptokinase and aspirin at the time of presentation and up to 24 hours after the onset of symptoms.

ISIS-3 evaluated the use of three different thrombolytic agents, streptokinase, tissue plasminogen activator (tPA) and anistreplase, and of aspirin plus heparin versus aspirin alone in 41 299 patients with suspected acute MI. All patients received aspirin, half also received 12 500 units of heparin subcutaneously twice daily for 7 days. In addition patients were randomized to one of the three thrombolytic agents. The end point of the trial was the assessment of survival after 35 days, although follow-up continued after this.

When comparing the use of heparin post MI, ISIS-3 showed that there were fewer deaths in the 7 days of treatment confirming earlier findings in GISSI-2. However, there was no difference in survival at 35 days with the overall mortality in both groups at this time being 10%. Heparin was associated with an excess of major non-cerebral bleeds and haemorrhagic strokes but the incidence of stroke overall was unchanged due to fewer non-haemorrhagic strokes.

Of the different thrombolytic therapies, anistreplase had the highest rate of allergic reactions, and tPA the lowest. The rate of haemorrhagic stroke was higher with both these agents compared to streptokinase. tPA, but not anistreplase, also had a higher rate of non-cerebral bleeds. Reinfarction rates were significantly lower in the tPA treated group. There was no significant difference between the three groups in terms of 35-day or 6-month mortality.

It is interesting that the 3-hr tPA infusion used in ISIS-3 did not appear to be superior to streptokinase. tPA activates tissue plasminogen efficiently only when bound to fibrin, which it does with great affinity. It therefore would be expected to exert its effects locally and effectively at the site of acute thrombosis with little action elsewhere. Faster recanalization and restoration of coronary artery patency should be produced. In 1993 the GUSTO investigators published their findings from a randomized trial of 41 021 patients with acute MI comparing four different thrombolytic strategies. The four strategies were as follows: streptokinase with subcutaneous heparin, streptokinase with intravenous heparin, accelerated tPA with intravenous heparin and streptokinase with tPA and intravenous heparin. Accelerated tPA refers to the rapid intravenous administration of tPA over 1.5 hours compared to the more conventional 3 hours used in ISIS-3. Two thirds of the dose is given in the first 30 minutes. The results showed that this method of tPA administration produced a reduction in risk of mortality of 1% compared to streptokinase. The use of accelerated tPA instead of streptokinase would prevent an additional 10 deaths per 1000 patients treated. The patients likely to benefit most from this regime were shown to be patients with anterior infarcts and patients under the age of 75. Although the combined end point of death plus disabling stroke was lower in the tPA groups compared to streptokinase, there was a significant excess of haemorrhagic strokes in the tPA group.

References

Anderson H V, Willerson J 1993 Thrombolysis in acute myocardial infarction. New England Journal of Medicine 329: 703-709

GISSI-2 1990 A factorial randomized trial of alteplase vs streptokinase plus heparin vs no heparin among 12 490 patients with acute myocardial infarction. Lancet 336: 65-71

The Global Utilization of Streptokinase and Tissue Plasminogen Activator for Occluded Coronary Arteries (GUSTO) investigators 1993 An international randomized trial comparing four thrombolytic strategies for acute myocardial infarction. New England Journal of Medicine 329: 673-682

Gruppo Italiano per lo Studio della Streptochinasi nell'Infarto Miocardio (GISSI) 1986 Effectiveness of intravenous thrombolytic therapy in acute myocardial infarction. Lancet i: 397-402

Horton R 1993 Thrombolysis: tPA fast by GUSTO. Lancet 341: 1188

First International Study of Infarct Survival (ISIS-1) Collaborative Group 1986 Randomized trial of intravenous atenolol among 16 027 cases of suspected acute myocardial infarction: Lancet ii: 57-66

ISIS-2 Collaborative Group 1988 Randomized trial of intravenous streptokinase, oral aspirin, both or neither among 17 187 cases of suspected acute myocardial infarction Lancet 2: 349-360

ISIS-3 Collaborative Group 1992 Randomized comparison of streptokinase vs tPA vs anistreplase and of aspirin plus heparin vs aspirin alone among 41 299 cases of suspected acute myocardial infarction. Lancet 339: 753-770

144. ISIS-2 (MI)

A. **T**　B. **F**　C. **F**　D. **F**　E. **T**

145. Contraindications to streptokinase

A. **T**　B. **T**　C. **F**　D. **T**　E. **F**

ISIS-2 evaluated the survival impact of a thrombolytic agent (streptokinase) and aspirin in acute myocardial infarction (MI). The trial developed from several smaller studies yielding different results from the use of streptokinase and the publication of the GISSI trial showing benefit with streptokinase in acute MI. Aspirin had been shown to improve survival in patients with a past history of MI and in unstable angina, but not in acute MI. 17 187 patients were recruited to receive streptokinase, aspirin, both or neither.

Streptokinase was given as an intravenous infusion of 1.5 MU over 1 hour and aspirin was given at a dose of 160mg per day for a month, with the first dose chewed. As well as showing a relative risk reduction in mortality of 23% in the aspirin group and 25% in the streptokinase group at 35 days, this trial also showed that, compared to placebo, when the two were added the relative reduction in risk of mortality was 42%. In terms of patient numbers the appropriate use of the two agents together may prevent up to 50 deaths per 1000 patients treated.

The trial showed that the absolute mortality reductions were greatest for those at greatest risk of death, i.e. women, older patients, and those with a past history of MI, anterior MI and systolic hypotension (BP<100mmHg). The benefits were greatest in patients treated early after symptom onset (within 4 hours) but a significant advantage, although much smaller, was seen up to 24hrs.

An excess of cerebral haemorrhage leading to death or disability in the first 24hrs was seen in patients receiving streptokinase. However, the overall incidence of major stroke was unaltered at 35 days due to a reduction in cerebral infarcts. Allergic reactions were noted and their incidence was not altered in the 22% of patients receiving hydrocortisone prophylaxis.

Streptokinase given alone was associated with an excess of reinfarctions, which was completely abolished by the addition of aspirin. This may be because streptokinase increases systemic platelet activity due to its fibrinolytic effect and this is negated by the antiplatelet effect of aspirin.

Contraindications to thrombolysis are listed in the *British National Formulary* as recent or current bleeding, peptic ulceration, trauma or surgery, oesophageal varices, acute pancreatitis, cavitating lung disease, severe liver disease, severe vaginal bleeding, parturition within 10 days, pregnancy up to 18 weeks, abnormal coagulation, bleeding diatheses and stroke within the past 6 months or with any residual deficit. Diabetic retinopathy is also listed but a recent British Medical Journal editorial suggests that this should be a relative rather than absolute contraindication.

References

GISSI 1986 Effectiveness of intravenous thrombolytic treatment in acute myocardial infarction Lancet. i: 397-402

ISIS-2 1988 Randomized trial of intravenous streptokinase, oral aspirin, both or neither among 17 187 cases of suspected acute myocardial infarction Lancet. ii: 349-360

Ward H, Yudkin J 1995 Thrombolysis in patients with diabetes. British Medical Journal 310: 3-4

---

146. ISIS-4 (MI)

A. F   B. F   C. F   D. T   E. F

ISIS-4 involved 58 050 patients admitted to 1086 hospitals up to 24 hours after the onset of a suspected myocardial infarction (MI). The main contraindications were cardiogenic shock or persistent severe hypotension. The patients were randomized in a '2 x 2 x 2 factorial' study. The treatment comparisons were: 1 month of oral captopril, 50 mg bd.; 1 month of oral controlled-release mononitrate titrated to a dose of 60 mg once per day; and 24 hours of intravenous magnesium sulphate (8 mmol as a bolus followed by 72 mmol).

Captopril produced a significant reduction in 5-week mortality of 7% or about five fewer deaths per thousand patients treated for one month. In certain high risk groups the benefits were even greater, with 18 lives saved in those with a previous history of MI, and 14 lives saved in patients with associated heart failure. It produced no increase in deaths during the first 24 hours even amongst those who had low blood pressure at entry. The dose of captopril was rapidly titrated to 50mg bd with the first dose given within 2 hours of thrombolysis. The final dose was reached in under 24 hours. Much lower doses with much slower rates of increase are used at many UK centres.

The results were in accordance with the results of several other studies including GISSI-3 (Gruppo Italiano per lo Studio della Streptochinasi nell'Infarto Miocardico) and CCS-1 (Chinese Captopril Study 1). These trials suggested that the early treatment with an ACE inhibitor in acute MI prevents about five deaths per 1000 in the first month. This is probably a class effect. Some authors recommend the use of ACE inhibitors in all cases of MI, while others suggest reserving them for high risk patients such as those with a history of previous MI or those in heart failure.

Isosorbide mononitrate produced no significant reduction in 5-week mortality. It was, however, safe with somewhat fewer deaths in the first 24 hr. Its continued use for symptomatic relief for both angina and heart failure is therefore recommended, but it is not indicated in the treatment of asymptomatic individuals post myocardial infarction.

Magnesium produced a small non-significant excess of deaths. Collectively the results of eight small randomized trials in a total of over 1000 patients showed a mortality reduction of approximately one half. The second Leicester Intravenous Magnesium Intervention Trial (LIMIT-2) of over 2000 patients showed a reduction in 28-day mortality of approximately one quarter but with very wide confidence intervals. When prepublication reports of the results from ISIS-4 were first released, there was speculation that the disparities in the results were because of differences in how the magnesium was used. It was suggested that the magnesium infusion was given too long after the onset of symptoms or that the magnesium infusion was given after thrombolysis and was therefore less effective in ISIS-4. Subgroup analysis of the results from ISIS-4 failed to show any benefit in those not receiving thrombolysis, or in those given magnesium rapidly after the onset of symptoms. The results of ISIS-4 do not support the routine use of intravenous magnesium in the treatment of acute MI.

References

Chinese Cardiac Study Collaborative Group 1995 Oral captopril vs placebo among 13 642 patients with suspected acute myocardial infarction: interim report from the Chinese Cardiac Study (CCS-1) Lancet 345: 686-687

GISSI-3 1994 Effects of lisinopril and transdermal glyceryl trinitrate singly and together on 6-week mortality and ventricular function after acute myocardial infarction. Lancet 343: 1115-1122

ISIS-4 Collaborative Group 1995 Randomized factorial trial assessing early oral captopril, oral mononitrate, and intravenous magnesium sulphate in 58 050 patients with suspected acute myocardial infarction. Lancet 345: 669-686

Woods K L, Fletcher S, Roffe C et al 1992 Intravenous magnesium sulphate in suspected acute myocardial infarction: results of the second Leicester Intravenous Magnesium Intervention Trial (LIMIT-2) Lancet 339: 1553-1558

Woods K L, Fletcher S 1994 Long-term outcome after intravenous magnesium in suspected acute myocardial infarction: the second Leicester Intravenous Magnesium Intervention Trial (LIMIT-2). Lancet 343; 816-819

147. Left ventricular remodelling

A. T   B. T   C. F   D. F   E. F

Left ventricular remodelling after acute MI is the process in which architectural changes in the ventricular size, shape and wall thickness occur both regionally and globally. It is now apparent that these pathophysiological changes have important negative prognostic implications and can be therapeutically manipulated.

The sudden occlusion of a coronary vessel starts the process. If reperfusion does not occur in time necrosis of myocardial cells occurs. An inflammatory response then ensues with resorption of cellular debris and the initiation of collagen deposition and fibroblast proliferation. In this early phase the tensile strength of the region involved is significantly reduced and a process called infarct expansion occurs. The affected area is permanently lengthened by wall tension stretching the weakened segment. This process occurs most markedly with large transmural infarcts especially when they affect the ventricular apex. The apex is the most vulnerable area because of its increased curvature and reduced wall thickness.

A small increase in the length of the wall of the ventricular apex will result in a relatively larger increase in effective ventricular radius than the same increase in wall length elsewhere in the ventricle. Likewise small increases in wall length at the apex produce proportionally greater reductions in wall thickness. These changes in the radius and the wall thickness both result in increased wall stress. Data from human studies using echocardiography confirm that the complication rate and mortality rate are higher with increasing degrees of infarct expansion.

The picture is further complicated by the fact that areas remote from the infarcted segment also undergo structural changes. These changes are not as marked or as fast in development but they have been confirmed in humans and they are important in the process of eventual ventricular functional impairment. Late remodelling appears to involve the remote areas more than the initial infarcted region.

Ventricular enlargement in the early phase can have beneficial effects. A 20% reduction in effective ventricular contractile circumference means that a normal stroke volume cannot be achieved without prior ventricular enlargement as the ejection fraction is reduced. In the longer term the enlargement leads to maladaptive changes as the increased load on the viable myocardium in the enlarged ventricle promotes further enlargement and hypertrophy. These changes also result in distortion in the ventricular shape which leads to a further reduction in cardiac efficiency.

Ventricular remodelling can be modified at three stages. Reduction in risk factors can reduce the initial risk of a MI. Reperfusion can reduce the early and late stages of ventricular enlargement and distortion. Drug therapies can reduce the late maladaptive changes. ACE inhibitors are known to be effective in reducing ventricular enlargement and improving prognosis post MI. They produce these effects through several different mechanisms. They reduce atrial filling pressures, which appears to be important. They also have direct negative trophic actions on the heart as well as reducing neurohormonal stimulation and altering intra-renal haemodynamics. All of these properties may be important in their beneficial effects.

Cardiac remodelling with progressive ventricular enlargement post MI can now be considered one of the modifiable risk factors in secondary prevention. A better understanding of this process may produce more successful therapeutic interventions in the future.

Reference

Pfeffer M A 1995 Left ventricular remodelling after acute myocardial infarction. Annual Review of Medicine 46: 455-466

148. Coronary artery bypass grafting (CABG)

A. **T**   B. **T**   C. **T**   D. **F**   E. **T**

From the results of randomized trials it has long been known that coronary artery bypass grafting (CABG) surgery is more effective than medical therapy for relieving anginal symptoms. An overview of randomized trials comparing CABG with medical therapy included 2500 patients and found that bypass surgery resulted in a significant reduction in mortality compared to initial medical therapy in patients with chronic coronary heart disease. The benefits were greatest in those patients at most risk of death.

Trials comparing angioplasty with medical therapy have shown that in patients with angina and exercise induced ischaemia, angioplasty leads to greater relief of symptoms.

A meta-analysis comparing CABG and angioplasty in patients with chronic coronary artery disease enrolled 3371 patients with a follow-up of 2.7 years. Cardiac death or non-fatal MI occurred in 9.9% of angioplasty patients and 9.3% of surgery patients. Relief from angina was greater in the surgery group. 34% of patients in the angioplasty group required a further revascularization procedure during the first follow-up year, including 18% who crossed over to CABG.

The mainstay of treatment of chronic coronary artery disease remains risk factor modification and, in those with symptoms, aspirin and anti-anginal drugs. In patients who remain symptomatic the choice of whether to perform a revascularization procedure, and whether this should be angioplasty or surgery, should be tailored to the individual patient and depend on local expertise.

One of the main drawbacks of angioplasty is restenosis. Two recent reports offer hope that the incidence of this outcome can be reduced. A meta-analysis of randomized studies using calcium channel blockers post-angioplasty, included five studies and 919 patients. It showed a 30% relative risk reduction of restenosis in patients receiving calcium channel blockers. Another approach using monoclonal antibody fragment directed against the platelet glycoprotein IIb/IIIa integrin, has recently been reported to reduce restenosis in high risk patients.

References

Hillegass W B, Ohman E M, Leimberger J D et al 1994 A meta-analysis of randomized trials of calcium antagonists to reduce restenosis after coronary angioplasty. American Journal of Cardiology 73: 835-839

Parisi A F, Folland E D, Hartigan P (for the Veterans Affairs ACME Investigators) 1992 A comparison of angioplasty with medical therapy in the treatment of single vessel coronary artery disease. New England Journal of Medicine 326: 10

Pocock S J, Henderson R A, Rickards AF et al 1995 Meta-analysis of randomized trials comparing coronary angioplasty with bypass surgery. Lancet 346: 1148-1149

Rihal C S, Yusuf S 1996 Chronic coronary artery disease: drugs, angioplasty, or surgery? British Medical Journal 312: 265-266

Topol E J, Califf R M, Weisman H F et al 1994 Randomized trial of coronary intervention with antibody against platelet IIb/IIIa integrin for reduction of clinical restenosis: results at 6 months. Lancet 343: 881-886

Yusuf S, Zucker D, Peduzzi P et al 1994 Effect of coronary artery bypass graft surgery on survival: overview of 10-year results from randomized trials by the Coronary Artery Bypass Graft Surgery Triallists Collaboration. Lancet 334: 563-570

149. Hibernating myocardium

A. **F**   B. **T**   C. **T**   D. **F**   E. **F**

When faced with a reduced blood supply, the myocardium may infarct. If, however, flow is above a critical level for a prolonged period it may downregulate to re-equilibrate with the reduced supply of oxygen and nutrients. This allows the tissue to remain viable but non-functioning. After months in this state, the myocardium shows a loss of myofibrillar content and accumulation of glycogen. Hibernating myocardium, therefore, is a state of persistently impaired myocardial function at rest due to reduced coronary blood flow that can be restored to normal by restoring blood flow or reducing oxygen demand. The phenomenon may be found in the context of unstable angina, chronic stable angina, acute MI, left ventricular failure and congestive cardiac failure. Hibernating myocardium should be contrasted with stunned myocardium. The latter term is used to describe the short-term myocardial dysfunction which follows temporary, total or near total interruption of coronary flow.

The therapeutic significance of the hibernating myocardium is its reversibility. If a patient undergoes revascularization, myocardial contractility improves. If, however, reduced coronary flow is persistent, there may be progressive cellular damage, ischaemia, infarction, heart failure or death.

Positron emission tomography, radionucleotide scanning and dobutamine echocardiography can all be used to detect non-functioning but viable (therefore hibernating) myocardium. In diagnosis they all have a sensitivity and specificity of about 85%. These techniques can be used to select patients who may have the best results from revascularization, either by coronary artery bypass grafting (CABG) or percutaneous transarterial coronary angioplasty (PTCA). Studies have shown that the best predictor of improved left ventricular function after CABG is the amount of hibernating myocardium before the procedure.

Hibernating myocardium is common in angina patients. In one study it was demonstrated in 75% of patients with unstable angina and 28% of patients with stable angina. Amongst patients with impaired left ventricular function, survival after CABG is significantly better in those with unstable compared to stable angina, reflecting the greater proportion of the unstable patients with hibernating myocardium.

Hibernating myocardium is also common in acute MI, and occurs both in the region of the infarct and in regions distant from it. In a randomized trial of PTCA 6 weeks post-MI, where there was no clinical or exercise induced evidence of ischaemia, the group receiving PTCA showed a significant increase in ejection fraction, whereas the nonPTCA group did not. These results clearly show the existence of hibernating myocardium in the post-MI patients. Another important finding is that further cardiac events are much more common in patients with hibernating myocardium post-MI than in patients where it is not found, suggesting that revasularization in this group is especially important.

Patients presenting with left ventricular failure or dilated cardiomyopathy are frequently found to have hibernating myocardium, even in the absence of ischaemic symptoms or a history of MI. There is, therefore, a case for screening this group.

Hibernating myocardium is described as acute, subacute or chronic depending on the time to recovery after revascularization. In the acute form recovery is almost immediate, whereas in the chronic form, which is associated with myocardial changes on biopsy, the myocardium may take up to a year to recover.

Reference

Rahimtoola S H 1995 From coronary heart disease to heart failure: role of hibernating myocardium. American Journal of Cardiology 75: 16E-22E

150. Syndrome X

A. F   B. F   C. F   D. F   E. F

Syndrome X is a term used to describe patients who suffer from the symptom of exertional angina pectoris but have normal coronary angiograms. Strict diagnostic criteria for the condition are not widely accepted which has lead to difficulties in comparing studies. Some define the syndrome as angina-like pain with normal coronary angiograms, whereas others argue that other known causes of chest pain have to be excluded, and some feel a positive exercise tolerance test is necessary to make the diagnosis. It is now thought that the syndrome probably consists of a heterogeneous group of pathophysiological entities.

Between 10 and 30% of patients undergoing angiography for chest pain have normal angiograms. Coronary angiography may miss early atherosclerotic disease and angina-like symptoms may result from oesophageal disorders, mitral valve prolapse, musculoskeletal disorders, cardiomyopathy, left ventricular hypertrophy, systemic hypertension, psychosomatic disorders and hyperventilation.

Patients with syndrome X usually present in their late forties and often have coronary risk factors. There is a female preponderance. Approximately 50% have associated breathlessness and a similar percentage have resting ST and T wave abnormalities. The life expectancy of most patients is little affected by the condition but the morbidity is often considerable, with 75% continuing to suffer from chest pain at follow-up. Often patients are not convinced that they do not suffer from a serious underlying heart condition.

There are many theoretical causes for the condition. Some studies have suggested that metabolic abnormalities such as insulin resistance or altered lactate metabolism may be involved. Abnormalities of ventricular function have been observed with up to 25% of patients showing a decline in left ventricular function over 4–5 years. The coronary artery flow reserve, which is the difference between resting and maximal flow, has been found to be reduced. Increased microvascular tone, endothelial cell dysfunction, altered pain perception, increased sympathetic tone and oestrogen deficiency have also been implicated in the pathogenesis.

Management consists of excluding other causes of chest pain, reassurance and drug therapy. Between 17 and 100% of cases in different studies have been found to be due to oesophageal disorders. The low risk of myocardial infarction should be stressed and counselling and simple advice may be helpful in those with anxiety disorders. Nitrates and other anginal therapies are found to be helpful in many patients. Hormone replacement therapy is useful in those with post-menopausal symptoms. Imipramine and other neuropathic pain treatments have also been used. Kaski and colleagues showed significant improvements in exercise induced ischaemia in patients treated with ACE inhibitors.

References

Chauhan A 1995 Syndrome X: angina and normal coronary angiography. Postgraduate Medical Journal 71: 341-345

Kaski J C, Rosano G, Gavrieledes S et al 1994 Effects of angiotensin converting enzyme inhibiting on exercise induced angina and ST segment depression in patients with microvascular angina. American Journal of Cardiology 23: 652-657

151. Hypertrophic cardiomyopathy (HCM)

A. T   B. F   C. F   D. F   E. F

Hypertrophic cardiomyopathy is an autosomal dominant disease with characteristic hypertrophy of the left ventricle particularly the interventricular septum. It is the most common cause of sudden death in the young.

The principal symptoms of clinical disease are exertional angina, dyspnoea, fatigue and syncope. Around 25% of patients with HCM have evidence of left ventricular outflow obstruction. Dynamic subaortic obstruction is a consequence of asymmetric septal hypertrophy and anterior movement of the mitral valve in systole. Relief of obstruction improves quality of life but has not been shown to reduce mortality. Ways of reducing the degree of obstruction include negatively inotropic drugs such as beta-blockers, dual chamber cardiac pacing to alter the pattern of septal contraction, and surgical reduction of the septal bulge. New techniques involving focal infarction of the septum using cardiac catheterization and balloon induced ischaemia have shown promising results. This technique is, however, in its infancy and the long-term sequelae are not known.

Linkage analysis techniques have been used to locate some of the genes which cause HCM. The first gene found was located on the long arm of chromosome 14 in the region of the myosin genes. This was subsequently found to be the beta myosin heavy chain gene (beta MHC). However other kindreds did not demonstrate genetic linkage to chromosome 14 suggesting genetic and phenotypic heterogenicity of the disease.

Genes have been identified on chromosome 1q3 – the troponin T gene, and on chromosome 15q2 – the alpha-tropomyosin gene; a fourth locus has been identified on chromosome 11q 11. Several families which do not link to any of these loci have also been identified, suggesting at least one more as yet undiscovered gene culprit.

All three of the identified genes code for sarcomeric proteins. The beta MHC protein forms the thick filaments of the sarcomeres which interact with the thin actin filaments to generate force through hydrolysis of ATP to ADP. The troponin T encoded protein links the troponin complex to tropomyosin. The alpha-tropomyosin gene codes for a protein that binds to actin to form the thin filaments. The mutant beta MHC gene produces a protein with impaired actomyosin interaction and in cats it has been shown to disrupt the sarcomere.

Analysis of the correlation between genotype and phenotype shows that particular mutations are associated with more or less severe forms of the disease in a consistent manner. This is especially important as some forms of the disease confer a normal life expectancy while others result in a high risk of sudden death in early adult life. This has obvious implications both for therapeutic intervention, and antenatal counselling and prenatal screening.

Hypertrophy and dilatation are common responses to cardiac injury. Hypertrophy would appear to be a secondary response to a variety of different genetic mutations. It is predominantly seen in the left ventricle despite the same protein defects being present in all the cardiac myocytes, implying that the hypertrophy is a result of excess workload. The development of hypertrophy does not take place until adolescence.

Unravelling of the molecular genetics behind HCM has already had clinical applications, both in preclinical screening of the young and in deciding which adults are most at risk of sudden death and thus would benefit from an automatic internal defibrillator. It is possible that in the future gene therapy, directed either at inhibiting expression of the defective gene or at overexpressing the wild type gene, may be effective treatment. Even in established hypertrophy, as long as irreversible fibrosis has not developed, regression of hypertrophy with remodelling of the left ventricle and a normalization of left ventricular function may be possible.

References

Knight C, Gunning M, Henein M et al 1996 Non-surgical septal reduction for hypertrophic cardiomyopathy. Journal of Invasive Cardiology (in press)

Marian A J, Roberts M D 1995 Molecular genetics of hypertrophic cardiomyopathy. Annual Review of Medicine 46: 213-222

152. Cardiac tumours

A. F   B. F   C. F   D. F   E. F

Primary cardiac tumours are rare. Metastatic tumours are 20–40 times more common, but these usually occur in the pericardium and only very rarely in the myocardium or endocardium. Unlike thrombi (the most common cause of an intracardiac mass) tumours are often accompanied by systemic features such as fever, fatigue, arthralgia, rash and weight loss. Blood tests show an anaemia with either a normochromic, normocytic or a haemolytic picture, a raised ESR, CRP and serum globulin. They can thus mimic infective, immunological and malignant processes.

Three quarters of the primary tumours are benign and nearly half of these are myxomas. Other primary tumours include rhabdomyomas and sarcomas. Most myxomas are sporadic but familial cases with an autosomal dominant pattern of inheritance have been reported.

75% of myxomas originate in the left atrium, and most arise in the interatrial septum at the border of the fossa ovalis. Most present either with embolism, which occurs in 40% of patients and is usually systemic, intracardiac obstruction or constitutional symptoms. The myxoma can obstruct filling of the left or right side of the heart resulting in cardiac failure. It can obstruct any of the cardiac valves although the mitral is the most commonly affected. Valve obstruction may cause syncope or sudden death and right atrial myxomas can mimic constrictive pericarditis by blocking the tricuspid valve. On auscultation about 50% of patients have either a diastolic or systolic murmur which is usually positional. In a third of patients prediastolic murmurs can be heard 100 msec after the second heart sound. This is known as the 'tumour plop'.

Diagnosis requires either echocardiography, CT or MRI. Two-dimensional echo can delineate the location, size, shape and attachment of the tumour, but transoesophageal echo gives an unimpeded view with better information about site of insertion and morphological features of the tumour. Angiography is performed in older patients to exclude coronary artery disease prior to surgery.

The treatment of choice is surgical resection. The root of the pedicle and full thickness of the intra-atrial septum must be excised and the atrial septal defect then repaired. Operative mortality is reported to be between zero and 3%. Recurrent tumours have been described, particularly in the familial myxomas.

Reference

Reynes K 1995 Cardiac myxomas. New England Journal of Medicine 333:1610-1617

---

153. Heart valve replacement

A. **T** B. **F** C. **T** D. **F** E. **T**

Valvular heart disease may remain asymptomatic for many years. Criteria for valve replacement have changed with advances such as reliable doppler echocardiography and mitral balloon valvotomy.

Patients with symptomatic aortic regurgitation are candidates for valve replacement. Occasionally the native valve can be repaired thus avoiding the need for a prosthesis. In asymptomatic patients there is increasing evidence that survival and cardiac function can be improved significantly by early valve replacement if there is echocardiographic evidence of left ventricular dysfunction.

In patients with aortic stenosis there is only a small decrease in survival whilst they remain asymptomatic. Sudden death in asymptomatic patients with congenital aortic stenosis is less rare. Without surgery symptomatic aortic stenosis carries a high mortality. Several studies have shown that between 50 and 70% of patients with an aortic pressure gradient of 50 mmHg or more will become symptomatic within 3 years. Only a few studies have looked at aortic valve replacement in asymptomatic patients. These conclude that the risks from surgery and complications of valve replacement outweigh any potential survival benefit. A possible exception is in patients without overt symptoms but with reduced exercise tolerance. Supervised exercise stress tests may allow these patients to be identified. Surgery may then be beneficial.

Sudden death in patients with asymptomatic mitral stenosis is very rare. Mildly symptomatic patients can be managed medically with no survival disadvantage. Exceptions include recent onset atrial fibrillation where restoration of valve function may allow conversion to sinus rhythm. Valvotomy is a useful alternative to surgery but may be complicated by mitral regurgitation.

Chronic mitral regurgitation is common and usually progresses slowly, resulting in no increased mortality. When left ventricular failure occurs, survival may be limited to 5 years. Valve function can sometimes be restored by native valve repair.

Complications of valve replacement include peri and postoperative mortality, valve failure, endocarditis, haemolysis, the complications of anticoagulation and thromboembolism.

Reference

Carabello B A 1995 Indications for valve surgery in asymptomatic patients with aortic and mitral stenosis. Chest 108: 1678-1682

154. Atrioventricular nodal re-entry tachycardia

A. T   B. T   C. F   D. T   E. T

Atrioventricular nodal re-entry tachycardia is probably the most common regular paroxysmal supraventricular tachycardia and it accounts for more than half the patients referred for diagnostic electrophysiology. Patients usually present in the fourth or fifth decades of life. Women are more commonly affected, making up 70% of patients with this arrhythmia.

In this type of arrhythmia there are usually two distinct conduction pathways in the AV node. One, referred to as the 'fast pathway', has a rapid conduction velocity and a relatively long refractory period. The other, referred to as the 'slow pathway', has a slow conduction velocity and a short refractory period. Atrioventricular re-entry is typically initiated by an atrial premature beat. This depolarization, typically, is blocked from anteriograde conduction in the fast pathway (because of its longer refractory period), whilst it is able to conduct slowly in the anteriograde direction of the slow pathway. If this is slow enough, the fast pathway will have recovered from its refractory period, enabling rapid conduction in the retrograde direction of the fast pathway to ensue. This is then followed by slow anteriograde conduction in the slow pathway again, allowing a continuous circuit to be set up.

The P waves are negative in the inferior ECG leads. The reason for this is that the atria are activated in a caudocranial direction with the impulses starting in the re-entrant nodal circuit. They are, however, rarely visible as they are usually superimposed on the QRS complexes. In 10% of cases the re-entry circuit is reversed with anteriograde conduction over the fast pathway and retrograde conduction over the slow pathway. This is referred to as uncommon atrioventricular nodal re-entrant tachycardia. In this situation the P waves are usually visible on the surface electrocardiogram as inverted waves in the inferior leads. This is normally precipitated by a ventricular premature beat rather than one of atrial origin.

Drugs which cause a temporary block in atrioventricular conduction, such as adenosine, are effective therapies. Adenosine is usually given as a rapid intravenous bolus in increasing doses until there is a response or a 12mg dose is reached. After this dose, 90% of such arrhythmias will have been terminated.

Reference

Ganz L I, Freidman P L 1995 Supraventricular tachycardia. New England Journal of Medicine 332: 162-174.

DERMATOLOGY
155. Paraneoplastic syndromes
A. T   B. F   C. T   D. T   E. T.

156. Paraneoplastic syndromes
A. T   B. F   C. F   D. F   E. T

A variety of cutaneous paraneoplastic syndromes have been described in association with solid tumours. They are clinically important as they may precede the diagnosis of the underlying malignancy. Often associated with a particular solid tumour, they may suggest a poor prognosis. They are also of considerable interest in that a variety of immune or cytokine mediated processes have been found to be involved in their pathogenesis.

Digital clubbing is perhaps the best known of these conditions and in about 10–20% there is associated hypertrophic osteoarthropathy. The most frequent malignant disorders associated with this sign are bronchogenic carcinoma and mesothelioma. Clubbing can also be hereditary or idiopathic and can be secondary to a variety of non-malignant disorders. Hypertrophic osteoarthropathy results from periostial new bone formation resulting in pain adjacent to the wrists, knees, ankles and elbows. At least 90% of such cases have or will develop a malignant condition, most commonly peripheral non-small cell lung cancer. Interestingly vagotomy can result in regression.

Dermatomyositis is associated with cancer in about 25% of cases. Its features include proximal myopathy, Gottron's papules (erythematous dermal papules over the phalangeal joints) and a heliotrope rash. The creatinine kinase is often markedly elevated and there are characteristic features on electromyography and muscle biopsy. Ovarian cancer has the strongest association with dermatomyositis.

Multi-centric reticulohistiocytosis is a condition in which approximately 25% of cases develop malignancy and in 75% of cases the diagnosis precedes that of the underlying malignant disorder. Its features include severe arthritis with nodular lesions most commonly affecting the upper half of the body. The arthritis may progress to arthritis mutilans. A variety of joints can be affected and systemic features such as weight loss and fever may be present. Characteristic histological features are found on skin biopsy.

A variety of reactive erythemas are associated with underlying malignancy. Erythema gyratum repens presents with scaly erythematous lesions that form concentric rings giving the skin a wood grain appearance. Underlying malignancies are found in over 75% of cases with cancers of the lung, oesophagus and breast being the most common. It may be associated with other disorders such as tuberculosis and the CREST (calcinosis, Raynaud's, oesophageal dysmotility, sclerodactyly and telangiectasia) syndrome. Other reactive erythemas include necrolytic migratory erythema which is strongly associated with glucagonoma and tends to respond to treatment with somatostatin analogues.

A variety of coagulation disorders can result from malignant disease. For example, a thrombotic state can result from alterations in the levels of fibrinogen, platelets, factor 5 and antithrombin III. Approximately 6% of cases of deep vein thrombosis are associated with underlying malignant conditions but this association is more marked in those under 50 without known risk factors, and rises to about 50% of cases of migratory thrombophlebitis. Migratory thrombophlebitis is a recurrent condition also known as Trousseau's syndrome. It is strongly associated with a variety of cancers especially those of the lung and pancreas (both body and tail).

Acanthosis nigricans in childhood is often benign but in adults is usually associated with malignancies or endocrinopathies. In paraneoplastic cases 80–90% are associated with abdominal adenocarcinoma. The skin is usually affected in the intertriginous areas such as the neck, groin, axillae and infra-mammary folds. There is hyperpigmentation with a moss-like or velvety texture which is caused by hyperkeratosis and papillomatosis. There may be mucosal involvement in up to 30% of cases. Tripe palms is a condition with thickening of the soles and palms giving a velvety appearance which is associated with underlying malignancies in 90% of cases.

Tylosis is diffuse hyperkeratosis of the palms and soles. There is an hereditary form in which individuals have an increased risk of developing oesophageal carcinoma, and an acquired form where there is an increased incidence of underlying carcinoma, particularly oesophageal carcinoma. Discrete palmar and plantar hyperkeratosis may be associated with underlying malignancy but this may be due in part to the common aetiological risk factor, arsenic exposure.

Bazex's syndrome is associated with malignancy in all reported cases and in about 60% of patients the skin lesions precede the underlying carcinoma. It is characterized by psoriaform lesions over sacral areas (helices of the ears, the nose, fingers and elbows); and also by nail abnormalities.

The sign of Leser-Trélat refers to a sudden increase in the size and number of solar keratoses and is associated with the development of a variety of internal malignancies such as intra-abdominal adenocarcinoma and lymphoproliferative disorders. A variety of growth factors, such as transforming growth factor alpha and epidermal growth factor, have been found to be elevated in such cases.

Florid cutaneous papillomatosis is the rapid onset of multiple wart-like lesions initially on the back of the hands and wrists which in all reported cases is associated with malignancy, most commonly gastric.

In pityriasis rotunda 6% of cases are associated with malignancies such as hepatocellular carcinoma and gastric carcinoma. It is a condition found in Far Eastern populations, and South African and West Indian blacks; and manifests with scaly, round, hyperpigmented lesions on the trunk, buttocks and thighs.

Hypertrichosis lanuginosa acquisita refers to the acquired development of fine non-pigmented hairs most commonly affecting the face. The most common associated carcinomas are those of the lung and colon. It is also associated with a variety of drug therapies such as cyclosporin, spironolactone, phenytoin, mindoxil and corticosteroids; and conditions such as thyrotoxicosis and porphyria.

There are a variety of known cutaneous paraneoplastic conditions. The detection of these conditions may predate the diagnosis of an associated malignancy and may help direct investigations to a particular organ or organs allowing earlier diagnosis.

Reference

Kurzock R, Cohen P R 1995 Cutaneous paraneoplastic syndromes in solid tumours. American Journal of Medicine 99: 662-671

157. Basal cell carcinoma (BCC)

A. **F**   B. **F**   C. **T**   D. **F**   E. **T**

In the UK the incidence of basal cell carcinoma (BCC) has risen by 238% in 14 years. It is believed that it is exposure to the sun in the years up to age 20 that sets off processes which result in malignant change 40–60 years later. The intermediate steps are likely to involve the activation of oncogenes, the deactivation of tumour suppressor genes and changes in p53 gene protection. With ageing the ability to repair DNA damage induced by sunlight is impaired, and in some individuals there are likely to be genetic factors which predispose them to the development of cancers at an earlier age.

The three main clinical types of BCC are superficial, nodular and infiltrative. There is also basosquamous carcinoma which has clinical and histological features of both BCC and squamous cell carcinoma (SCC). The basal cell naevus syndrome is an autosomal dominant disorder resulting from a defect on chromosome 9q. The condition is characterized by BCCs, bony abnormalities, epidermal cysts and odontogenic keratocysts on the jaw, palmar and plantar pits and other neoplasms.

Biopsy is advisable to confirm the diagnosis of BCC and to decide on the definitive treatment. The preferred treatment depends on the site and size of the lesion and the preferred techniques of the dermatologist or surgeon. BCCs may be treated with curettage, simple excision, cryosurgery with liquid nitrogen, or radiotherapy. Excision gives cure rates of 95–99%.

Newer treatments are under investigation. The intralesional injection of interferon alpha into small lesions has been shown to give an 85% cure rate with excellent cosmetic results. Oral retinoids are not curative but are used in patients with the basal cell naevus syndrome and xeroderma pigmentosum to induce tumour regression and suppression. Phototherapy has been used exploiting the fact that BCC cells take up haematoporphyrin in greater concentrations than normal surrounding cells. This makes them photosensitive to certain light frequencies. Subsequent treatment with monochromatic light will then selectively destroy the tumour cells. BCC only rarely metastasises. Cisplatin has been found to be the most useful chemotherapeutic agent at providing palliation and promoting regression in the few patients who do suffer metastasis.

Out-patient follow-up should involve the search for both recurrence and for new lesions, including melanomas which are more common in patients who have had a BCC. The aim is to treat lesions when they are small.

It is important that the public are made aware that sunlight is carcinogenic. There is evidence that sunscreens suppress actinic keratoses but no hard evidence that they protect against BCCs, so the wearing of hats and long sleeves in the sun should be promoted. The results of public health measures to reduce the epidemic of skin cancer in Australia will be of interest.

Reference

Goldberg L H 1996 Basal cell carcinoma. Lancet 347: 663-666

---

158. Stevens-Johnson syndrome

A. T   B. F   C. F   D. F   E. F

Erythema multiforme, Stevens-Johnson syndrome and toxic epidermal necrolysis form a spectrum of skin diseases with common aetiologies and similar histopathological features. At the mild end of the spectrum there are the classical target lesions without mucous membrane involvement, and at the other there are life threatening epidermal necroses with extensive skin detachment, erosions of the mucous membrane, severe constitutional symptoms and case fatalities of 30–40%. Drugs are usually the cause of toxic epidermal necrolysis but although they are important in the aetiology of erythema multiforme and Stevens-Johnson syndrome, infections such as herpes simplex and *Mycoplasma pneumoniae* are also common antecedents.

In case reports over a hundred drugs have been implicated as causes of these diseases. The incidence of Stevens-Johnson is estimated at only 1–6 cases per million person years, but the more severe forms are potentially fatal, and previous case reports have been responsible for the withdrawal of some drugs from the market.

A large retrospective case-control study was set up to look at the relative risks of developing Stevens-Johnson and toxic epidermal necrolysis associated with the use of various drugs. Significant excess risk was associated with the use of anti-bacterial sulphonamides, with 4.5 cases per million users per week. Interestingly there was no association with the structurally similar thiazide diuretics or the sulphonylureas. The NSAID isoxicam was withdrawn from the market in France after being associated with 13 cases of toxic epidermal necrolysis. The study found that the two currently marketed oxicam drugs had a significantly greater association with the disease than either diclofenac or proprionic acid derivatives. The aromatic anti-epileptic drugs (phenobarbitone, phenytoin and carbamazepine) were found to confer a risk that was no greater than that with sodium valproate, previously viewed as safer in this respect, and the risk was greatest in the first 2 months of use. Allopurinol and chlormethiazole were also found to be associated with the development of the conditions. More surprising was the association with corticosteroids.

The disease in its mild forms is usually self-limiting but the more severe forms confer significant morbidity and mortality. The prompt removal of the causative agent and supportive treatment of the complications of the syndromes is important. Corticosteroids are not thought to improve the outcome and may be deleterious to children.

Reference

Roujeau J C, Kelly J P, Naldi L et al 1995 Medication use and the risk of Stevens-Johnson syndrome and toxic epidermal necrolysis. New England Journal of Medicine 333: 1600-1607

159. Dermatological treatments
A. F   B. T   C. T   D. T   E. F

Topical calcipotriol is a new effective treatment for plaque-type psoriasis. The active ingredient vitamin D3 acts locally increasing the extracellular calcium concentration. This leads to the further differentiation of keratinocytes and thus reduces cell turnover and scaling. Calcipotriol has been shown to be better than placebo, coal tar and topical clobetasol proprionate in the treatment of chronic plaque-type psoriasis. It is not thought that routine measurements of serum calcium are needed in normocalcaemic patients.

Topical steroids, emollients and oral anti-histamines are the mainstay of treatment for pruritis, while ultraviolet light, cyclosporin and systemic steroids provide additional relief but are unsafe for long-term use. The tricyclic anti-depressant doxepin has anti-histamine activity and is known to be effective at relieving pruritis. A topical formulation of doxepin has been developed for the treatment of atopic dermatitis. In a placebo controlled double blind trial, topical doxepin 5% gave greater relief from itch than placebo. Side-effects include a localized burning sensation in 30% of patients and mild drowsiness for the first few days of use.

Reference

Lowitt M H, Lowitt N R 1995 Recent advances: dermatology. British Medical Journal 311: 1615-1616

160. Urticaria
A. T   B. T   C. T   D. F   E. T

An autoimmune mast cell mechanism has been proposed in the pathogenesis of chronic urticaria. Urticaria is an unpleasant and occasionally life threatening skin disease characterized by hives and angio-oedema. It can result from exposure to physical elements such as cold, pressure, sunlight, heat, and water. Other causal agents include drugs especially the non-steroidal anti-inflammatory drugs, foods, infections, and autoimmune connective tissue disorders. The majority of cases, however, are idiopathic. Recent reports from Greaves et al identify an IgG auto-antibody able to cross link IgE receptors on mast cells in the serum of up to 60% of patients with idiopathic chronic urticaria. The existence of these auto-antibodies may explain the chronic nature of the illness and the fact that treatment with plasmapheresis, intravenous immunoglobulin and immunosuppressive regimens is beneficial to some patients.

Reference

Greaves M W 1995 Chronic urticaria. New England Journal of Medicine 332: 1767-1772

---

161. Malignant melanoma

A. **F**   B. **T**   C. **T**   D. **T**   E. **T**

The incidence of melanoma in Caucasians in both the northern and southern hemispheres increased at a rate of 3–7% per year from the mid-1950s to the early 1980s. The rise in mortality has been smaller due to a reduction in case fatality to under 20%. Recent studies have shown steep increases in the incidence of melanoma and a study in New South Wales showed a doubling of histologically confirmed melanomas in a 2-year period. Whether this is a true epidemic or is a result of earlier diagnosis, changes in histopathological definitions, or an increase in the number of excised lesions sent for histological classification is under debate.

Clark & Breslow found the depth of dermal invasion to be the most important prognostic indicator of long-term survival. Breslow tumour thickness states that tumours more than 1 mm thick have a much higher mortality than those of less than 1 mm. Patients with tumours less than 1 mm deep have a 5-year survival of 90%. Prognosis not only depends on the absolute depth of the tumour but also on the level of dermis to which it extends. The Clark's level distinguishes tumours according to the level of dermis they extend to, with level III disease defined as extending beyond the papillary dermis into the reticular dermis and indicating a poor prognosis. Other independent indicators of a poor prognosis include male sex and anatomical location in the upper arms, thorax, scalp and neck. Evidence suggests that high continuous exposure to the sun is less dangerous than intermittent exposure as a trigger for the development of malignant melanoma.

In the familial atypical mole-melanoma syndrome patients with multiple large atypical moles have an increased risk of melanoma. Some families with this condition have been shown to have deletions of the P16 gene. The P16 gene is known to encode a protein which controls mitosis and DNA synthesis. The search for other genes or transcription-factors involved in the pathogenesis of malignant melanoma continues.

References

Lowitt M H, Lowitt N R 1995 Recent advances: dermatology. British Medical Journal 311: 1615-1616

Rees J L 1996 The melanoma epidemic: reality and artifact. British Medical Journal 312: 138

RESPIRATORY MEDICINE
162. Pulse oximetry

A. **T**   B. **T**   C. **F**   D. **F**   E. **F**

Pulse oximetry enables oxygenation to be measured continuously and non-invasively. The absorption spectra of oxyhaemoglobin and deoxyhaemaglobin differ, and the ratio of their concentrations can be determined by the ratio of the quantity of light absorbed at two different wavelengths. The light absorbed by the tissues and venous and capillary blood can be calculated by the oximeter measuring absorption at two points on the pulse waveform, the difference being due to arterial blood alone. The oximeter probe contains a red and infrared light emitter and a detector. Ambient light can be corrected for by the diodes rapidly switching on and off, and after this correction the oxyhaemoglobin saturation can be found from an empirically determined table. The displayed saturation is an average of the previous 3–6 seconds of recording.

Inaccuracies in recording can arise if perfusion is poor, if there is venous pulsation or motion artifact. Vital dyes and dyshaemoglobins interfere with accurate recording. For example carboxyhaemoglobin is detected as oxyhaemoglobin. Excessive ambient light may saturate the detector and give erroneous readings. A sharp waveform with a clear dicrotic notch indicates good perfusion, whereas a waveform resembling a sine wave indicates poor perfusion. Recordings can be improved by rubbing the skin, moving the probe site or applying a topical vasodilator.

Cyanosis is defined as the presence of more than 5 g/100 ml of reduced haemoglobin in capillary blood. Even a skilled observer cannot detect hypoxaemia until the oxyhaemoglobin saturation is under about 80%. For most clinical situations a saturation of above 90% is ideal. Below this level saturation falls rapidly as the oxygen tension declines due to the sigmoid shape of the oxygen dissociation curve. The default setting for most oximeters for low saturation is therefore 90%.

Pulse oximetry is indicated in any situation where hypoxia may occur. A great advantage is that measurement can be continuous.

Oximeters with memory facilities are particularly useful for the investigation of sleep disordered breathing. Oximetry can replace blood gas analysis in many situations, except where acid base analysis is sought, or where estimation of carbon dioxide is essential.

Although oximetry provides an accurate method for detection of hypoxaemia to saturations of 70%, it does not provide an absolute indicator of hyperoxia. This is particularly important in preventing oxygen toxicity in neonates.

Reference

Hanning C D, Alexander-Williams J M 1995 Pulse oximetry: a practical review. British Medical Journal 311: 367-370

---

163. Hypoxaemia

A. T   B. T   C. F   D. F   E. F

When exposed to prolonged hypoxia, the body induces several physiological responses designed to maintain adequate oxygen delivery. At a partial pressure of arterial oxygen (PaO_2) below 7.3 kPa ventilatory drive increases, leading to a higher PaO_2 and a fall in $PaCO_2$. In hypoxic tissues the vascular beds dilate, inducing a compensatory tachycardia that increases cardiac output and improves oxygen delivery. In response to alveolar hypoxia the pulmonary vascular bed constricts, thereby improving the match between ventilation and perfusion. In addition, hypoxia leads to the increased production of erythropoietin by the kidney resulting in erythrocytosis. This further increases the oxygen carrying capacity of the blood and therefore oxygen delivery to the tissues. In the long-term these physiological responses may be detrimental. Erythrocytosis can lead to a predisposition to thromboembolism, with a greater incidence of myocardial infarction and stroke. Erythrocytosis in combination with prolonged pulmonary vasoconstriction and increased cardiac output may lead to pulmonary hypertension, right heart failure (cor pulmonale), and death.

In addition to the cardiovascular effects of prolonged hypoxia, neuropsychological effects are often pronounced. In patients with chronic obstructive pulmonary disease (COPD) as well as in healthy individuals with experimentally induced hypoxia, low PaO_2 is associated with impaired judgment, learning, and short-term memory. In addition patients with chronic hypoxia are subjectively breathless and have poor exercise tolerance and capacity.

Reference

Tarpy S P, Celli B R 1995 Long-term oxygen therapy. New England Journal of Medicine 333: 710-714

164. Long-term oxygen therapy in chronic obstructive pulmonary disease

A. **T**   B. **F**   C. **T**   D. **T**   E. **F**

In patients with COPD who are hypoxic, oxygen supplementation improves pulmonary haemodynamics, exercise capacity and neuropsychological performance. It may also reduce the work involved in breathing and improve the quality of sleep.

Studies during the 1980s established that long-term oxygen therapy improves survival in these patients. The Medical Research Council study randomly assigned patients to receive 15 hours continuous oxygen or no oxygen. During 5 years of follow-up, 19 of 42 patients treated with oxygen died, compared to 30 of the 45 controls. In the USA, the Nocturnal Oxygen Therapy Trial Group randomly assigned patients to either 12 or 24 hours of daily oxygen. After 26 months mortality in the continuously treated group was half that in the 12-hour group.

Current indications for continuous oxygen therapy are a daytime PaO_2 of less than or equal to 7.3 kPa in a patient with a diagnosis of COPD, who usually has an FEV1 of less than or equal to 1.2 litres. The degree of hypoxia may be less severe if the patient has a history of cor pulmonale. The degree of hypoxia during an acute exacerbation of COPD does not necessarily reflect severe hypoxia between attacks, and long-term therapy should usually only be initiated when a patient is in a steady state and hypoxia is confirmed on two occasions 3 weeks apart. When initiating oxygen or changing dose, blood gas measurement should be used as a guide, aiming to increase the PaO_2 above 8 kPa without causing excessive CO_2 retention. Patients should be advised not to smoke because of the potential fire hazards, however smoking should not be regarded as a contraindication to long-term oxygen therapy.

Oxygen is available in concentrators which are bulky but inexpensive, or gas cylinders. Liquid oxygen is expensive and is not widely available in the UK. Most patients use nasal cannulae which are effective but inefficient. There is current interest in reservoir nasal cannulae, transtracheal catheters and electronic demand devices, all of which have the potential to increase the efficiency of oxygen delivery.

References

Medical Research Council Working Party 1981 Long-term domiciliary oxygen therapy in chronic hypoxic cor pulmonale complicating chronic bronchitis and emphysema. Lancet 1: 681-686

Nocturnal Oxygen Therapy Trial Group 1980 Continuous or nocturnal oxygen therapy in hypoxic chronic obstructive lung disease: a clinical trial. Annals of Internal Medicine 93: 391-398

Tarpy S P, Celli B R 1995 Long-term oxygen therapy. New England Journal of Medicine 333: 710-714

165. Nasal intermittent positive pressure ventilation
A. T   B. T   C. T   D. F   E. F

In both the acute and chronic setting, non-invasive ventilation is growing in popularity. This may be achieved either with negative, or positive pressure ventilation. Negative pressure can be applied to the chest wall by using a cabinet-type device which encloses the entire body below the neck, or by using a jacket or cuirass device. These techniques have been useful in patients with neuromuscular and chest wall disorders, as well as very young children. In COPD, however, this type of ventilation has been unsuccessful in normalizing blood gases because it provokes upper airway collapse and induces a form of obstructive sleep apnoea/hypopnoea syndrome. The other main drawback of these methods is that they are frequently unpopular with patients and are difficult to transport.

Positive pressure ventilation can be applied via a tracheostomy. This may be required for the chronic ventilation of patients with lesions of the cervical spinal chord and severe neuromuscular disease. These patient groups often require high levels of nursing support. The outcome depends on the underlying medical condition, but there is considerable morbidity and mortality associated with the tracheostomy itself.

Nasal intermittent positive pressure ventilation (NIPPV) was introduced into the UK in 1986 and has been applied to domiciliary use, in-patient use in acute ventilatory failure, and weaning of intensive care unit patients. Silicon masks or full face masks are commercially available, and small portable ventilators (e.g. BiPAP, Nippy) cost between £3000 and £6000. Face mask ventilation can be used in children as young as 2 years. The main disadvantages are discomfort, rhinitis and air leaks through the mouth.

Patients with chronic hypercapnic respiratory failure who do not respond to standard treatment should be considered for home ventilation, with the aim of controlling symptoms, improving quality of life, and reducing mortality. Nocturnal ventilatory support is advisable in symptomatic patients when oxygen saturation is below 90% for most of the night and the partial pressure of carbon dioxide exceeds 7 kPa. Home ventilation is suitable for patients with chest wall disease (e.g. scoliosis, thoracoplasty), respiratory muscle disorders (e.g. old polio, myopathies, muscular dystrophies) and neurological disorders (e.g. primary alveolar hypoventilation, central sleep apnoea, brain stem lesions, cervical cord lesions, neuropathies). French and UK studies of domiciliary NIPPV, show that 5-year survival in patients with scoliosis, stable neuromuscular disorders and old TB, who also have chronic ventilatory failure is around 80–100%. Quality of life in these groups is good and fewer hospital admissions are required. Many patients are able to return to full-time employment. Ventilation overnight often leads to normalization of blood gases which persists during the day when the patient is no longer on the ventilator. Some COPD patients with type II respiratory failure benefit from NIPPV. In contrast to negative pressure ventilation, NIPPV is more mechanically efficient and not associated with upper airway collapse. The relative benefits of long-term oxygen therapy and NIPPV are being investigated in a multi-centre European trial. Some patients with progressive neuromuscular disorders can be successfully ventilated with NIPPV, although some bulbar function is required to protect the airway against aspiration.

A recent randomized controlled study of NIPPV in acute COPD has shown that the mortality rate, need for intubation and hospital stay were reduced compared to a group receiving standard treatment. The type of ventilator used does not appear to be a major factor.

References

Brochard L, Mancebo J, Wysocki M et al 1995 Non-invasive ventilation for acute exacerbations of chronic obstructive pulmonary disease. New England Journal of Medicine 333: 817-822

Leger P, Bebicam J M, Cornette A et al 1994 Nasal intermittent positive pressure ventilation: long-term follow-up in patients with severe chronic respiratory insufficiency. Chest 105: 100-105

Simonds A K 1994 Sleep studies of respiratory function and home respiratory support. British Medical Journal 309: 35-40

Simonds A K, Elliott M 1995 Outcome of domiciliary nasal intermittent positive pressure ventilation in restrictive and obstructive disorders. Thorax 50: 604-609

166. Obstructive sleep apnoea

A. T   B. F   C. F   D. F   E. T

Obstructive sleep apnoea (OSA) is increasingly being recognized as a common cause of morbidity and mortality. Definitions vary, however many researchers use a working definition of five apnoeas (greater than 10 seconds) per hour. Prevalence among adults is estimated at between 1 and 4% depending on the population studied, the definition and screening method used. The condition is more common in men than women. Clinical features include repetitive apnoea, loud snoring and excessive daytime sleepiness. Less consistent features include daytime anxiety, nocturnal choking attacks, morning headaches, reflux oesophagitis, impotence, poor concentration and altered mood.

The primary pathology in OSA is either structural or functional obstruction of the upper airway during sleep. During sleep the muscles of the pharynx relax and this can then lead to collapse of the airway. Predisposing factors include obesity, anatomical abnormalities (large tonsils, nose and facial trauma), neuropathies and myopathies affecting the pharynx, acromegaly (50% of acromegalics in one study), myxoedema and Marfan's syndrome.

Central to accurate diagnosis is the sleep study. Protocols vary but most sleep laboratories monitor oxygen saturation and pulse during video recordings of sleep. Some laboratories also record EEG, body movements, oronasal airflow and intrathoracic pressure. The more sophisticated studies are particularly useful in difficult cases to differentiate obstructive from central or mixed apnoea syndromes.

The treatment of choice is nasal continuous positive airway pressure (nasal CPAP). The role of uvulopalatopharyngoplasty is yet to be defined. Early reports that up to 60% of patients responded to the operation have been criticized due to short follow-up and only partial resolution of symptoms. In some patients with severe OSA unable to tolerate nasal CPAP, tracheotomy has been used.

The long-term physiological effects of severe OSA are still being investigated. Right heart failure from pulmonary hypertension can occur particularly in patients with coexistent chronic airflow limitation, asthma, muscle weakness or lung fibrosis. Whether OSA can cause sustained daytime systemic hypertension remains controversial. An increased incidence of stroke, MI and driving accidents all cause mortality in OSA, although a causal relationship has not been proven.

References

McNamara S G, Grunstein R R, Sullivan C E 1993 Obstructive sleep apnoea. Thorax 48: 754-764

Simonds A K 1994 Sleep studies of respiratory function and home respiratory support. British Medical Journal 309: 35-40

Strollo P J, Rogers R M 1996 Current concepts: obstructive sleep apnoea. New England Journal of Medicine 334; 2: 99-104

167. British Thoracic Society asthma guidelines

A. T   B. T   C. F   D. F   E. F

The British Thoracic Society (BTS) published guidelines for the management of asthma in 1990, which were updated in 1993 in response to concern over increasing prevalence, morbidity, admissions and deaths from asthma. It is now agreed that the basic pathophysiology of asthma is of inflammation of the airways with secondary oedema, smooth muscle contraction and mucus secretion leading to reversible airways obstruction. It is this understanding of the pathophysiology as well as the results of large drug trials which have established steroids as the mainstay of preventative treatment in all but the most mild cases of asthma. The BTS guidelines outline a stepwise approach to the management of chronic asthma, with introduction of inhaled steroid early in treatment.

The guidelines stress the importance of objective measures of severity during an acute attack. Inability to complete sentences, a respiratory rate greater than 25 breaths per minute, tachycardia greater than 110 beats per minute or bradycardia, peak flow less than 50% predicted, a silent chest, cyanosis, hypotension or exhaustion can be indicaters of a severe attack. Blood gas analysis should always be performed and hypoxia, normocapnea, hypercapnea and acidosis can all be indications of a severe attack.

Beta 2 agonist therapy, oral and intravenous steroids and high dose oxygen are the mainstay of treatment, with theophylines, intravenous beta 2 agonists, and ipratropium bromide being second line agents.

Prior to discharge the peak flow should be more than 75% predicted with less than 25% diurnal variation. Inhaled steroids should be commenced 48 hours and nebulizers converted to inhalers at least 24 hours prior to discharge. Patients should have a written management plan, early follow-up and home peakflow monitoring.

Much controversy exists regarding a possible link between use of high dose inhaled beta 2 agonists and the increased death rate, particularly sudden death, from asthma. Beta 2 agonists may in high doses precipitate cardiac arrhythmias especially in hypoxic patients. These agents provide the best symptomatic relief from asthma but use should not exceed recommended doses, and excessive use should lead to a review of therapy and usually an increase in anti-inflammatory treatment.

References

British Thoracic Society 1990 Guidelines for management of asthma in adults I. British Medical Journal 301: 651-654

British Thoracic Society 1990 Guidelines for management of asthma in adults II. British Medical Journal 301: 797-800

British Thoracic Society 1993 Guidelines for the management of asthma: a summary. British Medical Journal 306: 776-782

Crane J, Pearce N, Burgess C et al 1995 Asthma and the beta agonist debate. Thorax 50 (Suppl 1): S5-S10

du Bois R M 1995 Respiratory medicine: recent advances. British Medical Journal 310: 1594-1598

168. Asthma and the environment

A. T   B. F   C. F   D. F   E. T

The prevalence of asthma in developed countries is increasing. This increase appears to persist even when changes in diagnostic criteria are accounted for. Migrants from areas of low to high asthma frequency adopt the increased levels of their new country. This suggests that environmental factors play an important role in asthma. Explanations for geographical and temporal changes in asthma have included an increase in allergen exposure, tobacco smoking by mothers of child bearing age, dietary differences, air pollution, occupational allergen exposure and viral respiratory infections.

The introduction of new allergens into a community has been linked to epidemics of asthma. A well documented example is the epidemic following the introduction of soya handling at Barcelona harbour. There seems to be a critical time for allergen sensitization in early infancy. Studies have documented that exposure to the house dust mite in early life is linked to the later development of allergy and asthma. Interestingly, sensitivity to the house dust mite is seasonal, with higher rates amongst children born in the autumn.

Tobacco smoking can increase total serum IgE concentrations. The rates of atopy, however, are lower in smokers possibly because atopic individuals are less likely to smoke. If asthma rates are studied in the work environment, smokers are more likely to develop occupational asthma.

The increase in asthma and allergic diseases has coincided with an increase in smoking amongst women. The rates of eczema and possibly asthma are higher in children born to mothers who smoke during pregnancy. This could reflect an effect of smoking on immune development or on lung development.

The effects of diet on asthma are most convincing for salt. In men but not women a strong association has been identified between table salt consumption and airway hyper-responsiveness. The effects of consumption of anti-oxidants on asthma have not yet been elucidated.

The increase in incidence of asthma has coincided with a fall in atmospheric concentrations of fossil-fuel combustion products (particulates and sulphur dioxide), and an increase in concentration of pollutants from burning motor fuel (oxides of nitrogen and ozone). A causal relationship between asthma and air pollution has not been proven. However, it is established that air pollution can cause falls in lung function in established asthmatics. The effects of air pollutants interact. For example, exposure to ozone reduces the dose of pollen required to induce an asthmatic response. There is no convincing evidence for a role for air pollution in inducing allergy or asthma. Indoor air pollution may have a more important effect on asthma than outdoor air pollution. There is some suggestion that improvements in insulation increase exposure to indoor allergens such as house dust mite and cat fur.

Viral infection leads to a deterioration of asthma in children. A causal relationship between viral infection and asthma induction in childhood has not been established, however, and it is possible that early virus exposure may actually be protective. Rates of hayfever and skin test allergy fall in children with many siblings, suggesting that early exposure to viral infection may protect against the development of atopy and asthma. It has been suggested that this may occur because viral infection reduces T-helper cell type 2 responses that would normally facilitate allergy development.

Reference

Newman-Taylor A 1995 Environmental determinants of asthma. Lancet 345: 296-299

169. Occupational asthma

A. **F**   B. **T**   C. **F**   D. **F**   E. **F**

Occupational asthma is a diagnosis which carries great socioeconomic implications for industry, the state and the individual. Irritant induced asthma and pre-existent idiopathic asthma aggravated by work are forms of occupational asthma which may require modifications to the workplace, but do not necessitate removal of the individual from their occupation. However, occupational asthma with latency (which is the most common form), once diagnosed, should be managed by prompt removal of the allergen or a change in occupation. The most important prognostic factor is the duration of symptoms prior to removal of the offending allergen. Because of this, early diagnosis following symptom onset is important.

Diagnosing occupational asthma is difficult as asthma is common within the general population. It should be suspected in all cases of new onset asthma in adults and in all cases where the patient is known to be working in an occupation with known causative agents, especially when symptoms improve at weekends or during holidays. Causative agents include cereals, enzymes, animal derived allergens, isocyanates, metals, formaldehyde and platinum salts.

A diagnosis of asthma requires a careful history and demonstration of variable airflow limitation or bronchial hyper-responsiveness to histamine or methacholine. Asthma has then to be related to work. Spirometry and peak flow evaluation before and after work are neither sensitive nor specific but have their place in diagnosis. They must be performed on more than one occasion. Serial measurements of forced expiratory volume over one second (FEV1) under supervision in the workplace is a more accurate method of diagnosis. For high molecular weight allergens like cereals, whose reactions are largely IgE mediated, immunological tests are simple and sensitive but not very specific. Specific inhalation challenges in a controlled laboratory environment will confirm a diagnosis. However, exposure has to be graded carefully to avoid high dose irritant effects and in 20% of cases of occupational asthma the results will be negative. Most occupational physicians use a combination of methods. Due to socioeconomic considerations and compensatory benefits, diagnosis must be confirmed by a specialist respiratory physician.

Reference

Chan-Yeung M, Malo J-L 1995 Occupational asthma. New England Journal of Medicine 333: 107-112.

170. Cystic fibrosis

A. F   B. F   C. T   D. T   E. T

171. Cystic fibrosis

A. F   B. F   C. T   D. F   E. F

Cystic fibrosis is a disorder of sodium and chloride excretion across epithelial cell membranes. It is an autosomal recessive disorder and is the commonest recessively inherited disorder in the UK with an incidence of 1 in 2000 live births reflecting a population carrier frequency of 1 in 25. The genetic locus is on the long arm of chromosome 7. There have been over 200 different genetic abnormalities described and this may account for the diverse spectrum of disease presentation and severity. The gene is composed of 250 000 base pairs coding for a 1480 amino acid protein called the cystic fibrosis transmembrane conductance regulator. In 70% of cases the defect is a three nucleotide deletion at the 508 position coding for phenylalanine.

The diagnosis is most commonly made in childhood but up to 3% of cases are first diagnosed over the age of 18. A family history should always be sought. Although chronic obstructive pulmonary disease is the most common cause of death in cystic fibrosis, patients are living longer and many now have a life expectancy of 20 to 30 years or longer. Presentation is diverse. In infants failure to thrive, diarrhoea, rectal prolapse and persistent cough should arouse suspicion. By childhood most patients have finger clubbing. They may have features of bronchiectasis with intermittent haemoptysis. Less common features include obstructive jaundice or signs of cirrhosis. In adolescence delayed puberty, and in adulthood infertility, become evident. Most, but not all, females are infertile. Males are invariably sterile. Adults may also present with nasal polyps and diabetes.

Diagnosis is by a pilocarpine induced sweat test. A sweat chloride of >60meq/l is suggestive of the diagnosis. False positives may be obtained in hypothyroidism, mucopolysaccharidoses, glycogen storage disorders and familial hypoparathyroidism. In addition respiratory disorders such as alpha-1-antitrypsin deficiency may cause false positive sweat test results.

The management of patients with respiratory complications of cystic fibrosis includes regular postural drainage of bronchial secretions. Bronchodilators may be of benefit and a trial of beta agonists is worthwhile in patients with asthmatic features. Viscous secretions contain DNA from inflammatory cells and there is evidence to suggest a role for inhaled human recombinant DNAse in improving lung function. Early in the disease acute respiratory decompensation is usually secondary to infection with *Staphylococcus aureus* and *Haemophilus influenzae*. Later colonization by *Pseudomonas aeruginosa* is common and requires treatment with intravenous and nebulized antibiotics. Pneumothorax is common in advanced disease.

In the future gene therapy may become a valid method of treating patients with cystic fibrosis. The principle of gene therapy in cystic fibrosis is to insert the cystic fibrosis transmembrane regulator (CFTR) gene into somatic gastrointestinal or respiratory cells of affected patients which would then express normal CFTR mRNA and manufacture the normal CFTR protein. A vector such as the adenovirus could be used for delivery. A small number of human studies have been conducted with encouraging results.

References

du Bois R M 1995 Respiratory medicine: recent advances. British Medical Journal 310: 1594-1598

Elborn J S 1994 Cystic fibrosis: prospects for gene therapy. Hospital Update 20: 13-20

Gaskin K J 1994 Gastrointestinal and hepatobiliary disease in cystic fibrosis. Medicine International. 22: 272-276

Rommens J M, Iannuzzi M C, Kerem B et al 1989 Identification of the cystic fibrosis gene: chromosome walking and jumping. Science 245: 1059-1065

172. Tuberculosis

A. **T**   B. **F**   C. **F**   D. **T**   E. **T**

173. Multi-drug-resistant tuberculosis

A. **T**   B. **T**   C. **F**   D. **F**   E. **F**

Before 1985 the industrialized world had experienced a steady decline in TB. The incidence of the disease is now increasing steadily. In 1992 the World Health Organization declared TB a global emergency. Worldwide 1.7 billion people have latent infection (one third of the world's population), with an annual toll of

8 million new cases and 2.9 million deaths. In terms of infectious diseases TB is the single biggest killer. HIV and TB co-infection have particularly devastating effects. TB leads to progression of HIV disease, and in HIV patients TB spreads rapidly, is often atypical, extrapulmonary and has a greater mortality. HIV is the most potent risk factor for TB. Currently the problem is most acute in Africa with 20–67% of TB patients being co-infected with HIV. The prospects for co-infection in Asia are daunting.

Primary resistance is defined as resistance to one or more drug in an individual who has not been previously treated for TB. Secondary resistance occurs in patients who have been on treatment for a fully sensitive organism. From an epidemiological stand-point, primary resistance implies that a TB control programmme has functioned poorly in the past whereas secondary resistance suggests that the current programme is failing. Multi-drug-resistant tuberculosis (MDRTB) is defined as resistance to at least rifampicin and isoniazid. These drugs form the backbone of most therapeutic regimens.

MDRTB is not new. In the 1950s when effective therapy was available, poor treatment programmes led to its development. The same is happening today. The brunt of the MDRTB epidemic has been in the USA, particularly in New York. In the USA, 3% of new cases, and 6.9% of recurrent cases are resistant to both rifampicin and isoniazid. Amongst those with HIV infection, transmission rates are high and death usually occurs in 1–4 months. Those without HIV have a 50% treatment-failure rate despite therapy for 18–24 months. Rates of MDRTB are increasing in Asia and Africa. The first UK cases have now been reported from an HIV centre in London.

The cause of the resurgence of TB is complex. Probably the most important factors are poverty and failure of strategies for TB control. Following the fall in incidence rates up to the mid-1980s, health planners in many nations drastically cut back on spending on TB programmes.

The mainstay of TB diagnosis is the identification of acid fast bacilli in clinical specimens. This does not distinguish *Mycobacterium tuberculosis* from atypical mycobacterial infection and gives no information on drug resistance. Culture to identify species and drug sensitivities can take 6–10 weeks. For this reason there has been interest in new methods for mycobacterial diagnosis and identification. These methods include use of the polymerase chain reaction to identify mycobacterial nucleic acid, radiometric culture, and liquid chromatography for mycolic acid. None of these techniques is widely available and all are expensive. An interesting technique to determine drug sensitivities rapidly is being developed. This involves the introduction of a gene coding for luciferase into mycobacteria. Only live mycobacteria emit light, so when antibiotics are added to the culture medium, if the bacillus is drug sensitive it stops emitting light.

Another interesting development which is particularly useful for studying the epidemiology of infection, has been the use of restriction fragment length polymorphism. A restriction enzyme cleaves certain sequences of the mycobacterial DNA, converting it into fragments which can be separated by gel electrophoresis to produce a strain specific fingerprint. Comparison of infecting strains between individuals gives information about route of transmission and whether reinfection or reactivation has led to disease.

Prevention of TB, and particularly MDRTB, depends on the implementation of effective control and treatment programmes. Combination preparations are important to prevent resistance. Where compliance is a concern, directly observed therapy should be instituted. For MDRTB as for sensitive TB nosocomial spread can be minimized by isolating smear positive cases for 2 weeks.

Patients co-infected with TB and HIV are treated in the UK with standard triple therapy. The treatment of MDRTB is difficult and mortality is high. Patients should be put on five or six chemotherapeutic agents which should be chosen on the basis of the laboratory sensitivity. Close contacts of patients with MDRTB should be considered for prophylaxis. One new therapeutic possibility is immunotherapy. By augmenting the immune response with, for example, cytokine therapy, patients with MDRTB may be cured of clinical infection despite the inadequacies of antimicrobial therapy.

References

Joint Tuberculosis Committee of the British Thoracic Society 1994 Control and prevention of tuberculosis in the United Kingdom: code of practice 1994. Thorax 49: 1193-1200

Malin A S, McAdam K P W J 1995 Escalating threat from tuberculosis: the third epidemic. Thorax 50 (Suppl 1): S37-S42

174. *Pneumocystis carinii*

A. **F**   B. **T**   C. **T**   D. **T**   E. **T**

Pneumocystis carinii was until recently considered to be a protozoa. Application of molecular biology techniques to its study have, however, established close gene homology with various fungal species, and most authors now consider the organism to be phenotypically and genetically an atypical fungus. Similar study techniques have established that different species of this fungus infect different host species, and at least in rats, one animal can be infected with more than one species. In studies on HIV negative health care workers it appears that pneumocystis can be carried asymptomatically, although most clinical infections appear to be caused by reinfection rather than reactivation. The organism is present in the environment, and amongst HIV positive individuals there is a marked seasonal variation in infection, with peaks in late spring and late summer. This probably reflects variation in temperature and humidity, factors which are important for fungal growth and sporulation.

P. carinii pneumonia (PCP) occurs most commonly in HIV patients with CD4 counts below 200. At seroconversion the CD4 count can fall dramatically, and PCP at this stage of infection is well documented. The classic clinical presentation in an HIV infected individual is shortness of breath on exertion or non-productive cough associated with diffuse bilateral interstitial shadowing on chest X-ray and arterial hypoxaemia. Atypical presentations include upper lobe shadowing, focal consolidation, nodular or cavitating lesions, hilar lymphadenopathy, small pleural effusions and gut and liver disease.

Many physicians empirically treat patients with a classic presentation, reserving bronchoscopy and bronchoalveolar lavage for those with atypical features or those who fail to respond to treatment. Exercise oximetry is a very sensitive screen for PCP. Failure to desaturate almost excludes the diagnosis. Measurement of transfer factor during lung function is non-specific, but if normal has a good negative predictive value. PCR on induced sputum for PCP is being used more often, having a sensitivity of about 80%. Indium-111 labelled human polyclonal immunoglobulin scanning can distinguish between infection with pulmonary Kaposi's sarcoma, and infection with pulmonary lymphoma. It is particularly useful for excluding PCP in a patient with pre-existing pulmonary Kaposi's sarcoma.

The treatment of choice for PCP is a 3-week course of high dose co-trimoxazole. Intravenous pentamidine is equally effective and dapsone and trimethoprim, clindamycin and primaquine and atovaquone are second line choices. Adjuvant steroids have been shown in trials to reduce morbidity and mortality in patients with a PaO_2 of less than 9.3 kPa. Nebulized pentamidine is now not recommended for the treatment of PCP because of its low response rate as well as an increased incidence of upper lobe and extrapulmonary relapse. Primary prophylaxis should be given to any patient with a CD4 count below 200 or any patient with an AIDS defining diagnosis regardless of their CD4 count. Secondary prophylaxis should be given to all patients. Co-trimoxazole is the prophylaxis of choice, but if not tolerated nebulized pentamidine, dapsone, dapsone with pyrimethamine and sulfadoxine with pyrimethamine are alternatives. 5% of patients with PCP die from the acute infection. Poor prognostic indicators include severe hypoxia, widespread X-ray shadowing and a prolonged history.

Reference

Miller R F, Mitchell D M 1995 *Pneumocystis carinii* pneumonia. Thorax 50: 191-200

175. The adult respiratory distress syndrome (ARDS)

A. F   B. T   C. T   D. F   E. T

ARDS is the term used to describe a pulmonary condition characterized by progressive hypoxaemia, chest X-ray infiltrates and reduced lung compliance in the presence of a normal left atrial pressure. The condition occurs in a wide variety of conditions. Sepsis accounts for as many as half of all cases. Other causes include drugs, smoke inhalation, acute pancreatitis, aspiration and trauma.

Early pathogenic changes in ARDS include neutrophil sequestration in the lungs and aggregation of intravascular fibrin-platelet aggregates. Injury to the capillary-alveolar barrier leads to increased pulmonary vascular permeability with lung inflammation and pulmonary oedema. Progressive obliteration of the pulmonary microvasculature occurs. Ventilation-perfusion mismatch leads to severe hypoxaemia. This is worsened by alveolar and small airway collapse. Lung injury is most prominent in dependant regions of the lung. There is a marked deficiency of surfactant and this probably adds to the abnormal lung mechanics. Decreased lung compliance in ARDS may be due to oedema, inflammation, or fibrosis. It may also reflect the reduced lung volume available for ventilation. Inflammation and oedema of the airways leads to increased airways resistance. Pulmonary hypertension occurs secondary to endothelial dysfunction which leads to thrombosis, perivascular oedema and eventual interstitial fibrosis. Overt right ventricular dysfunction may develop if pulmonary dysfunction is severe.

A number of mediators contribute to the pathology of ARDS. Complement activation with subsequent neutrophil activation and aggregation are major factors in injury to the lung. Activated neutrophils release cytokines, particularly tumour necrosis factor and interleukin-1, which participate in the inflammatory response. These processes lead to a coagulopathy, platelet activating factor and prostenoid release, platelet aggregation, induction of NO synthase and enhanced cellular oxidant production. Leucocyte adhesion molecules are expressed with enhanced neutrophil migration and activation. Hypoxic cellular injury also occurs. Reactive oxygen species overwhelm endogenous anti-oxidant defences leading to cellular damage. Cyclo-oxygenase and lipoxygenase products also play a role in the inflammatory process.

The current management for patients with ARDS involves identification and treatment of any underlying condition precipitating or perpetuating the ongoing acute lung injury, and supportive care involving mechanical ventilation, haemodynamic management and prevention of secondary complications.

Supplemental oxygen and positive pressure mechanical ventilation are critical supportive therapies to maintain adequate gas exchange and provide rest for the ventilatory muscles. There is convincing evidence that both prolonged high dose oxygen therapy and positive pressure ventilation can produce significant lung injury. Established strategies used to try and overcome these problems include use of a small tidal volume, optimizing positive end expiratory pressure and varying the inspiratory and expiratory time strategy.

ECMO is a technique by which blood is continuously removed from the circulation, passed through a membrane oxygenator and then returned. The results of controlled trials of ECMO in ARDS are discouraging and further technical advances will be necessary before this can be considered a realistic treatment option. A new experimental ventilatory support approach is the use of liquid fluorocarbons as a substitute for gas to maintain functional residual capacity. This is still in early clinical development.

Many other agents have been tried in ARDS. These include corticosteroids, anti-endotoxin monoclonal antibodies, tumour necrosis factor and interleukin-1 blockers, non-steroidal anti-inflammatory agents, inhaled surfactant, anti-oxidants and vasodilators such as inhaled nitric oxide. Despite promising anecdotal reports and supportive laboratory and animal model data, none of these agents has shown a survival benefit in well run trials of patients with ARDS. The groundwork has now been laid, however, for additional clinical trials to investigate new ways to reduce severe acute lung injury.

The outlook for patients with ARDS remains poor. There is a 50–70% mortality, and if failure of an organ in addition to the lungs supervenes, most patients will die. Of those who survive, most recover normal or near normal lung function. Only a small proportion, usually those that have required ventilatory support for many weeks, develop bronchiectasis or pulmonary fibrosis.

References

Fulkerson W J, MacIntyre N, Stamler J et al 1996 Pathogenesis and treatment of the adult respiratory distress syndrome. Archives of Internal Medicine 156: 29-38

Kooef M H, Schuster D P 1995 The acute respiratory distress syndrome. New England Journal of Medicine 332: 27-36

Strieter R M, Kunkel S L 1994 Acute lung injury: the role of cytokines in the elicitation of neutrophils. Journal of Investigative Medicine 42: 640-650

GASTROENTEROLOGY

176. Risk factors for hepatocellular carcinoma

A. T   B. T   C. T   D. T   E. T

177. Management of hepatocellular carcinoma

A. F   B. F   C. F   D. F   E. F

Hepatocellular carcinoma is the second most common malignancy in South-East Asia and its frequency is increasing in the West. Recent studies suggest that the prognosis can be markedly improved with early detection and treatment.

Studies have shown that cirrhosis is present in 60–90% of cases of hepatocellular carcinoma and the annual risk of developing malignant transformation in cirrhotics is about 3%. Hepatitis B viral infection is another major risk factor. One study from Taiwan revealed that the risk in HBsAg positive people is 390 times greater than in those who were HBsAg negative. Hepatitis B core antibody positivity in those who are HBsAg negative is also a major risk factor. It is thought that hepatitis C viral infection may increase the risk even more than hepatitis B. Alcoholics have a four fold increased incidence but it may be that it is the development of cirrhosis rather than the alcohol consumption per se which is causative. The mycotoxin aflatoxin produced by the mould *Aspergillus flavus* which contaminates ground nuts and grain is another important risk factor in some tropical countries. Other known aetiological factors include haemochromatosis, alpha-1-antitrypsin deficiency, glycogen storage diseases and porphyria cutanea tarda. Cirrhosis caused by autoimmune hepatitis, Wilson's disease and primary biliary cirrhosis are all rarely associated with primary hepatocellular carcinoma.

A variety of treatments have been shown to be beneficial. Orthotopic liver transplantation may produce a favourable outcome. In one study the survival rate at 4 years following liver transplantation for small non-resectable tumours without metastases in cirrhotics was 73% (small tumours being defined as one tumour less than 5 cm or three tumours not greater than 3 cm). In another study no recurrence was detected in the 14 patients who underwent transplantation for single tumours less than 4 cm in size with a mean follow-up of 23 months. Liver transplantation has the additional advantage of curing the underlying cirrhosis.

The results for resection are not as good, with 3-year survival rates of about 35% in cirrhotics with small tumours. Resection does not prevent progression of the underlying liver disease or the risk of malignant transformation in the remaining liver tissue. The results are more encouraging in those without cirrhosis.

Another useful technique is percutaneous ultrasound guided ethanol injection. One large series reported a 71% 3-year survival in well compensated cirrhotics with tumours less than 5 cm in diameter randomized to treatment compared with 26% in those not treated. Interferon treatment in cirrhotics with viral hepatitis may substantially reduce the risk of malignant change.

Primary prevention strategies aim to reduce the alcohol consumption and incidence of cirrhosis in the population as a whole. Those with cirrhosis should be regularly screened with alpha-fetoprotein measurement and ultrasound scanning, so that, more treatable tumours can be detected early. More sensitive techniques such as lipiodol angiography and enhanced MRI imaging can be used in equivocal cases. Other treatments such as chemoembolization, hormone manipulation and radioactive lipiodol treatment are used as adjuvant therapies and for the treatment of those unsuitable for surgical intervention.

References

Beasley R P 1982 Hepatitis B virus as an aetiological agent in hepato-cellular carcinoma-epidemiological considerations. Journal of Hepatology 2: 215

Hardell L, Bengtsson N O, Jonson U et al 1984 Aetiological aspects of primary liver cancer with special regard to alcohol, organic solvents and acute intermittent porphyria – an epidemiological investigation. British Journal of Cancer 50: 380

Livraghi T, Bolondi L, Buscarini L et al 1995 Treatment, resection and ethanol injection in hepatocellular carcinoma: a retrospective analysis of survival in 391 patients with cirrhosis. Journal of Hepatology 22: 522-526

McPeake J R, O'Grady J G, Zaman S et al 1993 Liver transplantation for primary hepatocellular carcinoma: tumour size and number determine outcome. Journal of Hepatology 18: 226-234

Mazzaferro V, Regalia E, Doci R et al 1996 Liver transplantation for the treatment of small hepatocellular carcinomas in patients with cirrhosis. New England Journal of Medicine 334: 693-699

Williams R, Rizzi P 1996 Treating small hepatocellular carcinomas. New England Journal of Medicine 334: 728-729

178. Colorectal cancer

A. T   B. T   C. T   D. T   E. F

Molecular biology has greatly increased our understanding of the pathogenesis of malignant transformation. The identification of genetic defects in tumour cells from a variety of different tissues has led to the discovery that many tumours arise as a result of multiple changes in a cell's genetic make-up. The loss of a tumour suppressor gene or the activation of an oncogene alone, are often insufficient triggers for malignant change.

In the West colonic cancer is very common with approximately a 6% lifetime risk. Both genetic and environmental factors are involved in its pathogenesis. The Western diet with its high fat and low fibre content has been implicated as an environmental risk factor. The inheritance of any single genetic defect appears to be insufficient on its own to effect malignant transformation. Additional somatic mutations are required.

Sporadic forms of the disease account for over 90% of cases. Similar genetic defects are seen in the tumour cells of sporadic and hereditary cases. The hereditary non-polyposis colorectal cancer syndromes (HNPCC), also called the Lynch or family cancer syndromes, account for 5–10%, and the hereditary polyposis syndromes account for approximately 1% of the annual incidence of colorectal carcinoma.

The hereditary polyposis syndromes familial adenomatous polyposis (FAP), Gardner's syndrome and Turcot's syndrome all carry a greatly increased risk of colorectal carcinoma. The gene which is abnormal in these conditions is thought to be the same. It is the adenomatous polyposis gene (APC) located on chromosome 5. It is a tumour suppressor gene, the protein product of which is able to suppress growth in malignant cells. The introduction of wild type APC into colonic cancer cell lines has been shown to suppress tumour growth. APC gene mutations can also be identified in nearly 70% of sporadic colorectal carcinomas and adenomatous polyps.

In HNPCC families several mismatch repair gene abnormalities have been discovered. Abnormalities in the function of these genes leads to genetic instability with the increased risk of oncogene activation or defective tumour suppressor gene production. This increases the risk of environmental genetic damage leading to oncogenesis.

Persons with inherited or familial colorectal cancer syndromes involving the APC gene have a constitutional or germ line lesion involving one allele of this gene. Aberrations in the APC gene lead to increased or abnormal colonic epithelial cell proliferation. As an individual gets older more cells are affected by somatic mutations as a result of free radical and other environmental damage. The descendants of such cells produce adenomatous polyps. Further somatic genetic mutations may eventually lead to malignancy. This theory of pathogenesis helps to explain why 90% of colonic tumours are thought to develop from adenomatous polyps. Individuals with no constitutional defect are less likely to develop a carcinoma but can do so as a result of progressive genetic damage occurring with increasing age.

Several genetic defects are known to be involved in colorectal cancer including K-ras point mutations, DCC (deleted in colorectal carcinoma) mutations and p53 deletions or mutations. Often oncogene over-expression is combined with defective or absent tumour suppressor gene activity.

Analysis of the precise genetic abnormalities involved in adenoma formation may prove to be an accurate guide to the future risk of developing carcinoma. It could then be used to give an indication of the need for colonoscopic screening. Certain genetic abnormalities are markers for poor prognosis whilst other defects suggest a better prognosis. This information can be used as a guide for the need for adjuvant chemotherapy after surgery. PCR has been used successfully to look for ras point mutations in patients' stool samples which may be useful for screening in the future. Gene therapy with the introduction of functional p53 or APC genes into colonic cancers in vivo may lead to improved prognosis if suitable well targeted vectors can be developed.

References

Groden J, Thliverrs A, Samowitz W et al 1991 Identification and characterization of the familial polyposis coli gene. Cell 66: 589-600

Groden J 1995 Colon-cancer genes and brain tumours. New England Journal of Medicine 332: 884-886

Hamilton S R, Liu B, Parsons R E et al 1995 The molecular basis of Turcot's syndrome. New England Journal of Medicine 332: 13; 839-847

Jen J, Kim H, Piantadosi S et al 1994 Allelic loss of chromosome 18q and prognosis in colorectal cancer. New England Journal of Medicine 331: 213-221

Rustgi A K 1994 Hereditary gastrointestinal polyposis and non-polyposis syndromes. New England Journal of Medicine 331: 1694 - 1703

Toribara N W and Sleisenger M H 1995 Current concepts: screening for colorectal cancer. New England Journal of Medicine 332: 861-868

179. Familial adenomatous polyposis

A. F   B. T   C. F   D. T   E. T

180. Extra-colonic features of familial adenomatous polyposis

A. T   B. T   C. T   D. F   E. T

The hereditary polyposis syndromes consist of familial adenomatous polyposis (FAP), Gardner's syndrome, Turcot's syndrome and the hamatomatous syndrome – Peutz-Jeghers syndrome.

FAP is an autosomal dominant condition characterized by the presence of hundreds to thousands of adenomatous polyps present throughout the large intestine which have usually become apparent by the third decade. About 20% of cases have no family history, suggesting that a spontaneous mutation has occurred. There is a high incidence of malignant transformation with the polyps, with nearly 80% of the cancers developing in the distal or left side of the colon.

A variety of extra-colonic features are well recognized in FAP including mandibular osteomas, polyps of the upper gastrointestinal tract, congenital hypertrophy of the retinal pigment epithelium, increased risk of peri-ampullary tumours and increased risk of carcinoma of the gastric antrum amongst Japanese families.

Gardner's syndrome produces the same colonic features as FAP but the extra-colonic features tend to be more apparent and varied. Carcinomas of the thyroid, adrenal glands, biliary tree and liver occur along with multiple lipomas. Non-steroidal drugs have been shown to lead to regression of polyps, but surgical resection is necessary once colonic polyps have developed, to prevent the development of carcinoma.

Gardner's syndrome, FAP and Turcot's syndrome (a condition in which colonic polyps are associated with an increased risk of colonic carcinoma and brain tumours) all result from mutations of the adenomatous polyposis coli (APC) gene. They have many similarities. The differences in phenotypic expression may depend on the nature and site of the mutation in the APC gene.

References

Groden J, Thliverrs A, Samowitz W et al 1991 Identification and characterization of the familial polyposis coli gene. Cell 66; 589-600

Rustgi A K 1994 Hereditary gastrointestinal polyposis and non-polyposis syndromes. New England Journal of Medicine 331: 1694-1703

Toribara N W and Sleisenger M H 1995 Current concepts: screening for colorectal cancer. New England Journal of Medicine 332: 861-868

181. Ulcerative colitis

A. F   B. T   C. T   D. F   E. T

182. Ulcerative colitis

A. T   B. F   C. F   D. F   E. F

Ulcerative colitis affects about 80 in 100 000 of the population. In 70% of cases the course of disease is of a relapsing colitis sometimes with long disease-free intervals. About 10% of cases have severe fulminant disease and about 10% only ever have one attack.

Presentation is usually with bloody diarrhoea, abdominal pain or weight loss. Occasionally the first presentation is with extra-gastrointestinal manifestations such as erythema nodosum. Associations exist between ulcerative colitis and ankylosing spondylitis, sacroiliitis and sclerosing cholangitis. These do not reflect disease activity. This is in contrast to skin and eye abnormalities such as pyoderma gangrenosum and iritis. There is an increased incidence of cholangiocarcinoma.

Severe disease is indicated by a tachycardia, fever, increased bowel frequency, anaemia and hypoalbuminaemia. Sometimes toxic dilatation of the colon may cause a reduction in the frequency and severity of diarrhoea. Toxic dilatation can be precipitated by the use of anti-diarrhoeal agents and their use is not recommended for symptom control. Hospital admission is advisable for severe attacks and failure of symptoms to settle with medical management in hospital is an indication for early surgical intervention.

Most patients are managed medically with 5-aminosalicylic acid (5-ASA) preparations and corticosteroids. Azathioprine is useful as a steroid sparing agent for troublesome disease. Cyclosporin has also been used with varying degrees of success. Most of the studies have been small and uncontrolled and in patients with severe ulcerative colitis. Side-effects of sulphasalazine are common and are mostly related to the sulphapyridine component. These include headaches, rash, haematological abnormalities and reduced male fertility which is reversible on stopping the drug. Preparations such as mesalazine and olsalazine do not have the sulphapyridine component. Rare side-effects of 5-ASA preparations include fibrosing alveolitis and interstitial nephritis. Uncommonly 5-ASA based agents exacerbate colitic symptoms.

A proportion of patients with ulcerative colitis will develop abnormal liver function tests. This may reflect fatty change in the liver or may be a result of progressive primary sclerosing cholangitis (PSC).

A long-term complication of ulcerative colitis is an increased incidence of colorectal carcinoma. Colitics with extensive disease are at risk and most centres offer carcinoma surveillance after 10 years of extensive disease. At 15 years the incidence of colon cancer is 3%, at 20 years it is 5% and at 35 years 30%. Persistent dysplasia on colonic biopsies is an indication for proctocolectomy.

References

Ferguson A 1994 Ulcerative colitis and Crohn's disease. British Medical Journal 309: 355

Forgacs I 1995 Clinical gastroenterology: recent advances. British Medical Journal 310: 113-116

Lee Y-M, Kaplan M M 1995 Primary sclerosing cholangitis. New England Journal of Medicine 332: 924-933

Mayberry J F, Rhodes J, Williams G T 1994 Ulcerative colitis. Medicine International 22: 314-320

Mills P R 1993 Management of ulcerative colitis. Prescribers Journal 33: 1-7

Nightingale J M D, Rathbone B J 1995 Inflammatory bowel disease. Update 52: 13-24

183. Crohn's disease

A. T   B. T   C. F   D. F   E. T

Crohn's disease is a chronic relapsing inflammatory disease which can affect any part of the gastrointestinal tract. It is equally common in men and women. It is exacerbated by smoking and can occur at any age. The incidence of Crohn's disease is increasing, affecting approximately 40 in 100 000 of the population. There is a familial incidence but the aetiology remains unclear. Recent studies have identified the persistence of the measles paramyxoma virus within the small bowel of some patients with Crohn's disease but whether this is related to the aetiology remains to be identified. There is an increased incidence in some genetic syndromes such as Turner's syndrome and tyrosine-positive albinism (Hermansky-Pudlak syndrome).

The inflammation seen in Crohn's disease is transmural and granulomata are characteristic histological abnormalities. Presentation is varied depending on the site of the disease. Oral ulceration is common, the rectum is often spared. Small bowel disease needs to be differentiated from yersinia infection, tuberculosis, carcinoma or lymphoma. Common presentations include abdominal pain, diarrhoea which may be bloody, fever and weight loss. Vitamin B12 deficiency may result if the terminal ileum is affected and inflammatory masses, bowel strictures and fistulae may complicate the disease.

Treatment can be medical or surgical. In general, strictures, masses or fistulae are treated surgically. The mainstay of medical treatment involves nutritional support, corticosteroids and 5-aminosalicylic acid preparations. For steroid dependent disease azathioprine is a useful steroid sparing agent, but side-effects such as pancreatitis and bone marrow suppression may limit its use. Elemental diets may be useful. Tolerance of these diets is poor and nasogastric administration may be required. Another useful treatment is long-term metronidazole. Peripheral neuropathy can complicate this but is usually reversible on discontinuing the drug.

Extra-gastrointestinal manifestations of Crohn's disease are less common than in ulcerative colitis and include episcleritis, iritis, arthropathy, venous thrombosis and erythema nodosum. The lifetime risk of colorectal carcinoma is small. Gallstones are common, especially following small bowel resection.

References

Jewell D 1994 Crohn's disease. Medicine International 22: 321-326

Lewin J, Dhillon A P, Sim R et al 1995 Persistent measles virus infection of the intestine: confirmation by immunogold electron microscopy. Gut 36: 564-569

Nightingale J M D, Rathbone B J 1996 Inflammatory bowel disease. Update 52: 13-24

Pearson D C, May G R, Fick G H et al 1995 Azathioprine and 6-mercaptopurine in Crohn's disease: a meta-analysis. Annals of Internal Medicine 122: 132-142

184. Whipple's disease

A. T B. T C. T D. T E. T

Whipple's disease classically presents with a malabsorption syndrome. Many patients, however, will have had arthralgia, cardiac or central nervous system involvement for many years before the onset of weight loss or diarrhoea. The disease most commonly affects middle aged men. The causative organism is thought to be *Tropheryma whippelii*. This organism has a characteristic appearance on electron microscopy, and polymerase-chain-reaction-based tests have been shown to be both sensitive and specific. These tests may facilitate earlier diagnosis in difficult cases.

Central nervous system involvement is relatively common. Dementia, ophthalmoplegia, myoclonus, and hypothalamic signs such as insomnia, hyperphagia and polydypsia are the most common manifestations. Oculomasticatory myorhythmia although rare is virtually pathognomonic. This consists of convergent nystagmus associated with palatal tongue and mandibular movements.

Patients may present with a variety of non-specific features such as pyrexia of unknown origin, a wasting syndrome or a sarcoidosis-like syndrome. Late diagnosis can lead to a less marked clinical response to antibiotic therapy. The PCR based tests use primers to amplify a known sequence coding for bacterial ribosomal RNA.

A duodenal biopsy showing periodic acid schiff (PAS) positive material remains the diagnostic test of choice. False negative biopsies do occur and false positive results can occur in the immunocompromised with atypical mycobacterial infections. The PCR based tests can be useful if the index of suspicion is high or if other tissues have been biopsied. Peripheral blood leucocytes are often PCR positive and this may prove to be a useful investigation.

References

Dobbins III W O 1995 The diagnosis of Whipple's disease. New England Journal of Medicine 332: 390-392

Rickman A L, Freeman W R, Green W R et al 1995 Uveitis caused by *Tropheryma whippelii* (Whipple's bacillus). New England Journal of Medicine 332: 363-367

185. Oesophageal achalasia

A. F   B. T   C. F   D. F   E. F

Achalasia of the oesophagus is a disease of unknown aetiology characterized by a lack of peristalsis in the body of the oesophagus, an increased lower oesophageal sphincter pressure with a failure of the lower oesophagus to relax during swallowing. This leads to stasis of food in the oesophagus with gradual dilatation over time. The incidence is around 1 in 100 000 in Western populations with both sexes being affected equally. There is degeneration of the myenteric plexus, vagal nerves and the dorsal vagal nuclei in the brain stem.

Dysphagia for both liquids and solids, active regurgitation, weight loss and pain are the most common symptoms. Regurgitation can also occur during sleep, and nocturnal cough and respiratory symptoms can be troublesome. Characteristic radiological features on barium swallow along with manometric findings are used to establish the diagnosis. Endoscopy is necessary to exclude a malignant stricture.

Drug therapies such as nitrates and calcium channel blockers have both been shown to reduce the lower oesophageal sphincter pressure in the short term. Their benefits tend to be minimal and short-lived and they are usually only used whilst awaiting more effective therapeutic measures. The current therapies of pneumatic balloon dilatation and surgical myotomy both have their disadvantages such as gastro-oesophageal reflux, stricture formation or oesophageal perforation.

Botulinum toxin is a potent neurotoxin which has been used to reduce skeletal muscle tone in a variety of clinical settings. In skeletal muscle it causes paralysis by binding to presynaptic nerve terminals and thereby inhibiting the release of acetylcholine at the neuromuscular junction. Direct injection of the toxin has been used successfully in the treatment of skeletal muscle disorders such as strabismus, blepharospasm, and laryngeal dystonia.

Botulinum toxin has been shown to reduce the lower oesophageal sphincter (LOS) pressure after direct injection directly into the LOS in patients with oesophageal achalasia, and this is thought to be due to a decrease in the excitatory cholinergic innervation of the sphincter muscle. It has been shown to be an effective therapy in oesophageal achalasia with benefits lasting for several months.

The long-term safety and efficacy of this treatment remain to be determined but this early work suggests it will prove to be a highly effective treatment. It is worth considering in patients with contraindications to either balloon dilatation or surgical myotomy. The indications for this therapy need to be established.

References

Cohen S and Parkman H P 1995 Treatment of achalasia - whalebone to botulinum toxin. New England Journal of Medicine 332: 815-817

Pasricha P J, Ravich W J, Hendrix T R et al 1995 Intrasphincteric botulinum toxin for the treatment of achalasia. New England Journal of Medicine 332: 774

186. *Helicobacter pylori* infection
A. **F**   B. **F**   C. **F**   D. **F**   E. **T**

187. *Helicobacter pylori* detection
A. **F**   B. **T**   C. **F**   D. **F**   E. **T**

The discovery of the spiral organism *Helicobacter pylori* in 1984 by Warren and Marshall has revolutionized the treatment of peptic ulcer disease. A strong association was discovered between *H. pylori* colonization of the gastric antral mucosa and duodenal ulceration and antral gastritis. There is now strong evidence to suggest a causative role for this organism in the pathogenesis of peptic ulcer disease and probably in gastric carcinoma and lymphoma. Prior to its discovery peptic ulcers could be successfully treated with H2 antagonists or proton pump inhibitors but the relapse rate was over 50%. With successful eradication of *H. pylori* relapse rates of under 5% per year can be achieved.

H. pylori is extremely common with a prevalence of about 50% in Western countries and much higher rates in many developing countries. The prevalence increases with age with around 20% of 20-year-olds and over 50% of the over 50s infected. The prevalence is also dependent on geographical location. In West Africa, for example, as many as 80% of 5-year-olds are infected. Infection is much more common in the socially deprived.

Many of those infected remain asymptomatic throughout life and high national or regional prevalence rates do not always correlate with a high rate of peptic ulcer disease. The high prevalence in developing countries does not translate into a catastrophic incidence of peptic ulcer disease. *H. pylori* infection is found in over 95% of patients with duodenal ulcers and in 80% of those with gastric ulcers with no history of recent non-steroidal anti-inflammatory (NSAID) usage.

There are many ways to test for *H. pylori* infection, none of which is 100% sensitive or specific. The invasive tests which require biopsy samples of gastric mucosa, usually taken at endoscopy include histology, culture, gram stain and urease based tests. These tests are 80–95% sensitive and between 93–100% specific. The urease based tests often become positive in less than 2 hours allowing the endoscopist to initiate appropriate therapy on the same day. Most physicians recommend that such tests be performed on all patients with evidence of current or previous peptic ulcer disease at endoscopy.

Non-invasive tests include those which detect *H. pylori* antibodies in the serum, whole blood or saliva and radiolabelled carbon-urea breath tests. The antibody based tests have a high sensitivity of 85% or over, but their specificity depends upon the population studied as they cannot reliably distinguish between past and present infection, and can remain positive for years after successful eradication. The radiolabelled carbon-urea breath test is positive in ongoing infection in over 85% of cases.

The urease test and the breath test both detect *H. pylori* by demonstrating the activity of its urease enzyme. This enzyme catalyses the conversion of urea to ammonia and carbon dioxide. In the urease tests a sample of gastric mucosa is mixed in a small container with urea and a pH indicator. If *H. pylori* is present in the sample a colour change occurs. With the breath test the subject swallows a sample of urea which contains radiolabelled carbon 13 or 14. In the presence of *H. pylori*, the urea is broken down in the stomach and the carbon dioxide is absorbed and can subsequently be detected in the subject's breath.

H. pylori eradication is recommended in all cases of peptic ulcer disease and successful eradication has been shown to reduce symptoms and rates of relapse and complications. Eradication is not of proven value in the treatment of non-ulcer dyspepsia. Growing evidence suggests it is indicated in those at high risk of developing gastric carcinoma and in those with low grade mucosa associated lymphoid tissue (MALT) lymphoma. A variety of *H. pylori* eradication regimens have been studied. Dual therapy, triple therapy and quadruple therapy have been used in clinical trials with regimens lasting between 7 and 14 days. They all have their advantages and disadvantages with varying success rates, side-effects and costs. Triple therapy with colloidal bismuth subcitrate, metronidazole and either amoxycillin or tetracyline orally for 7–14 days has been most extensively used. These regimens have been shown to achieve high rates of eradication of 70–92%. Newer regimens incorporating proton pump inhibitors and H2 antagonists may achieve higher eradication rates.

References

Ching C K, Lam S K 1995 Drug therapy of peptic ulcer disease. British Journal of Hospital Medicine 54: 101-106

Gibaldi M. 1995 *Helicobacter pylori* and gastrointestinal disease. Journal of Clinical Pharmacology 35: 647-654

Marshall B J, Warren J R 1984 Unidentified curved bacilli in the stomach of patients with gastritis and peptic ulceration. Lancet i: 1311-1315

Walsh J H, Peterson W L 1995 The treatment of *Helicobacter pylori* in the management of peptic ulcer disease. New England Journal of Medicine 333: 984-991

188. Gallstones

A. F.   B. F   C. T   D. F   E. T

Gallstone disease is very common in the West and is becoming more common in developing countries. Gallstones become more prevalent with increasing age. Women are three times more commonly affected than men. Gallstones consist of cholesterol or pigment and many are mixed. Only 10% are calcified and therefore detectable on plain X-ray. The least invasive diagnostic test is ultrasound scanning which is also very sensitive. Stones in the common bile duct are more difficult to detect with ultrasonography, but duct dilatation, particularly in the presence of jaundice or abnormal liver function tests, indicates the need for further investigation. Endoscopic retrograde cholangiopancreatography (ERCP) or endoscopic ultrasound in these cases can clarify the diagnosis.

Many gallstones do not cause symptoms and are detected incidentally. If symptomatic, the most common history is of intermittent right upper quadrant pain often after a meal and lasting from 1 to several hours. The disease can be quiescent for prolonged periods between attacks. Stones obstructing the cystic duct can cause cholecystitis and those obstructing the common bile duct can cause cholangitis or progressive jaundice. Acute cholecystitis can be further complicated by gall bladder perforation, empyema or mucocoele. Gallstones can lead to acute pancreatitis. Gall bladder cancer is an uncommon long-term complication of gallstones. It is thought to be caused by bile stasis and recurrent infection rather than the presence of gallstones themselves. Recurrent infection is an indication for treatment. Asymptomatic disease does not warrant treatment.

The usual treatment for gallstones is surgery. Some medical therapies are also available for patients unwilling or unfit to undergo surgery. The oral bile salts, ursodeoxycholic acid and chenodeoxycholic acid can be used for non-calcified cholesterol stones of less than 1 cm in diameter if the gall bladder retains contractility and the gallstone volume is less than 50% of the gall bladder volume. Bile salts work slowly, achieving maximal effect after 6 months with no evidence of a continued benefit beyond 12 months. Extracorporeal shockwave lithotripsy may be used in conjunction with bile salt therapy but it is less effective when used on its own and is best suited to small stones. Pain during therapy is common. Complete clearance of stones with this treatment may take up to a year. Methyl-tert butylether infusion directly into the gall bladder via percutaneous access can dissolve 90% of gallstones within 4–10 hours but is not available in the UK. Although complementary and herbal remedies are widely used for symptom relief, there is little evidence to support their efficacy from controlled trials. The usual medical treatment for common bile duct stones is ERCP with stone retrieval, sphincterotomy and occasionally stenting. About 50% of patients treated non-surgically for gallstones develop recurrent symptoms within five years.

References

Managing patients with gallstones 1994 Drugs and Therapeutics Bulletin 32: 33-35

Tait N, Little J M 1995 The treatment of gallstones. British Medical Journal 311: 99-105

189. Primary sclerosing cholangitis

A. F   B. T   C. F   D. F   E. F

190. Treatment of primary sclerosing cholangitis

A. F   B. F   C. F   D. F   E. T

Sclerosing cholangitis results from progressive inflammation and loss of the intra-hepatic or extra-hepatic bile ducts. In the early stages the disease primarily affects the biliary system with little damage to hepatocytes. Eventually there is progression to biliary cirrhosis and liver failure. The condition has several causes. It can occur secondary to recurrent or persistent bacterial infection usually in the presence of biliary obstruction, secondary to impaired hepatic arterial supply, or secondary to opportunistic infections in the immunocompromised. Primary sclerosing cholangitis (PSC) is the name for this chronic cholestatic liver disease when the aetiology is unknown. It has a strong association with inflammatory bowel disease.

PSC is the third commonest indication for liver transplantation amongst adults in the UK. The prevalence is about 3 cases in 100 000. Males are twice as commonly affected as females. In 75% of cases there is inflammatory bowel disease of which over 80% is ulcerative colitis. In patients with a diagnosis of ulcerative colitis 2.5–7.5% have or will develop PSC. The mean age at diagnosis is 40 years. The pathogenesis is poorly understood. There is an association with other autoimmune diseases and there are HLA associations. Animal models suggest an infectious aetiology.

25% of cases of PSC are diagnosed following the detection of abnormal liver function tests during follow-up for inflammatory bowel disease. Some present with established cirrhosis and portal hypertension and others with weight loss, right upper quadrant pain, pruritus or fatigue.

There is no specific diagnostic test. The diagnosis is most commonly made at ERCP which characteristically reveals a beaded appearance with strictures and dilatations affecting the intra-hepatic, extra-hepatic or the whole biliary system. Where there is a dominant stricture cholangiocarcinoma must be excluded. Liver biopsy is usually performed but the characteristic onion skin appearance in the portal tracts with fibrous tissue surrounding small bile ducts is relatively rarely seen. The common histological features include reduced numbers of bile ducts, copper deposition and piecemeal necrosis. Histology is used to stage the disease. Other causes of sclerosing cholangitis should be excluded.

The medical treatment consists of giving fat-soluble vitamin supplements, symptomatic treatment for pruritus and antibiotic therapy for recurrent cholangitis. Prophylactic antibiotic therapy with ciprofloxacin is given to reduce the incidence of ascending cholangitis. No specific medical therapy has been shown to halt the progression of the disease process or prolong life. Corticosteroids are of no benefit. Combination therapies using agents such as methotrexate and ursodeoxycholic acid are being studied. Dominant strictures can be treated surgically or endoscopically with or without stents. Frequently there is no biliary response to treatment of any associated inflammatory bowel disease and the condition can even present many years after total colectomy.

Usually the disease slowly progresses until cirrhosis or cholangiocarcinoma develop. Cholangiocarcinoma is difficult to diagnose for several reasons. Bile duct cytology from ERCP brushings often gives false negative results. CT or MRI scanning can be helpful but are not diagnostic and may miss small lesions. The tumour marker CA19-9 is often elevated but it is also elevated in PSC without cholangiocarcinoma. Cholangiocarcinoma has been found unexpectedly in the explanted liver in around 10% of cases in some studies. It is a difficult condition to treat with a poor prognosis but small incidental tumours may be cured by transplantation.

The treatment of choice for advanced disease is liver transplantation. The 3-year survival post-transplantation is 60–85%. The timing can be difficult, and the risks of the operation should be weighed against the risks of end stage liver disease and the development of cholangiocarcinoma.

Reference

Lee Y-M, Kaplan M 1995 Primary sclerosing cholangitis. New England Journal of Medicine 332: 924-933

---

191. Hepatitis E virus infection

A. **F**   B. **T**   C. **F**   D. **T**   E. **T**

Hepatitis E is a 27–34 nm diameter unenveloped, single stranded, positive sense RNA virus. The true incidence of this infection is unknown. In some Western countries more than 2% of blood donors are seropositive but it would appear a much lower percentage have suffered from symptomatic hepatitis E infection. Most of the world's recognized outbreaks and sporadic cases have occurred in developing countries. Those aged between 15 and 40 seem to be the most likely to develop symptomatic infection.

The incubation period is 2–9 weeks. Overall the mortality rate is thought to be between 0.5% and 4.0% but in pregnant women some studies have found it to be as high as 25%. These figures are based on outbreaks in developing countries and the contribution of malnutrition and coexistent disease to these mortality rates is unknown. The natural history in the majority of cases is of a self-limiting viral hepatitis.

Large water-borne outbreaks have occurred such as in the Xinjang Uighar region of China, which resulted in more than 100 000 cases of jaundice. Similar outbreaks have also occurred in India, Pakistan, Africa, and Mexico. Hepatitis E can also be transmitted vertically and by the faecal-oral route. There is at present inadequate data regarding transmission in body fluids such as semen and saliva. No animal hosts have yet been identified. Further research is needed to increase our knowledge and improve our management of this viral infection.

Reference

Scharschmidt B F 1995 Hepatitis E: a virus in waiting. Lancet 346: 519-520.

192. Hepatitis C virus infection
A. T   B. T   C. F   D. F   E. T

193. Treatment of hepatitis C virus infection
A. F   B. F   C. F   D. F,   E. T

Hepatitis C virus is a positive stranded RNA virus of just over 9000 nucleotides. It can cause a benign, asymptomatic disorder but it can also progress to chronic liver disease with serious consequences. The disease progression and the response to therapy is affected by host and viral factors.

The virus is found in 0.5–8.0% of blood donors world-wide. The disease follows a chronic course in more than 60% of those infected. The acute infection is often asymptomatic with only about 25% suffering from an icteric illness. Approximately 20% of patients develop cirrhosis after 20 years. As many as 10% of those with cirrhosis will develop hepatocellular carcinoma. The most common forms of transmission are through blood products and intravenous drug abuse. It is rarely transmitted through sexual contact and can be vertically transmitted only where there is significant viraemia.

Hepatitis C viral infection is often diagnosed in asymptomatic patients who have been found to have elevated transaminases during routine screening. It is also found in a high proportion of those previously diagnosed as suffering from non-A, non-B transfusion related hepatitis and in those previously diagnosed as having cryptogenic cirrhosis. Infection with hepatitis C virus can be diagnosed using assays which detect the presence of antibodies to a variety of hepatitis C antigens. The second and third generation assays are highly sensitive and specific.

The polymerase chain reaction can be used to detect the presence of hepatitis C virus RNA. It may be positive in those with normal transaminases and can be negative in those with elevated transaminases. It is also occasionally positive in patients who are negative on antibody testing. This usually occurs in immuno-suppressed, haemodialysed or agammaglobulinaemic individuals with chronic non-A non-B hepatitis. Quantitative assays are available for assessing the level of viraemia and are useful in predicting the prognosis and response to treatment.

Hepatitis C virus is made up of a heterogeneous group of RNA viruses which are members of the flavivirus family. The classification of hepatitis C virus is based on genetic sequencing with each strain having characteristic, relatively conserved sequences. The current system of nomenclature consists of six main groups with each group having subtypes. These different genotypes demonstrate a geographical variation in distribution.

Certain genotypes may be more pathogenic with a greater incidence of subsequent cirrhosis and hepatocellular carcinoma. The genotype also seems to influence response to medical therapy and the lag time to recurrent hepatitis following liver transplantation.

Interferon alpha is the treatment of choice for hepatitis C infection. The precise indications for therapy and the ideal dose and duration are still open to debate. Raised transaminases, detectable viraemia, and hepatitic features on liver biopsy are all features which suggest the need for treatment. Genotyping when available can also be helpful. Overall about 50% of patients will demonstrate a response by 6 months and the majority of these will have detectable falls in transaminase activity by 2–3 months (no response at this stage is an indication for withdrawal of therapy). In relatively unselected patient groups 80–85% relapse when interferon therapy is stopped.

Factors predicting a poor response to medical therapy include old age, the presence of cirrhosis, high titres of viral RNA, alcohol consumption and male sex.

Ribavirin is an oral guanosine analogue which produces little sustained effect on its own. Interferon alpha plus ribavirin seems to produce a better response than interferon alpha alone but further trial data is awaited. A variety of other medical treatments are being investigated including the use of ursodeoxycholic acid, iron depletion and N-acetylcysteine.

If the patient fails to respond to medical treatment, cirrhosis, liver failure or hepatocellular carcinoma may ensue. Following liver transplantation, more than 90% of cases show recurrence of hepatitis C virus infection within 3 months, but the 2-year post transplant survival seems to be similar in cases of hepatitis C virus infection to that of cirrhosis due to other causes.

References

Dusheiko G M, Khakoo S, Soni P et al 1996 A rational approach to the management of hepatitis C infection. British Medical Journal 312: 357-363

Report of meeting of physicians and scientists, Royal Free Hospital and School of Medicine, London 1995 Genetic diversity of hepatitis C virus: implications for pathogenesis, treatment, and prevention. Lancet 345: 562-567

194. Variceal haemorrhage in patients with cirrhosis
A. T   B. F   C. F   D. F   E. F

195. Prevention of recurrent variceal haemorrhage
A. F   B. F   C. F   D. F   E. T

Bleeding from oesophageal varices is a major life threatening complication of portal hypertension usually resulting from underlying liver cirrhosis. Management involves identification of the at risk population so that prophylactic measures can be instituted, and the treatment of acute bleeding episodes and prevention of recurrent haemorrhage.

Merkel and colleagues found the major risk factors predicting variceal haemorrhage in those with oesophageal varices were large varices, hepatic venous wedge pressure gradients (HVPG) greater than 12 mmHg, previous variceal haemorrhage and a high Pugh's score. Variceal size is usually assessed endoscopically. The HVPG is the difference between the hepatic venous pressure and the hepatic wedge pressure which approximates to the portal pressure. Variceal bleeding is unusual with gradients below 12 mmHg.

Child's classification of the severity of cirrhosis giving a grade A, B or C was modified by Pugh. Pugh's score is used to quantify the degree of cirrhosis looking at five parameters. It gives a value between 5 and 15, and the higher the score the more severe or advanced the cirrhosis. The Child–Pugh grading also influences prognosis after a first bleed with those classified as grade A having a mortality of less than 10% and those with grade C having a mortality of over 50%. Continued drinking confers a significant risk to those with alcoholic cirrhosis, increasing the risk of rebleeding from 10 to 50%.

The risk of a first bleed can be reduced significantly with non-selective beta blockade, if this reduces the HVPG. The dose should be adjusted so that the resting pulse rate is reduced by 25%. Some studies have also shown reduced bleeding and mortality rates after prophylactic endoscopic sclerotherapy but this is a more costly and potentially dangerous procedure and is not widely used as primary prophylaxis of variceal haemorrhage. Surgical shunts such as portocaval shunts are not widely used prophylactically as early studies showed no survival advantage.

Acute bleeding can be treated in a variety of ways. Most centres use drug treatment and endoscopic therapy, either with endoscopic sclerotherapy or band ligation as first line. Treatments with balloon tamponade, transjugular intra-hepatic portosystemic shunts (TIPS) and surgery are reserved for those who fail to respond to first line therapy.

Vasopressin causes splanchnic arterial vasoconstriction and therefore reduces portal flow. It also causes systemic vasoconstriction and reduced coronary arterial blood flow, and should be used with caution in those with ischaemic heart disease. Intravenous nitrates reduce portal pressures further and improve coronary flow and are therefore useful as combination treatment with vasopressin. Somatostatin decreases splanchnic flow without the systemic hypertension and reduced coronary flow but has a very short half-life. Ocreotide is a synthetic analogue of somatostatin with a longer half-life. Both have been shown to be as effective at controlling bleeding as injection sclerotherapy.

Sclerotherapy achieves adequate haemostasis in approximately 70% of acute cases. Further sessions are then required to achieve variceal obliteration. Complications include oesophageal ulceration and subsequent stricture formation, local or systemic sepsis and oesophageal perforation. Endoscopic variceal band ligation is a newer alternative which appears to be as effective and may have fewer side-effects.

Balloon tamponade using devices such as the Sengstaken-Blackemore tube controls bleeding in 70–80% of cases. About 50% rebleed when the balloons are deflated and there is a high complication rate with up to15–20% suffering severe adverse events.

Interventional radiological procedures such as the transjugular intra-hepatic shunt (TIPS) and surgical intervention in the acute setting are usually reserved for those who have failed to respond to medical therapy. The surgical procedures include portosystemic shunts and oesophageal transection.

The prevention of rebleeding can be achieved by endoscopic sclerotherapy, band ligation, drug therapy and surgery. Beta-blockers and sclerotherapy have been shown to be equally efficacious in reducing the incidence of rebleeding. Neither therapy has been shown to improve mortality. Surgical shunts and TIPS significantly reduce the incidence of rebleeding but do not improve survival. These can be very useful as holding procedures prior to liver transplantation.

References

Burroughs A K 1991 Somatostatin and ocreotide for variceal bleeding. Journal of Hepatology 13: 1-4

Merkel C, Bolognesi M, Bellon S et al 1992 Prognostic usefulness of hepatic vein catheterisation in patients with cirrhosis and portal oesophageal varices. Gastroenterology 102: 973-979

Pagliaro L, D'amico G, Sorensen T et al 1992 Prevention of first bleeding in cirrhosis. Annals of Internal Medicine 117: 59-70

Sandord N L, Kerlin P 1995 Current management of oesophageal varices. Australian and New Zealand Journal of Medicine 25: 528-534.

196. Transjugular intra-hepatic portosystemic shunt (TIPS)

A. F   B. F   C. F   D. F   E. F

The transjugular intra-hepatic portosystemic shunt (TIPS) is a percutaneous technique for reducing portal hypertension. It is most commonly used for treating bleeding oesophageal varices. It can also be used to treat intractable ascites and the hepatorenal syndrome.

A specifically designed needle called a Colapinto needle is introduced via the internal jugular vein. It is used to create an artificial tract through the liver parenchyma, between the portal vein and the right hepatic vein. This is performed with fluoroscopy or ultrasound guidance. The portal pressure is then measured directly before a balloon catheter is used to dilate the tract. A stent is then inserted to prevent stenosis of the tract. It is often a lengthy procedure taking several hours.

Technical success, defined as the placement of a stent between the portal and hepatic venous systems with a reduction in the pressure gradient between the portal and hepatic vein to below 15 mmHg is achieved in 75–100% of cases. The mortality rate and technical success of the procedure are dependent upon the level of operator expertise and patient selection.

The most serious complications include internal haemorrhage, puncture site haematoma, fever, haemobilia, bacteraemia, transient oliguric renal failure and myocardial infarction. The procedure can precipitate portosystemic encephalopathy by increasing the volume of blood which bypasses the liver parenchyma. Reducing the diameter of the stent by placing a second stent inside the first is usually effective at controlling this.

The procedure has a high success rate in controlling variceal haemorrhage with initial control in up to 93% of cases. Rebleeding does occur but usually follows stent stenosis or blockage. Doppler ultrasound scanning can screen for changes in flow through the stent, enabling early stent dilatation to be arranged.

The control of ascites is another indication for the procedure with significant improvement in over 80% of cases. The high success rate has to be weighed against the significant mortality and morbidity associated with this procedure.

There has been little comparison with surgical shunts. There is no evidence that the procedure leads to any significant reduction in mortality. Patients requiring TIPS for uncontrolled variceal haemorrhage often fall into poor prognostic groups because of the severity of their underlying liver disease. Most deaths are not due to procedural complications or technical failure but are due to the complications of the underlying liver disease.

Debate still continues about the precise indications for TIPS. It can be very useful in controlling complications whilst a patient is being prepared for liver transplantation. Patients with low grade cirrhosis who do not require emergency intervention may be better treated with surgical shunts.

Reference

Skeens J, Semba C, Dake M 1996 Transjugular portosystemic shunts. Annual Review of Medicine 46: 95-102

EMERGENCY MEDICINE
197. Advanced cardiac life support
A. F   B. F   C. F   D. F   E. F

The European Resuscitation Council guidelines for advanced life support were updated in 1992. They attempted to base their recommendations on evidence and produce algorithms which were simple to follow. The importance of minimizing delay in delivering defibrillating shocks in ventricular fibrillation (VF) was stressed, as this offers the best chance of a successful outcome. Defibrillation should be attempted if there is any possibility that the underlying rhythm could be VF. If cardiac monitoring equipment is not available and VF is a possibility, defibrillation should be attempted.

Adrenaline is the first drug given in an arrest, whether it is due to VF, electromechanical dissociation or asystole. It is given because of its actions as a peripheral vasoconstrictor which redirects blood flow to vital organs. Lignocaine is not included in the guidelines as a first line agent in VF. It may be used, however, as it is an effective agent at suppressing malignant arrhythmias, but this needs to be balanced against its negatively inotropic effect.

If a patient has unreactive pupils during an arrest this suggests a poor prognosis. It does not, however, always reflect the presence of irreversible brain damage. It should be remembered that drugs used during an arrest as well as pre-existing eye disease could be responsible for pupillary signs.

Basic and advanced life support has already featured in MRCP Part two exams and is likely to be included in Part one in the near future. Perusal of the guidelines is strongly recommended.

Reference

European Resuscitation Council guidelines 1992 (abridged) 1993 British Medical Journal 306: 1589-1593

198. Hypothermia

A. F.   B. F   C. T   D. F   E. T

Hypothermia is defined as a fall in core body temperature below 35°C. The diagnosis may be missed, as hypothermia can cause many physical signs, particularly central nervous system abnormalities ranging from mild confusion to deep coma. The elderly and neonatal populations are most at risk.

Management is focused on basic life support measures and more advanced measures based on recognition of the complications of hypothermia. Hypocapnia, alkalosis and hypothermia all shift the oxygen haemoglobin dissociation curve to the left which causes reduced oxygen delivery to the tissues. A lactic acidosis is generated by tissue hypoxia and shivering, and is complicated by impaired hepatic and renal function. Acidosis should be corrected gradually as the rewarming process will itself increase the efficiency of normal acid-base control.

Fluid shifts are common and accurate fluid balance management is required. Tissue perfusion may be compromized by vasodilation during rewarming, decreased oral intake and cold induced diuresis. Colloid plasma expansion may then be required. Nasogastric intubation is indicated because of the risk of ileus and aspiration.

Hyperkalaemia resulting from acidosis, rhabdomyolysis and renal failure may occur, and electrocardiographic changes indicating cardiotoxic effects may be masked by the hypothermia. Hypoglycaemia may be a cause of accidental hypothermia. Hyperglycaemia may indicate diabetic ketoacidosis as a cause or pancreatitis as a complication of accidental hypothermia.

Coagulopathies are common and cannot be predicted by normal coagulation profiles which are only accurate at 37ºC. Decreased platelet activity occurs due to impaired thromboxane B2 production and cold will directly suppress the bone marrow causing thrombocytopenia. Conversely, hypercoagulable states also occur with a rising haematocrit.

Septicaemia should be treated if there is a clinically apparent focus or empirically if the patient is vulnerable as in the elderly, neonates or immunocompromised. White cell function is impaired in hypothermia and the white cell count is an unreliable marker of infection.

In the event of cardiac arrhythmias many drugs are ineffective, particularly digoxin. In general it is preferable to avoid using anti-arrhythmic agents if possible. The arrhythmia reflects the effect of cold on the heart and with rewarming it will usually resolve. Life threatening arrhythmias are best treated by rapid rewarming, extracorporeally if available. If an anti-arrhythmic is required bretylium should be considered.

Rewarming methods may be active or passive. If there is a perfusing rhythm present then passive rewarming can be used for cardiovascularly stable patients with a temperature greater than 32°C. In all other cases active methods are advisable. Methods include airway rewarming which is simple but slow. Countercurrent warming of colloids used in volume expansion is another method. More efficient methods are peritoneal lavage resulting in a rewarming rate of 2–4° per hour using 6 1 per hour exchanges with heated crystalloid dialysate. This also has the advantage of allowing dialysis in hyperkalaemic patients. In district general hospitals this is the most readily available method of faster rewarming and it can be used in the absence of a perfusing rhythm. The best method of active rewarming is extracorporeal rewarming using haemodialysis circuits or cardiac bypass circuits.

Reference

Danzl D F, Pozos R S 1994 Accidental hypothermia. New England Journal of Medicine 331: 1756-1760

---

199. ECG abnormalities in cocaine users

A. T   B. T   C. T   D. T   E. T

Cocaine is an alkaloid derived from the erythroxylin cocoa plant. Cocaine hydrochloride is water soluble, the free base form, 'crack', is not. Crack vaporizes at higher temperatures than the salt and can therefore be smoked. Peak effect and duration of action depend on the route of administration. Metabolism is liver dependent and cocaine metabolites are excreted in the urine.

The commonest presentations of cocaine use to the emergency departments are due to its cardiovascular effects. They are variable and may be fatal. Cocaine has both adrenergic and local anaesthetic action and its toxic effects are therefore complex. The commonest serious consequence on the cardiovascular system is acute myocardial infarction. Most patients develop chest pain within minutes. The mechanism is unclear but may be related to thrombus formation, increased oxygen demand and vaso-constriction. Cocaine may cause accelerated atherosclerosis.

Cocaine can also suppress myocardial activity and left ventricular dysfunction is well described, as is cardiomyopathy in association with prolonged use. Cardiac arrhythmias are common and many ECG abnormalities are recognized. These include ventricular tachycardia and fibrillation, supraventricular tachycardia, atrioventricular nodal block, complete heart block and asystole. Other changes supporting the diagnosis of cardiotoxicity in suspected cases include a prolonged PR interval, a wide QRS complex and a prolonged QT interval. Reports of cocaine-associated aortic rupture, endocarditis, pneumopericardium and left ventricular hypertrophy have been published.

Reference

Mouhaffel A H, Madu E C, Satmary W A et al 1995 Cardiovascular complications of cocaine. Chest 107: 1426-1434.

200. Paracetamol overdose

A. **F.**   B. **T**   C. **T**   D. **T**   E. **T**

Paracetamol is the most commonly used drug in deliberate overdose. Liver failure due to paracetamol overdose accounts for half of tertiary liver unit referrals and for up to 150 deaths each year in the UK.

Several normograms are available for the management of paracetamol poisoning. These were developed using retrospective observations on untreated patients before the effective antidotes N-acetyl cysteine (NAC) and methionine were introduced. They predict the likelihood of developing transaminase levels > 1000 iu/l. Their value in treating children has never been evaluated.

Certain groups of patients are much more sensitive to the toxic effects of paracetamol. These include patients with anorexia nervosa and alcoholics, both of whom are glutathione depleted. These patients should be treated at much lower thresholds than the standard normograms suggest. For patients on enzyme inducing drugs such as anticonvulsants or isoniazid it is suggested that antidote administration should be commenced even if paracetamol is only just detectable.

60% of untreated patients with paracetamol levels > 200 mg/l at 4 hours will develop hepatotoxicity. As many as 90% will do so if the level is > 300 mg/l and it is in this group that most deaths occur. There is evidence to suggest that gastric lavage or activated charcoal have some use in reducing blood levels up to 1 hour post overdose. Activated charcoal seems to be the more effective. Available evidence suggests that when treatment is commenced less than 10 hours after the overdose it is highly likely to prevent death, although a significant proportion of patients will develop liver failure. NAC should be started before levels are available in all patients who have increased vulnerability to the toxic effects of paracetamol or who have ingested > 150 mg/kg. This also applies if there is doubt about the quantity of paracetamol taken.

Although both oral NAC and methionine are effective antidotes, in practice intravenous NAC is used as it induces less vomiting and is therefore likely to be more effective. Data from King's College Hospital liver unit strongly supports the use of NAC in overdoses that present late and continued use beyond the standard 20 hour regime in fulminant liver failure. Adverse reactions are uncommon and severe reactions such as hypotension, wheeze and urticaria can usually be managed by stopping the infusion temporarily and giving an anti-histamine.

In patients developing severe hepatic damage, younger patients with high peak bilirubin concentrations have the best prognosis, whereas those with prothrombin times >180 s, creatinine > 300 umol/l or uncorrectable acid-base abnormalities have the least favourable prognosis.

Reference

Vale J A, Proudfoot A T 1995 Paracetamol (acetaminophen) poisoning. Lancet 346: 547-552

Viva questions

1. A patient presents to your clinic for a second opinion. He gives a history of right arm and face weakness lasting 6 hours. At another hospital he has had investigations including carotid doppler studies, which revealed a 70% stenosis of the left internal carotid artery. How would you manage the patient?

2. Your consultant asks you to confirm a diagnosis of brain death on a patient in intensive care who has suffered a severe head injury. How would you go about this task, and what special tests may be necessary?

3. Do you think it is safe to eat British beef?

4. What genetic risk factors do you know for ischaemic heart disease?

5. A 45-year-old man is referred to clinic by his GP. He is increasingly muddled and has started to lose things. His mother and maternal aunt suffered from Alzheimer's disease in middle age. He is concerned about his risk of developing Alzheimer's disease, what advice would you give him?

6. A 35-year-old woman comes to see you. Her mother died at the age of 40 from carcinoma of the breast. What advice would you give her to minimize her chances of developing this disease?

7. What is hereditary haemorrhagic telangectasia? What are its complications? Do you know any recent discoveries about its genetic basis?

8. Animal models have proven very useful in studying the mechanisms of human diseases. Do you know of any examples?

9. There has been much written in the journals about gene therapy. What do you understand by this term, and do you know of any conditions where gene therapy might be useful?

10. Other than gene therapy, do you know of any methods that experimenters can use to manipulate the expression of genes?

11. Do viruses cause cancer?

12. What are oncogenes? How in the future might we fight cancer by combating their effects?

13. What do you understand by the term xenotransplantation?

14. Do you know of any relationship between particular human leucocyte antigens and disease? Can testing patients for particular antigens be useful clinically?

15. How do you think a cancer manages to maintain a blood supply as it grows and expands?

16. What do you understand by the terms, Western blotting, Southern blotting and polymerase chain reaction?

17. Vitamin K is required to synthesize factors involved in clotting. Do you know any vitamin K dependent proteins that are not involved in clotting?

18. A patient being investigated for anaemia has a blood film and bone marrow aspirate consistent with chronic myeloid leukaemia. How might analysis of the patient's chromosomes help confirm the diagnosis? Describe your approach to the management of such a patient.

19. A 34-year-old woman presents with pleuritic chest pain. A ventilation perfusion scan suggests a high probability of a pulmonary embolus. How would you manage the patient? Would any further investigations be indicated in the light of recent discoveries about the causes of venous thrombosis and embolism?

19. In patients requiring chemotherapy, myelosuppression is often a dose limiting side-effect. What are the risks associated with myelosuppression, and do you know of any recent developments in its treatment?

20. What is graft-versus-host disease? Can it ever be advantageous? What diseases can be treated with bone marrow transplantation?

21. A 70-year-old patient presents with shortness of breath on exertion. The full blood count reveals a haemoglobin of 9, platelets of 150 and a total white cell count of 56. What is the likely diagnosis? How would you treat this condition in the light of recent trials?

22. Should all patients with ischaemic heart disease be offered coronary artery by-pass grafting?

23. Do you think that plenty of vitamin C and E in the diet are important? Do you know of any data suggesting that their consumption may reduce the risk of ischaemic heart disease?

24. What do you understand by the term hibernating myocardium?

25. Do you know anything about the physiology of vitamin A? Do you know any conditions where its derivatives may have therapeutic potential?

26. Do you think calcium channel blockers have a role in acute myocardial infarction?

27. Amiodarone has many side-effects. What are they? When might you consider using this drug, and can you support your practice with any evidence?

28. What are the advantages and disadvantages of meta-analysis?

29. Do you think clinical medicine should be evidence-based?

30. What nosocomial infections have complicated your patients' treatment and what measures should we adopt to reduce these complications?

31. HIV infection has until recently been considered a terminal illness. Many now consider it a chronic disease. Do you know of any therapeutic measures which might improve the outlook for an HIV patient? Can you back up your suggestions with any trial data?

32. How would you reduce the vertical transmission of HIV?

33. What advice would you give to a traveller visiting a country where malaria is endemic?

34. Influenza is a major cause of morbidity and mortality. What strategies would you employ during an epidemic? Has any treatment been shown to be effective?

35. What are the advantages of tight glycaemic control in diabetics?

36. A diabetic patient presents to your clinic with oedema. Investigations reveal that he has heavy proteinuria hypoalbuminaemia and renal impairment. How could you have avoided this situation developing, and how would you continue to manage the patient?

37. What are the British Thoracic Society guidelines for the management of asthma? What are the markers of a severe asthma attack?

38. A 30-year-old man presents with a 3-week history of increasing shortness of breath on exertion and fever. He is HIV positive. What is your differential diagnosis and how would you manage the patient?

39. What causes asthma? Do you think air pollution plays a role? Can you back up your opinion with any evidence?

40. An obese 50-year-old man is referred to your clinic. He complains of being constantly tired and often waking with a headache. His new wife (his third), complains that his snoring can be heard from the other end of the house. How would you investigate this patient? Is any treatment available?

41. Tuberculosis is becoming more common. Why do you think this is? Do you know of any recent advances which can facilitate diagnosis? Why might a patient not respond to treatment?

42. What are the advantages and disadvantages of pulse oximetry?

43. What are the main priorities in cardiopulmonary resuscitation?

44. How would you diagnose Paget's disease? How would you treat a patient with bone pain caused by Paget's disease?

45. A 28-year-old patient suffered a head injury 4 weeks ago in a motor bike accident. He is unconscious, but does not require respiratory support. He is unresponsive to all external stimuli, but has cycles of eye opening and closing. What are the possible diagnoses? What are the criteria for diagnosing the persistent vegetative state?

46. A 40-year-old bus driver is referred to you having had one witnessed grand mal seizure. How would you assess him? When can he drive again?

47. What do you understand by the genetic term anticipation? Do you know of any diseases in which it occurs?

48. What is the role of thrombolysis in the treatment of acute stroke?

49. How is Duchenne muscular dystrophy inherited? Which tests would you perform if the sister of an affected patient wanted to know if she was a carrier?

50. Do you know what the prevalence of multiple sclerosis (MS) is in the UK? What is the natural history of the disease? What do you know about the recent advances in the treatment of MS?

51. A 30-year-old nurse presents with weakness and shortness of breath. She has recently had a diarrhoeal infection. What diagnosis do you suspect? How would you diagnose and manage this disease?

52. A 50-year-old university lecturer recently stopped driving at night because of problems with blurred vision. He now finds it difficult to keep his eyes open while reading in the evenings and has noticed his speech slurring towards the end of his lectures. What is the differential diagnosis? How would you investigate and manage this patient?

53. What is the active moiety of glyceryl trinitrate? What do you know about this molecule?

54. What is the cause of the hypercalcaemia seen in malignancy?

55. It is said that there is an epidemic of malignant melanoma. What do you know about this disease?

56. The surgical registrar phones you for the current guidelines on how to manage a patient who has had his spleen removed following traumatic rupture. What can you tell her?

57. An 85-year-old patient has a blood pressure of 160/100. Is treatment warranted?

58. A 35-year-old man is seen in your clinic. A recent routine health check at work showed him to have a cholesterol of 6.5. How do you manage him? What evidence can you cite to support your management?

59. Do you think selegiline has a role in the early treatment of Parkinson's disease? What other treatments do you know of?

60. What are the risks and benefits of the oral contraceptive pill?

61. What is the role of ACE inhibitors in the treatment of patients with myocardial infarction?

62. How would you advise a young woman who is on an anti-epileptic for grand mal seizures but wants to start a family?

63. How would you advise a woman who asks about getting pregnant while on warfarin for recurrent pulmonary emboli?

64. What are the classical articular features of rheumatoid arthritis? What extra-articular complications do you know of? What treatments are available?

65. How would you assess and manage a patient with acute gout? What is the important diagnosis to exclude when faced with an acute monoarthritis?

66. What is the audit cycle?

67. What are the criteria that make a disease suitable for a screening programme? How would you go about assessing the possible impact of this programme on the health of the population?

68. What is meant by the terms sensitivity and specificity?

69. How are doctors alerted to possible adverse drug reactions? Which drugs have you recently been made aware of through this system? How would you report a suspected adverse drug reaction or interaction?

70. What do you know about the natural history of hepatitis C virus infection? How would you treat it?

71. What are low-molecular-weight heparins and how do they work?

72. A 26-year-old woman who is taking the oral contraceptive pill presents with a swollen, red, painful calf. What questions would you like to ask and how would you investigate her?

73. A 54-year-old man is referred with a systolic blood pressure of 190 mmHg. You notice purpura, a centropetal fat distribution and cushingoid facies. How would you investigate? What is your differential diagnosis?

74. What is the role of magnesium in the treatment of acute myocardial infarction and why? Are nitrates useful in the treatment of acute myocardial infarction?

75. A 65-year-old smoker with a history of two previous myocardial infarctions presents with 2 hours of retrosternal chest pain and significant new anterior ST elevation. Discuss the trial evidence which would influence your management.

76. What do you understand about the term ventricular remodelling?

77. What is somatostatin? In which disorders are somatostatin analogues known to be of therapeutic benefit?

78. A 44-year-old woman is referred to your clinic with a history of left sided chest pain. She has a positive exercise test and a normal angiogram. What is your differential diagnosis and what further investigations would you recommend?

79. How is mitochondrial DNA passed from one generation to the next? Which disorders do you know of which are caused by abnormalities of mitochondrial DNA?

80. What do you know about hepatitis E virus infection?

81. A 58-year-old man with a long history of excessive alcohol consumption presents with haematemesis and melaena. Whilst you resuscitate him you notice stigmata of chronic liver disease. What is your differential diagnosis? Endoscopy reveals actively bleeding oesophageal varices. How would you manage him?

82. What are G proteins and how do they work?

83. *Helicobacter pylori* infection has radically altered the management of peptic ulcer disease. Do you agree with this statement and why?

84. A 65-year-old Egyptian gentleman presents with right upper quandrant pain and recent onset of ascites. The blood tests revealed a markedly elevated alpha-fetoprotein and a low albumin with abnormal clotting. What is the most likely diagnosis? What risk factors do you know of for this condition?

85. A 69-year-old lady presents with 10 kg weight loss and you notice multiple solar keratoses over her trunk. What is your diagnosis and how would you investigate further? Do you know any other cutaneous manifestations of malignant disease?

86. What are the features of Whipple's disease and how would you confirm the diagnosis?

87. Do you know of any diseases which are transmitted by ticks? Can you describe the main features of one of these conditions?

88. What is the electrophysiological mechanism of paroxysmal atrioventricular nodal re-entrant tachycardia? Describe the action of any drug which can be helpful in this disorder.

89. *Escherichia coli* can lead to severe complications. Do you know of any serotypes of particular concern? What are the major complications of infection with this organism?

90. What are the endothelins? How do you think a better understanding of their physiology may be helpful in the future?

91. What are the clinical uses of botulinum toxin?

92. The polymerase chain reaction (PCR) will be described as one of the greatest advances in science of the 20th century. What is it and what are some of its uses?

References

MOLECULAR BIOLOGY

Askari F K, McDonnell W M 1996 Antisense oligonucleotide therapy. New England Journal of Medicine 334: 316-319

Clark B, Gooi H C 1994 The polymerase chain reaction (PCR) and its clinical applications. Hospital Update 20: 278-286

Housman D 1995 Human DNA polymorphism. New England Journal of Medicine 332: 318-321

Huang Y Q, Li J J, Kaplan M H et al 1995 Human herpes virus-like nucleic acid in various forms of Kaposi's sarcoma. Lancet 345: 759-761

Johns D R 1995 Seminars in medicine of the Beth Israel Hospital, Boston: mitochondrial DNA and disease. New England Journal of Medicine 333: 638-644

Kientopf M, Esquivel E L, Brach M A et al 1995 Clinical applications of ribozymes. Lancet; 345; 8956: 1027-1031.

Latchman D S 1996 Mechanisms of disease: transcription-factor mutations and disease. New England Journal of Medicine 334: 28-33

Lerner R A, Benkovic S J, Schultz P G 1991 At the crossroads of chemistry and immunology: catalytic antibodies. Science 252: 659-667

Lodish H, Baltimore D, Berk A et al (eds) 1995 Molecular cell biology. W H Freeman, New York

Majzoub J A, Muglia L J 1996 Knockout mice. New England Journal of Medicine 334: 904-907.

McDonnell W M, Askari F K 1996 DNA vaccines. New England Journal of Medicine 334; 1: 42-45.

Milner J 1995 DNA damage, p53 and anticancer therapies. Nature Medicine 1; 9: 879-880

Morris J D H, Eddleston A L W F, Crook T 1995 Viral infection and cancer. Lancet 346: 754-758

Rady P L, Yen A, Rollefson J L et al 1995 Herpes-like DNA sequences in non-Kaposi's sarcoma skin lesions of transplant patients. Lancet 345: 1339-1340

Rooney C M, Smith C A, Ng C Y, et al 1995 Use of gene-modified virus-specific T lymphocytes to control Epstein-Barr-virus-related lymphoproliferation. Lancet 345: 9-13

Rosenthal N 1994 Regulation of gene expression. New England Journal of Medicine 331: 931-934

Rosenthal N 1994 Tools of the trade – recombinant DNA. New England Journal of Medicine 331: 315-318

Rosenthal N 1995 Recognising DNA. New England Journal of Medicine 333: 925-928

Shuldiner A R 1996 Transgenic animals. New England Journal of Medicine 334: 653-655

Southern E M 1975 Detection of specific sequences among DNA fragments separated by gel electrophoresis. Journal of Molecular Biology 98: 503-515

Stein C A, Cheng Y C 1993 Antisense oligonucleotides as therapeutic agents – is the bullet really magic? Science 261: 1004-1012

Wagner R W 1994 Gene inhibition using antisense oligodeoxynucleotides. Nature 372: 333-335

Wicks I 1995 Human gene therapy. Australian and New Zealand Journal of Medicine 25: 280-283

GENETICS

Cambien F, Poirier O, Lecerf L et al 1992 Deletion polymorphism in the gene for angiotensin-converting enzyme is a potent risk factor for myocardial infarction. Nature 359: 641-644

Collins F S 1996 BRCA1: Lots of mutations, lots of dilemmas. New England Journal of Medicine 334: 186-189

Harrison P J 1995 S182: from worm sperm to Alzheimer's disease. Lancet 346: 388.

Hughes J M B 1994 Intra-pulmonary shunts: coils to transplantation. Journal of the Royal College of Physicians 28; 3: 247-253

Hulka B S, Stark A T 1995 Breast cancer: cause and prevention. Lancet 346: 883-887

Hyman B T, Tanzi R 1995 Molecular epidemiology of Alzheimer's disease. New England Journal of Medicine 333: 1283-1284

Kastan M 1995 Ataxia-telangiectasia: broad implications for a rare disorder. New England Journal of Medicine 333: 662-663

Katsuya T, Koike G, Yee T W et al 1995 Association of angiotensinogen gene T235 variant with increased risk of coronary heart disease. Lancet 345: 1600-1603

McAllister K A, Grogg K M, Gallione C J et al 1994 Endoglin, a TGF-beta binding protein of endothelial cells, is the gene for hereditary haemorrhagic telangiectasia type 1. Nature Genetics 8: 345-351

McDonald M T, Papenberg K A, Ghosh S et al 1994 A disease locus for hereditary haemorrhage telangiectasia maps to chromosome 9q33-34. Nature Genetics 6: 197-204

Samani N, Martin D S, Brack M et al 1995 Insertion/deletion polymorphism in the angiotensin converting enzyme gene and risk of restenosis after coronary angioplasty. Lancet 345: 1013-1016

Savitsky K, Bar-Shira A, Gilad S et al 1995 A single ataxia telangiectasia gene with a product similar to PI-3 kinase. Science 268: 1749-1753

Selkoe D J 1995 Missence on the membrane. Nature 375: 734-735

Sherrington R, Rogaev E I, Liang Y et al 1995 Cloning of a gene bearing missence mutations in early-onset familial Alzheimer's disease. Nature 375: 754-760

Shovlin C L, Hughes J M B, Scott J et al 1994 A gene for hereditary haemorrhagic telangiectasia maps to chromosome 9q3. Nature Genetics 6: 205-209

St. Jacques S, Cymerman U, Pece N et al 1994 Molecular characterization of murine endoglin. Endocrinology 134; 6: 2645-2657

Swift M, Chase C L, Morrell D 1990 Cancer predisposition of ataxia-telangiectasia heterozygotes. Cancer Genet Cytogenet 46: 21-27

Swift M, Morrell D, Massey R B et al 1991 Incidence of cancer in 161 families affected by ataxia-telangiectasia. New England Journal of Medicine 325: 1831-1836

Teo K K 1995 Angiotensin converting enzyme genotypes and disease. British Medical Journal 311: 763-764

IMMUNOLOGY

Bevilacqua M P, Nelson R M, Mannori G et al 1994 Endothelial-leucocyte adhesion molecules in human disease. Annual Review of Medicine 45: 361-378

Drachman D B 1994 Myasthenia gravis. New England Journal of Medicine 330: 1797-1807

Klareskog L, Ronnelid J, Holm G 1995 Immunopathogenesis and immunotherapy in rheumatoid arthritis: an area in transition. Journal of Internal Medicine 238: 191-206

Nepom G T 1995 Class II antigens and disease susceptibility. Annual Review of Medicine 46: 17-25

Rosen F S, Cooper M D, Wedgwood R J 1995 Medical progress: the primary immunodeficiencies. New England Journal of Medicine 333: 431-440

Steele D J R, Auchincloss Jr H 1995 Xenotransplantation. Annual Review of Medicine 46: 345-360

BASIC SCIENCE

Agre P, Brown D, Nielsen S 1995 Aquaporin water channels: unanswered questions and unresolved controversies. Current Opinion in Cell Biology 7: 472-483

Burnett A L, Lowenstein C J, Bredt D S et al 1992 Nitric oxide: a physiological mediator of penile erection. Science 257: 401-403

Connolly D L, Shanahan C M, Weissberg P L 1996 Water channels in health and disease. Lancet 347: 210-212

Folkman J 1995 Angiogenesis in cancer, vascular, rheumatoid, and other diseases. Nature Medicine 1: 27-35

Folkman J 1995 Clinical applications of research on angiogenesis. New England Journal of Medicine 333; 6: 1757-1763

Fraser D R 1995 Vitamin D. Lancet 345; 8942: 104-108

Golding J, Greenwood R, Birmingham K et al 1992 Childhood cancer, intramuscular vitamin K, and pethidine given during labour. British Medical Journal 308: 341-346

Imaizumi T, Stafforini D M, Yamada Y et al 1995 Platelet-activating factor: a mediator for clinicians. Journal of Investigative Medicine 238: 5-20

Lefkowitz R L 1995 G proteins in medicine. New England Journal of Medicine 332: 186-188.

Levin E R 1995 Mechanisms of disease: endothelins. New England Journal of Medicine 333: 356-363

Martin T J, Grill V 1995 Hypercalcaemia. Clinical Endocrinology 42: 535-538

Moncada S, Higgs A 1993 Mechanisms of disease: the L-arginine-nitric oxide pathway. New England Journal of Medicine 329: 2002-2012

Ong A C M 1996 Surprising new roles for endothelins. British Medical Journal 312: 195-196

Report of a meeting of physicians and scientists, University College Medical School, London 1995 Raynaud's phenomenon. Lancet 346: 283-290

Shearer M J 1995 Vitamin K. Lancet 345: 229-234

Spector T D, Keen R W, Arden N K et al 1995 Influence of vitamin D receptor genotype on bone mineral density in postmenopausal women: a twin study in Britain. British Medical Journal 310: 1357-1360

Struthers A D 1994 10 years of natriuretic peptide research: a new dawn for their diagnostic and therapeutic use? British Medical Journal 308: 1615-1619

Vallance P, Collier J 1994 Biology and clinical relevance of nitric oxide. British Medical Journal 309: 453-457

Walshe J M 1995 Copper: not too little, not too much, but just right. Journal of the Royal College of Physicians London 29; 4: 280-288

STATISTICS AND EPIDEMIOLOGY

Clarke M J, Stewart L A 1994 Obtaining data from randomized controlled trials: how much do we need for reliable and informative meta-analysis? British Medical Journal 309: 1007-1010

Coggon D 1995 Statistics in clinical practice. British Medical Journal, London

Coggon D, Rose G , Barker D J P 1993 Epidemiology for the uninitiated. 3rd edn. British Medical Journal, London

Counsell C E, Fraser H, Sandercock P A G 1994 Archie Cochrane's challenge: can periodically updated reviews of all randomized controlled trials relevant to neurology and neurosurgery be produced? Journal of Neurology, Neurosurgery, and Psychiatry 57: 529-533

Doll R, Peto R, Hall E et al 1994 Mortality in relation to consumption of alcohol: 13 years' observations on male British doctors. British Medical Journal 309: 911-918

Doll R, Peto R, Wheatley K et al 1994 Mortality in relation to smoking: 40 years' observations on male British doctors. British Medical Journal 309: 901-911

Eysenck H J 1994 Meta-analysis and its problems. British Medical Journal 309: 789-792

Flournoy N, Olkin I 1995 Do small trials square with large ones? Lancet 345; 8952: 741-742

Gore S M, Altman D G 1982 Statistics in practice. British Medical Journal, London

Gronbaek M, Deis A, Sorensen T I et al 1995 Mortality associated with moderate intake of wine, beer, or spirits. British Medical Journal 310: 1165-1169

Hein H O, Suadicani P, Gyntelberg F 1996 Alcohol consumption, serum low density lipoprotein cholesterol concentration, and risk of ischaemic heart disease: 6 year follow up in the Copenhagen male study. British Medical Journal 312: 736-741

Rimm E B, Klarsky A, Grobbee D et al 1996 Review of moderate alcohol consumption and reduced risk of coronary heart disease: is the effect due to beer, wine, or spirits? British Medical Journal 312: 731-736

Sackett D L, Rosenberg W M C, Muir Gray J A et al 1996 Evidence based medicine: what it is and what it isn't. British Medical Journal 312: 71-72

PHARMACOLOGY AND THERAPEUTICS

Bauer J H, Reams G P 1995 The angiotensin II type 1 receptor antagonists. A new class of anti-hypertensive drugs. Archives of Internal Medicine 155: 1361-1368

Brodie M J, Dichter M A 1996 Anti-epileptic drugs. New England Journal of Medicine 334: 168-17

Burkart F, Pfisterer M, Kiowski W et al 1990 Effect of anti-arrhythmic therapy on mortality in survivors of myocardial infarction with asymptomatic complex ventricular arrhythmias: Basel anti-arrhythmic study of infarct survival (BASIS). Journal of the American College of Cardiology 16: 1711-1718

The Cardiac Arrest in Seattle: conventional amiodarone drug evaluation study (CASCADE) investigators 1993 Randomized anti-arrhythmic drug therapy in survivors of arrest (the CASCADE study). American Journal of Cardiology 72: 1295-1300

The CONSENSUS trial study group 1987 Effects of enalapril on mortality in severe congestive heart failure: results of the cooperative north Scandinavian enalapril survival study. New England Journal of Medicine 316: 1429-1435

Crofford O B 1995 Metformin. New England Journal of Medicine 333: 588-589

DeFronzo R A, Goodman A M 1995 Efficacy of metformin in patients with non-insulin-dependent diabetes mellitus. New England Journal of Medicine 333: 541-549

Department of Health 1995 New advice on oral contraceptives. Department of Health, London

Doval H C, Nul D R, Grancelli H O et al 1994 Randomized trial of low dose amiodarone in severe congestive heart failure. Grupo de ettudio de la sobrevida en la insuficienca cardiaca en Argentina (GESICA). Lancet 344: 493-498

Drugs for Parkinson's disease reviewed. 1995 Drug and Therapeutics Bulletin 33 (7): 49-52

Early E, Dmitrovsky E 1995 Acute pro-myelocytic leukaemia: retinoic acid response and resistance. Journal of Investigative Medicine 43: 337-344.

Engel J 1996 Surgery for seizures. New England Journal of Medicine 334: 647-652

Farley T M M, Meirik O, Chang C L et al 1995 Effect of different progestagens in low oestrogen oral contraceptives on venous thromboembolic disease. Lancet 346: 1582-1588

Ferner R E, Moss C 1996 Minocycline for acne. British Medical Journal 312: 138

Ganz L I, Freidman P L 1995 Supraventricular tachycardia. New England Journal of Medicine 332: 162-174.

Gough A, Chapman S, Wagstaff K et al 1996 Minocycline induced autoimmune hepatitis and systemic lupus erythematosus-like syndrome. British Medical Journal 312: 169-172

Green H L, Roden D M, Katz R J et al 1992 The cardiac arrhythmia suppression trial: first CAST... then CAST-II. Journal of the American College of Cardiology 19: 894-898

Gruppo Italiano per lo Studio della Soprawivenza nell'Infarto Miocardio (GISSI-3) 1994 Effects of lisinopril and transdermal glyceryl trinitrate singly and together on 6-week mortality and ventricular function after acute myocardial infarction. Lancet 343: 1115-1122

Horton R 1995 Spinning the risks and benefits of calcium antagonists. Lancet 346: 586-587

Jick H, Jick S S, Gurewich V et al 1995 Risk of idiopathic cardiovascular death and non-fatal venous thromboembolism in women using oral contraceptives with differing progestagen components. Lancet 346: 1589-1593

Johnston C I 1995 Angiotensin receptor antagonists: focus on losartan. Lancet 346: 1403-1407

Kendall M J, Lynch K P, Hjalmarson A et al 1993 Beta-blockers and sudden cardiac death. Annals of Internal Medicine 123: 358-367

Koopman M W, Prandoni P, Piovella F et al 1996 Treatment of venous thrombosis with intravenous unfractionated heparin administered in the hospital as compared with subcutaneous low-molecular-weight heparin administered at home. New England Journal of Medicine 334: 682-687

Kostis J B 1988 Angiotensin converting enzyme inhibitors. II: clinical use. American Heart Journal 116: 1591-1605

Lamberts S W J, Van Der Lely A, De Herder W W et al 1996 Drug therapy: Ocreotide. New England Journal of Medicine 334: 246-254.

Lees A J 1995 (on behalf of the Parkinson's Disease Research Group of the United Kingdom) Comparison of therapeutic effects and mortality data of levodopa, and levodopa combined with selegiline in patients with early, mild Parkinson's disease. British Medical Journal 311: 1602-1607

Leizorovicz A, Simonneau G, Decousus H et al 1994 Comparison of the efficacy and safety of low-molecular-weight heparins and unfractionated heparins in the initial treatment of deep vein thrombosis: a meta-analysis. British Medical Journal 309: 299-304

Lensing A W, Prins M H, Davidson B L et al 1995 Treatment of deep vein thrombosis with low-molecular-weight heparins: a meta-analysis. Archives of Internal Medicine 155: 601-607

Levine M, Gent M, Hirsh J et al 1996 A comparison of low-molecular-weight heparin administered primarily at home with unfractionated heparin administered in the hospital for proximal deep-vein thrombosis. New England Journal of Medicine 334: 677-681

Lewis A L, Spitzer W O, Heinemann L A J et al 1996 Transnational research group on oral contraceptives and the health of young women. Third generation oral contraceptives and risk of myocardial infarction: an international case-control study. British Medical Journal 312: 88-90

Lip G Y H, Metcalfe M J, Dunn F G 1993 Diagnosis and treatment of digoxin toxicity. Postgraduate Medical Journal 69: 337-339

Losartan– a new anti-hypertensive 1995 Drugs and Therapeutics Bulletin 33: 73-74

Mackie M A, Davidson J 1995 Prescribing of quinine and cramp inducing drugs in general practice. British Medical Journal 311: 541

McPherson K 1996 Third generation oral contraceptives and venous thromboembolism. British Medical Journal 312: 68-69

Man-Son-Hing M, Wells G 1995 Meta-analysis of efficacy of quinine for the treatment of nocturnal leg cramps in elderly people. British Medical Journal 310: 13-16

Nelson H S 1995 Drug therapy: B-adrenergic bronchodilators. New England Journal of Medicine 333: 499-506.

Nicorandil for angina 1995 Drugs and Therapeutics Bulletin 33(12): 89-92

Parkinson's study group 1989 Effect of deprenyl on the progression of disability in early Parkinson's disease. New England Journal of Medicine 321: 1364-1371

Parkinson's study group 1993 Effects of tocopherol and deprenyl on the progression of disability in early Parkinson's disease. New England Journal of Medicine 328: 176-183

Podrid P J 1995 Amiodarone: re-evaluation of an old drug. Annals of Internal Medicine 122: 689-700

Poulter N R, Chang C L, Farley T M M et al 1995 Venous thromboembolic disease and combined oral contraceptives: results of international multicentre case-control study. Lancet 346: 1575-1582

Psaty B M, Heckbert S R, Koepsell T D et al 1995 The risk of myocardial infarction associated with anti-hypertensive drug therapies. Journal of the American Medical Association 274: 620-625

Schafer A I 1996 Low-molecular heparin – an opportunity for home treatment of venous thrombosis. New England Journal of Medicine 334: 724-726

Siebels J, Cappato R, Ruppel R et al 1993 Preliminary results of the cardiac arrest study Hamburg (CASH). CASH investigators. American Journal of Cardiology 72: 109F-113F

Singh S N, Fletcher RD , Fisher S et al 1993 Veterans affairs congestive heart failure anti-arrhythmic trial. CHF STAT Investigators. American Journal of Cardiology 72: 99F-102F

Smyth R L, Van Velzen D, Smyth A R et al 1994 Strictures of ascending colon in cystic fibrosis and high-strength pancreatic enzymes. Lancet 343: 85-86

The SOLVD Investigators 1991 Effect of enalapril on survival in patients with reduced left ventricular ejection fractions and congestive heart failure. New England Journal of Medicine 325: 293-302

The SOLVD Investigators 1992 Effect of enalapril on mortality and the development of heart failure in asymptomatic patients with reduced left ventricular ejection fractions. New England Journal of Medicine 327: 685-691

Spitzer W O, Lewis A L, Heinemann L A J et al 1996 Transnational research group on oral contraceptives and the health of young women. Third generation oral contraceptives and risk of venous thromboembolic disorders: an international case-control study. British Medical Journal 312: 83-88.

Stumvoll M, Nurjhan N, Perriello G et al 1995 Metabolic effects of metformin in non-insulin-dependent diabetes mellitus. New England Journal of Medicine 333: 550-554

Treating hypertension in patients with diabetes mellitus 1994 Drugs and Therapeutics Bulletin 32: 79-80

Who needs nine ACE Inhibitors? 1995 Drugs and Therapeutics Bulletin 33: 1-3

HAEMATOLOGY

Allan N C, Richards S M, Shepherd P C A 1995 UK Medical Research Council randomized, multicentre trial of interferon-alpha n1 for chronic myeloid leukaemia: improved survival irrespective of cytogenetic response. Lancet 345: 1392-1397

Baglin T 1996 Disseminated intravascular coagulation: diagnosis and treatment. British Medical Journal 312: 683-687

Bociek R G, Stewart D A, Armitage J O 1995 Bone marrow transplantation – current concepts. Journal of Investigative Medicine 43; 2: 127-141

Dale C D 1995 Where now for colony-stimulating factors? Lancet 346: 135-136

Greengard J S, Eichinger S, Griffin J H et al 1994 Variability of thrombosis among homozygous siblings with resistance to activated protein C due to an arg to gln mutation in the gene for factor V. New England Journal of Medicine 331: 1559-1562

Hamblin T J 1995 The CME lecture. Chronic lymphocytic leukaemia – new drugs and management. Journal of the Royal College of Physicians, London 29; 5: 419-421

Hughes G R V, Khamashta M A 1994 The antiphospholipid syndrome. Journal of the Royal College of Physicians 28: 301-304

Power J P, Lawlor E, Davidson F et al 1995 Molecular epidemiology of an outbreak of infection with hepatitis C in recipients of anti-D immunoglobin. Lancet 345: 1211-1213.

Rees D C, Cox M, Clegg J B 1995 World distribution of factor V Leiden. Lancet 346: 1133-1135

Ridker P M, Hennekens C H, Lindpaintner K et al 1995 Mutation in the gene coding for coagulation factor V and the risk of myocardial infarction, stroke and venous thrombosis in apparently healthy men. New England Journal of Medicine 332: 912-917

The risks and uses of donated blood 1993 Drugs and Therapeutics Bulletin 33: 89-92

Schafer A I 1995 Hypercoagulable states: molecular genetics to clinical practice. Lancet 344: 1739-1742

Schulman S, Rheiden A, Lindmater P et al 1995 Anticoagulant therapy after a first episode of venous thromboembolism. New England Journal of Medicine 332: 1661-1665

Stewart W P 1993 Granulocyte and granulocyte-macrophage colony-stimulating factors. Lancet 342: 153-157

Weinmann E E, Salzman E W 1994 Deep-vein thrombosis. New England Journal of Medicine 311: 1630-1640

Wetzler M, Kantarjian H, Kurzrock R et al 1995 Interferon alpha therapy for chronic myelogenous leukemia. American Journal of Medicine 99: 402-411

Working party of the British committee for standards in haematology clinical haematology task force 1996 Guidelines for the prevention and treatment of infection in patients with an absent or dysfunctional spleen. British Medical Journal 312: 430-433

Young N S 1995 Aplastic anaemia. Lancet 346: 228-232

Zahavi J, Charach G, Schafer R et al 1993 Ischaemic necrotic toes associated with antiphospholipid syndrome and treated with iloprost. Lancet 342: 862

INFECTIOUS DISEASES

Bisno A L, Stevens D L 1996 Streptococcal infections of skin and soft tissues. New England Journal of Medicine 334: 240-245

Brabley D J, Warhurst D C 1995 Malaria prophylaxis: guidelines for travellers from Britain. British Medical Journal 319: 709-714

Bridges S H, Saryer N 1995 Gene therapy and immune restoration for HIV disease. Lancet 345: 427-432

Burge T S, Watson J D 1994 Necrotizing fasciitis. British Medical Journal 308: 1453-1454

Campbell G L, Hughes J M 1995 Plague in India: A new warning from an old nemesis. Annals of Internal Medicine 122; 2: 151-153

Choo V 1995 Combination superior to Zidovudine in Delta trial. Lancet 346: 895.

Cohen B 1995 Parvovirus B19: an expanding spectrum of disease. British Medical Journal 311: 1549-1552

Concorde Coordinating Committee 1994 Concorde: MRC/ANRS randomized double blind controlled trial of immediate and deferred Zidovudine in symptom-free HIV infection. Lancet 343: 871-881

Diagnosis and treatment of streptococcal sore throat. 1995 Drugs and Therapeutic Bulletin 33; 2: 9-12

Emery S, Cooper D A 1995 Anti-retroviral therapy of human immunodeficiency virus type-1 infection. Australian and New Zealand Journal of Medicine 25: 344-349

Fishbein D B, Dennis D T 1995 Tick-borne diseases: a growing risk. New England Journal of Medicine 333: 452-453

Friedland J S 1993 Uncommon infections: brucellosis. Prescribers Journal 33: 24-28.

Ip M, Osterberg L G, Chau P Y et al 1995 Pulmonary meliodosis. Chest 108:1420-1424

Klein N J, Heyderman R S, Levin M 1993 Management of meningococcal infections. British Journal of Hospital Medicine 50: 42-49

Letter from the Chief Medical Officer Feb 1994 Meningococcal infection: meningitis and septicaemia.

Levine A M 1990 Lymphoma in acquired immunodeficiency syndrome. Seminars in Oncology 17: 104-112

Lipsky J J 1994 Concorde lands. Lancet 343: 866-867

Lipton S A, Gendelman H E 1995 Dementia associated with the acquired immunodeficiency syndrome. New England Journal of Medicine 332: 934-939

Molyneux M, Fox R 1993 Diagnosis and treatment of malaria in Britain. British Medical Journal 306: 1175-1180

Nathavitharana K A, Tarlow M J 1995. Advances in treating bacterial meningitis. Update 51: 69-76

O'Connell S 1995. Lyme disease in the United Kingdom. British Medical Journal 310: 303-309

Outbreak of Ebola viral haemorrhagic fever – Zaire 1995 Morbidity Mortality Weekly Report 44: 381

The Paediatric AIDS Clinical Trials Group Protocol 076 Study Group 1995 Reduction of maternal-infant transmission of human immunodeficiency virus type 1 with Zidovudine treatment. New England Journal of Medicine 331; 18: 1173-1180

Pattison J R 1994 Human parvovirus B19. British Medical Journal 308: 149-150

Peckham C, Gibb D 1995 Current concepts: mother-to-child transmission of the human immunodeficiency virus. New England Journal of Medicine 333: 298-302

Pfister H, Wilske B, Weber K 1994 Lyme borreliosis: basic science and clinical aspects. Lancet 343: 1013-1020

Pinching A J 1996 Managing HIV disease after Delta. British Medical Journal 312: 521-522

Rogers F M, Jaffe H W 1995 Reducing the risk of maternal-infant transmission of HIV: a door is opened. New England Journal of Medicine 331; 18: 1222-1223

Schaad U B, Lips U, Gnehm H E et al 1993 Dexamethasone therapy for bacterial meningitis in children. Lancet 342: 457-461

Simpson D I H 1995 The filovirus enigma. Lancet 345: 1252-1253

Simpson D M, Tagliati M 1994 Neurologic manifestations of HIV infection. Annals of Internal Medicine 121: 769-785

Strandaert S M, Dawson J E, Schaffner W et al 1995 Ehrlichiosis in a golf-orientated retirement community. New England Journal of Medicine 333: 420-425

Sweeney B J, Miller R F, Harrison M J G 1993 Progressive multifocal leucoencephalopathy. British Journal of Hospital Medicine 50: 187-192

Tabaqchali S, Jumaa P 1995 Diagnosis and management of *Clostridium difficile* infection. British Medical Journal 310: 1375-1381.

Thomson H, Cartwright K 1995 Streptococcal necrotizing fasciitis in Gloucestershire: 1994. British Journal of Surgery 82: 1444-1445

Tunkel A R, Scheld W M 1995 Acute bacterial meningitis. Lancet 346: 1675-1680

Wiselka M 1994 Influenza: diagnosis, management and prophylaxis. British Medical Journal 308: 1341-1345.

RHEUMATOLOGY

Compston J E 1994 The therapeutic use of bisphosphonates. British Medical Journal 309: 711-715

Doherty M, Deighton C, Compston J 1994 Osteoporosis. Medicine International. 22: 209-212

Emmerson B T 1996 The management of gout. New England Journal of Medicine 334: 445-451

Francis R M 1995 Oral bisphosphonates in the treatment of osteoporosis: a review. Current Therapeutic Research 56: 831-851

Goodacre J A, Carson Dick W 1995 Treatment of gout. Prescribers Journal 35: 105-110

Hosking D, Meunier P J, Ringe J D et al 1996 Paget's disease of bone: diagnosis and management. British Medical Journal 312: 491-494

Isenberg D A, Black C 1995 ABC of rheumatology. Raynaud's phenomenon, scleroderma and overlap syndromes. British Medical Journal 310: 795-798

Klareskog L, Ronnelid J, Holm G 1995 Immunopathogenesis and immunotherapy in rheumatoid arthritis: an area of transition. Journal of Investigative Medicine 238: 191-206

Peel N, Eastell R 1995 ABC of Rheumatology. Osteoporosis. British Medical Journal 310: 989-992

Report of a meeting of physicians and scientists 1995. Raynaud's phenomenon. University College Medical School, London. Lancet 346: 283-290

Snaith M C 1995 ABC of rheumatology: gout, hyperuricaemia and crystal arthritis. British Medical Journal 310: 521-524

RENAL MEDICINE

Almdal T, Norgaard K, Feldt-Rasmussen B et al 1994 The predictive value of microalbuminuria in IDDM: a 5-year follow-up study. Diabetes Care 17: 20-25

Boyce T G, Swerdlow D L, Griffin P M 1995 Escherichia coli O157: H7 and the haemolytic-uraemic syndrome. New England Journal of Medicine 333: 364-368

Clark C M, Lee D A 1995 Prevention and treatment of the complications of diabetes mellitus. New England Journal of Medicine 332: 1210-1217

The Diabetes Control and Complication Trial Research Group 1993 The effect of intensive treatment of diabetes on the development and progression of long-term complications in insulin-dependent diabetes mellitus. New England Journal of Medicine 329; (14): 977-986

Floege J, Ehlerding G 1996 Beta-2-microglobulin-associated amyloidosis. Nephron 72: 9-26.

Grantham J J 1995 Polycystic kidney disease – there goes the neighbourhood. New England Journal of Medicine 333: 56-57

Krolewski A S, Lattel L M B, Krolewski M et al 1995 Glycosylated haemoglobin and the risk of microalbuminuria in patients with insulin-dependent diabetes mellitus. New England Journal of Medicine 332: 1251-1255

Lewis E J, Hunsicker L G, Bain R P et al 1993 The effects of ACE inhibition on diabetic nephropathy. New England Journal of Medicine 329: 1456-1462

Mason P D, Pusey C D 1994 Glomerulonephritis: diagnosis and treatment. British Medical Journal 309: 1557-1563

Microalbuminuria Collaborative Study Group 1995 Intensive therapy and progression to clinical albuminuria in patients with insulin-dependent diabetes mellitus and microalbuminuria. British Medical Journal 311: 973-977

Moake J L 1994 Haemolytic-uraemic syndrome: basic science. Lancet 343: 393-397

Nield G H 1994 Haemolytic-uraemic syndrome in practice. Lancet 343: 398-401

Ponticelli C, Zucchelli P, Imbusciati E et al 1984 A controlled trial of methylprednisolone and chlorambucil in idiopathic membranous nephropathy. New England Journal of Medicine 310: 946-950

Riley L W 1983 Haemorrhagic colitis associated with a rare Escherichia serotype. New England Journal of Medicine 308: 681-685

Robertson S, Isles C, More I 1995 Glomerular disease made easier: 2. British Journal of Hospital Medicine 53: 323-326

Saggar-Malik A K, Jeffrey S, Patton M A 1994 Autosomal dominant polycystic kidney disease. British Medical Journal 308: 1183-1184

Viberti G, Mogensen C E, Groop L C et al 1994 Effect of captopril on progression to clinical proteinuria in patients with insulin dependent diabetes mellitus and microalbuminuria. Journal of the American Medical Association 271: 275-279

Woo D 1995 Apoptosis and loss of renal tissue in polycystic kidney diseases. New England Journal of Medicine 333: 18-25

ENDOCRINOLOGY

Atkinson M A, Maclaren N K 1994 The pathogenesis of insulin-dependent diabetes mellitus. New England Journal of Medicine 331: 1428-1435.

Braunstein G D 1993 Gynaecomastia. New England Journal of Medicine 328: 490-495

Clark C M, Vinicor F 1996 In: risks and benefits of intensive management in non-insulin-dependent diabetes mellitus. Annals of Internal Medicine 124; 1 pt 2: 81-85

The Diabetes Control and Complication Trial Research Group 1993 The effect of intensive treatment of diabetes on the development and progression of long-term complications in insulin-dependent diabetes mellitus. New England Journal of Medicine 329 (14): 977-986

Garner P 1995 Type 1 diabetes mellitus and pregnancy. Lancet 346: 157-161

Hall R, Besser M 1989 Fundamentals of clinical endocrinology, 4th edn. Churchill Livingstone, Edinburgh

Jones T H 1995 The management of hyperprolactinaemia. British Journal of Hospital Medicine 53: 374-378

Kanz N K, Herman W H, Becker M P et al 1995 Diabetes and pregnancy: factors associated with seeking pre-conception care. Diabetes Care 18: 157-165

Kendall-Taylor P 1995 Investigation of thyrotoxicosis. Clinical Endocrinology 42: 309-313.

New drugs for hyperprolactinaemia 1995 Drugs and Therapeutics Bulletin 33: 65-67

Orth D N 1995 Medical progress: Cushing's syndrome. New England Journal of Medicine 332: 791-803

Pandha H S, Waxman J 1995 Tumour markers. Quarterly Journal of Medicine 88: 233-241

White P C 1994 Disorders of aldosterone biosynthesis and action. New England Journal of Medicine 331: 250-258

NEUROLOGY

Almond J W, Brown P, Gore S M 1995 Creutzfeldt-Jakob disease and bovine spongiform encephalopathy: any connection? British Medical Journal 311: 1415-1421

Amar K, Wilcock G 1996 Vascular dementia. British Medical Journal 312: 227-231

Boston area anticoagulation trial for atrial fibrillation investigators 1990 The effect of low dose warfarin on the risk of stroke in patients with non-rheumatic atrial fibrillation. New England Journal of Medicine 323: 1505-1511

Carolei A, Marini C, Nencini P et al 1995 Prevalence and outcome of symptomatic carotid lesions in young adults. British Medical Journal 310: 1363-1366

Chief Medical Officer's Update 5 March 1995

Conference of the medical royal colleges and their faculties in the United Kingdom 1979 Diagnosis of death. British Medical Journal i: 332.

Drachman D B 1994 Myasthenia gravis. New England Journal of Medicine 330: 1797-1807

European Atrial Fibrillation Trial Study Group 1993 Secondary prevention in non-rheumatic atrial fibrillation after transient ischaemic attack or minor stroke. Lancet 342: 1255-1262

European Carotid Surgery Trialists Collaborative Group 1991 MRC European carotid surgery trial. Lancet 337: 1235-1243

Executive Committee for the Asymptomatic Carotid Atherosclerosis Study 1995 Endarterectomy for asymptomatic carotid artery stenosis. Journal of the American Medical Association 273: 1421-1428

Ezekowitz M D, Bridgers S L, James K E et al 1992 Warfarin in the prevention of stroke associated with non-rheumatic atrial fibrillation. New England Journal of Medicine 327: 140-141

Goldfarb L G, Brown P 1995 The transmissible spongiform encephalopathies. Annual Review of Medicine 46: 57-65

Gore S M 1996 Bovine Creutzfeldt-Jakob disease? British Medical Journal 312: 791-793

Gusella J F, MacDonald M E 1994 Huntington's disease and repeating trinucleotides. New England Journal of Medicine 330: 1450-1451

Gusella J F, Wexler N S, Coneally P M et al 1983 A polymorphic DNA marker genetically linked to Huntington's disease. Nature 306: 234-238

Havard C W H, Fonseca V 1990 New treatment approaches to myasthenia gravis. Drugs 39(1): 66-73

Hughes R A C, Rees J H 1994 Guillain-Barré syndrome. Current opinion in neurology 7: 386-392

Humphrey P R D 1995 Management of transient ischaemic attacks and stroke. Postgraduate Medical Journal 71: 577-584

The Huntington's Disease Collaborative Research Group 1993 A novel gene containing a trinucleotide repeat that is expanded and unstable on Huntington's disease chromosomes. Cell 72: 971-983

The IFNB Multiple Sclerosis Study Group, the University of British Columbia MS/MRI Analysis Group 1995 Interferon beta-1b in the treatment of multiple sclerosis: final outcome of the randomized controlled trial. Neurology 45: 1277-1285

Interferon beta-1B = hope or hype? 1996 Drug and Therapeutics Bulletin 34: 9-11

Kaminski H J, Mass E, Spiegel P et al 1990 Why are eye muscles frequently involved in myasthenia gravis? Neurology 40: 1663-1669

Kremer B, Goldberg P, Andrew S E et al 1994 A world-wide study of Huntington's disease mutation: the sensitivity and specificity of measuring CAG repeats. New England Journal of Medicine 330: 1401-1406

Leigh P N, Ray-Chaudhuri K 1994 Motor neurone disease. Journal of Neurology, Neurosurgery, and Psychiatry 57: 886-896

Multicentre Acute Stroke Trial–Italy Group 1995 Randomized controlled trial of streptokinase, aspirin, and combination of both in treatment of acute ischaemic stroke. Lancet 346: 1509-1514

North American Symptomatic Endarterectomy Trial Collaborators 1991 Beneficial effect of carotid endarterectomy in symptomatic patients with high-grade carotid stenosis. New England Journal of Medicine 325: 445-453

Oxfordshire Community Stroke Project 1983 Incidence of stroke in Oxfordshire: first year's experience of a community stroke project. British Medical Journal 287: 713-716

Petersen P, Boysen G, Godtfredsen J et al 1989 Placebo controlled, randomized trial of warfarin and aspirin for prevention of thromboembolic complications in chronic atrial fibrillation. (AFASAK). Lancet i: 175-179

Sawle G V 1995 Imaging the head: functional imaging. Journal of Neurology, Neurosurgery, and Psychiatry 58: 132-144

Smith R G, Appel S H 1995 Molecular approaches to amyotrophic lateral sclerosis. Annual Review of Medicine 46: 133-145

Stroke Prevention in Atrial Fibrillation (SPAF) Investigators 1991 Stroke prevention in atrial fibrillation study: final results. Circulation 84: 527-539

SPAF Investigators 1994 Warfarin versus aspirin for prevention of thromboembolism in atrial fibrillation: SPAF II study. Lancet 343: 687-691

Working Group of the Royal College of Physicians 1995 Criteria for the diagnosis of brain stem death. Journal of the Royal College of Physicians, London 29; (5): 281-282

Working Group of the Royal College of Physicians 1996 The permanent vegetative state. Journal of the Royal College of Physicians, London. 30: 119-121

Worton R 1995 Muscular dystrophies: diseases of the dystrophin-glycoprotein complex. Science 270: 755-756

CARDIOLOGY

Anderson H V, Willerson J 1993 Thrombolysis in acute myocardial infarction. New England Journal of Medicine 329: 703-709

Carabello B A 1995 Indications for valve surgery in asymptomatic patients with aortic and mitral stenosis. Chest 108: 1678-1682

Chauhan A 1995 Syndrome X: angina and normal coronary angiography. Postgraduate Medical Journal 71: 341-345

Chinese Cardiac Study Collaborative Group 1995 Oral captopril vs placebo among 13 642 patients with suspected acute myocardial infarction: interim report from the Chinese Cardiac Study (CCS 1) Lancet 345: 686-687

Dahlof B, Lindholm L H et al 1991 Morbidity and mortality in the Swedish trial in old patients with hypertension (STOP-Hypertension) Lancet 338: 1281-1285

Ganz L I, Freidman P L 1995 Supraventricular tachycardia. New England Journal of Medicine 332: 162-174.

GISSI-2 1990 A factorial randomized trial of alteplase vs streptokinase plus heparin vs no heparin among 12 490 patients with acute myocardial infarction. Lancet 336: 65-71

GISSI-3 1994 Effects of lisinopril and transdermal glyceryl trinitrate singly and together on 6-week mortality and ventricular function after acute myocardial infarction. Lancet 343: 1115-1122

The Global Utilization of Streptokinase and Tissue Plasminogen Activator for Occluded Coronary Arteries (GUSTO) investigators 1993. An international randomized trial comparing four thrombolytic strategies for acute myocardial infarction. New England Journal of Medicine 329: 673-682

Gruppo Italiano per lo Studio della Streptochinasi nell'Infarto Miocardio (GISSI) 1986 Effectiveness of intravenous thrombolytic therapy in acute myocardial infarction. Lancet i: 397-402

Hillegass W B, Ohman E M, Leimberger J D et al 1994 A meta-analysis of randomized trials of calcium antagonists to reduce restenosis after coronary angioplasty. American Journal of Cardiology 73: 835-839

Hoffman R M, Garewal H S 1995 Anti-oxidants and the prevention of coronary heart disease. Archives of Internal Medicine 155: 241-246

Horton R 1993 Thrombolysis: tPA fast by GUSTO. Lancet 341: 1188

First International Study of Infarct Survival (ISIS-1) Collaborative Group 1986 Randomized trial of intravenous atenolol among 16 027 cases of suspected acute myocardial infarction: Lancet ii: 57-66

ISIS-2 1988 Randomized trial of intravenous streptokinase, oral aspirin, both or neither among 17 187 cases of suspected acute myocardial infarction Lancet. ii: 349-360

ISIS-2 Collaborative Group 1988 Randomized trial of intravenous streptokinase, oral aspirin, both or neither among 17 187 cases of suspected acute myocardial infarction Lancet ii: 349-360

ISIS-3 Collaborative Group 1992 Randomized comparison of streptokinase vs tPA vs anistreplase and of aspirin plus heparin vs aspirin alone among 41 299 cases of suspected acute myocardial infarction. Lancet 339: 753-770

ISIS-4 Collaborative Group 1995 Randomized factorial trial assessing early oral captopril, oral mononitrate, and intravenous magnesium sulphate in 58 050 patients with suspected acute myocardial infarction. Lancet 345: 669-686

Kaplan N M 1995 Hypertension in the elderly. Annual Review of Medicine 46: 27-35

Kaski J C, Rosano G, Gavrieledes S et al 1994 Effects of angiotensin converting enzyme inhibiting on exercise induced angina and ST segment depression in patients with microvascular angina. American Journal of Cardiology 23: 652-657

Knight C, Gunning M, Henein M et al 1996 Non-surgical septal reduction for hypertrophic cardiomyopathy. Journal of Invasive Cardiology (in press)

Marian A J, Roberts M D 1995 Molecular genetics of hypertrophic cardiomyopathy. Annual Review of Medicine 46: 213-222

MRC Working Party 1992 Medical Research Council trial of treatment of hypertension in older adults: principal results. British Medical Journal 304: 405-412

Parisi A F, Folland E D, Hartigan P (for the Veterans Affairs ACME Investigators) 1992. A comparison of angioplasty with medical therapy in the treatment of single vessel coronary artery disease. New England Journal of Medicine 326: 10

Pedersen T R 1995 Lowering cholesterol with drugs and diet. New England Journal of Medicine 333: 1350-1351

Pfeffer M A 1995 Left ventricular remodelling after acute myocardial infarction. Annual Review of Medicine 46: 455-466

Pocock S J, Henderson R A, Rickards AF et al 1995 Meta-analysis of randomized trials comparing coronary angioplasty with bypass surgery. Lancet 346: 1148-1149

Rahimtoola S H 1995 From coronary heart disease to heart failure: role of hibernating myocardium. American Journal of Cardiology 75: 16E-22E

Reynes K 1995 Cardiac myxomas. New England Journal of Medicine 333: 1610-1617

Riemersma R A 1996 Coronary heart disease and vitamin E. Lancet 347: 776

Rihal C S, Yusuf S 1996 Chronic coronary artery disease: drugs, angioplasty, or surgery? British Medical Journal 312: 265-266

Scandinavian Simvastatin Survival Study 1994 Randomized trial of cholesterol lowering in 4444 patients with coronary heart disease. Lancet 344: 1383-1389

Shepherd J, Cobbe S M, Ford I et al (for the West of Scotland Coronary Prevention Study) 1995 Prevention of coronary heart disease with pravastatin in men with hypercholesterolaemia. New England Journal of Medicine 333: 1301-1307

Stephens N G, Parsons A, Schofield P M et al 1996 Randomized controlled trial of vitamin E in patients with coronary disease: Cambridge Heart Anti-oxidant Study (CHAOS). Lancet 347: 781-786

Systolic Hypertension in the Elderly Program (SHEP). Cooperative Research Group 1991 Prevention of stroke by anti-hypertensive drug treatment in older persons with isolated systolic hypertension in the elderly. Journal of the American Medical Association 265: 3255-3264

Topol E J, Califf R M, Weisman H F et al 1994 Randomized trial of coronary intervention with antibody against platelet IIb/IIIa integrin for reduction of clinical restenosis: results at 6 months. Lancet 343: 881-886

Ward H, Yudkin J 1995 Thrombolysis in patients with diabetes. British Medical Journal 310: 3-4

Winder T 1994 Lipid profiles. British Journal of Hospital Medicine 51: 102-104

Woods K L, Fletcher S 1994 Long-term outcome after intravenous magnesium in suspected acute myocardial infarction: the second Leicester Intravenous Magnesium Intervention Trial (LIMIT-2). Lancet 343; 816-819

Woods K L, Fletcher S, Roffe C et al 1992 Intravenous magnesium sulphate in suspected acute myocardial infarction: results of the second Leicester Intravenous Magnesium Intervention Trial (LIMIT-2) Lancet 339: 1553-1558

Yusuf S, Zucker D, Peduzzi P et al 1994 Effect of coronary artery bypass graft surgery on survival: overview of 10-year results from randomized trials by the Coronary Artery Bypass Graft Surgery Triallists Collaboration. Lancet 334: 563-570

DERMATOLOGY

Goldberg L H 1996 Basal cell carcinoma. Lancet 347: 663-666

Greaves M W 1995 Chronic urticaria. New England Journal of Medicine 332: 1767-1772

Kurzock R, Cohen P R 1995 Cutaneous paraneoplastic syndromes in solid tumours. American Journal of Medicine 99: 662-671

Rees J L 1996 The melanoma epidemic: reality and artifact. British Medical Journal 312: 138

Roujeau J C, Kelly J P, Naldi L et al 1995 Medication use and the risk of Stevens-Johnson syndrome and toxic epidermal necrolysis. New England Journal of Medicine 333: 1600-1607

RESPIRATORY MEDICINE

British Thoracic Society 1990 Guidelines for management of asthma in adults I. British Medical Journal 301: 651-654

British Thoracic Society 1990 Guidelines for management of asthma in adults II. British Medical Journal 301: 797-800

British Thoracic Society 1993 Guidelines for the management of asthma: a summary. British Medical Journal 306: 776-782

Brochard L, Mancebo J, Wysocki M et al 1995 Non-invasive ventilation for acute exacerbations of chronic obstructive pulmonary disease. New England Journal of Medicine 333: 817-822

Chan-Yeung M, Malo J-L 1995 Occupational asthma. New England Journal of Medicine 333: 107-112.

Crane J, Pearce N, Burgess C et al 1995 Asthma and the beta agonist debate. Thorax 50(Suppl 1): S5-S10

du Bois R M 1995 Respiratory medicine: recent advances. British Medical Journal 310: 1594-1597

Elborn J S 1994 Cystic fibrosis: prospects for gene therapy. Hospital Update 20: 13-20

Fulkerson W J, MacIntyre N, Stamler J et al 1996 Pathogenesis and treatment of the adult respiratory distress syndrome. Archives of Internal Medicine 156: 29-38

Gaskin K J 1994 Gastrointestinal and hepatobiliary disease in cystic fibrosis. Medicine International. 22: 272-276

Hanning C D, Alexander-Williams J M 1995 Pulse oximetry: a practical review. British Medical Journal 311: 367-370

Joint Tuberculosis Committee of the British Thoracic Society 1994 Control and prevention of tuberculosis in the United Kingdom: code of practice 1994. Thorax 49: 1193-1200

Kooef M H, Schuster D P 1995 The acute respiratory distress syndrome. New England Journal of Medicine 332: 27-36

Leger P, Bebicam J M, Cornette A et al 1994 Nasal intermittent positive pressure ventilation: long-term follow-up in patients with severe chronic respiratory insufficiency. Chest 105: 100-105

Malin A S, McAdam K P W J 1995 Escalating threat from tuberculosis: the third epidemic. Thorax 50 (Suppl 1): S37-S42

McNamara S G, Grunstein R R, Sullivan C E 1993 Obstructive sleep apnoea. Thorax 48: 754-764

Medical Research Council Working Party 1981 Long-term domiciliary oxygen therapy in chronic hypoxic cor pulmonale complicating chronic bronchitis and emphysema. Lancet 1: 681-686

Miller R F, Mitchell D M 1995 *Pneumocystis carinii* pneumonia. Thorax 50: 191-200

Newman-Taylor A 1995 Environmental determinants of asthma. Lancet 345: 296-299

Nocturnal Oxygen Therapy Trial Group 1980 Continuous or nocturnal oxygen therapy in hypoxic chronic obstructive lung disease: a clinical trial. Annals of Internal Medicine 93: 391-398

Rommens J M, Iannuzzi M C, Kerem B et al 1989 Identification of the cystic fibrosis gene: chromosome walking and jumping. Science 245: 1059-1065

Simonds A K 1994 Sleep studies of respiratory function and home respiratory support. British Medical Journal 309: 35-40

Simonds A K, Elliott M 1995 Outcome of domiciliary nasal intermittent positive pressure ventilation in restrictive and obstructive disorders. Thorax 50: 604-609

Strieter R M, Kunkel S L 1994 Acute lung injury: the role of cytokines in the elicitation of neutrophils. Journal of Investigative Medicine 42: 640-650

Strollo P J, Rogers R M 1996 Current concepts: obstructive sleep apnoea. New England Journal of Medicine 334; 2: 99-104

Tarpy S P, Celli B R 1995 Long-term oxygen therapy. New England Journal of Medicine 333: 710-714

GASTROENTEROLOGY

Beasley R P 1982 Hepatitis B virus as an aetiological agent in hepatocellular carcinoma-epidemiological considerations. Journal of Hepatology 2: 215

Burroughs A K 1991 Somatostatin and ocreotide for variceal bleeding. Journal of Hepatology 13: 1-4

Ching C K, Lam S K 1995 Drug therapy of peptic ulcer disease. British Journal of Hospital Medicine 54: 101-106

Cohen S and Parkman H P 1995 Treatment of achalasia – whalebone to botulinum toxin. New England Journal of Medicine 332: 815-817

Dobbins III 1995 The diagnosis of Whipple's disease. New England Journal of Medicine 332: 390-392

Dusheiko G M, Khakoo S, Soni P et al 1996 A rational approach to the management of hepatitis C infection. British Medical Journal 312: 357-363

Ferguson A 1994 Ulcerative colitis and Crohn's disease. British Medical Journal 309: 355

Forgacs I 1995 Clinical gastroenterology: recent advances. British Medical Journal 310: 113-116

Gibaldi M 1995 *Helicobacter pylori* and gastrointestinal disease. Journal of Clinical Pharmacology 35: 647-654

Groden J 1995 Colon-cancer genes and brain tumours. New England Journal of Medicine 332: 884-886

Groden J, Thliverrs A, Samowitz W et al 1991 Identification and characterization of the familial polyposis coli gene. Cell 66: 589-600

Hamilton S R, Liu B, Parsons R E et al 1995 The molecular basis of Turcot's syndrome. New England Journal of Medicine 332: 13; 839-847

Hardell L, Bengtsson N O, Jonson U et al 1984 Aetiological aspects of primary liver cancer with special regard to alcohol, organic solvents and acute intermittent porphyria – an epidemiological investigation. British Journal of Cancer 50: 380

Jen J, Kim H, Piantadosi S et al 1994 Allelic loss of chromosome 18q and prognosis in colorectal cancer. New England Journal of Medicine 331: 213-21

Jewell D 1994 Crohn's disease. Medicine International 22: 321-326

Lee Y-M, Kaplan M 1995 Primary sclerosing cholangitis. New England Journal of Medicine 332: 924-933

Lewin J, Dhillon A P, Sim R et al 1995 Persistent measles virus infection of the intestine: confirmation by immunogold electron microscopy. Gut 36: 564-569

Livraghi T, Bolondi L, Buscarini L et al 1995 Treatment, resection and ethanol injection in hepatocellular carcinoma: a retrospective analysis of survival in 391 patients with cirrhosis. Journal of Hepatology 22: 522-526

Managing patients with gallstones 1994 Drugs and Therapeutics Bulletin 32: 33-35

Marshall B J, Warren J R 1984 Unidentified curved bacilli in the stomach of patients with gastritis and peptic ulceration. Lancet i: 1311-1315

Mayberry J F, Rhodes J, Williams G T 1994 Ulcerative colitis. Medicine International 22: 314-320

Mazzaferro V, Regalia E, Doci R et al 1996 Liver transplantation for the treatment of small hepatocellular carcinomas in patients with cirrhosis. New England Journal of Medicine 334: 693-699

McPeake J R, O'Grady J G, Zaman S et al 1993 Liver transplantation for primary hepatocellular carcinoma: tumour size and number determine outcome. Journal of Hepatology 18: 226-234

Merkel C, Bolognesi M, Bellon S et al 1992 Prognostic usefulness of hepatic vein catheterisation in patients with cirrhosis and portal oesophageal varices. Gastroenterology 102: 973-979

Mills P R 1993 Management of ulcerative colitis. Prescribers Journal 33: 1-7

Nightingale J M D, Rathbone B J 1995 Inflammatory bowel disease. Update 52: 13-24

Pagliaro L, D'amico G, Sorensen T et al 1992 Prevention of first bleeding in cirrhosis. Annals of Internal Medicine 117: 59-70

Pasricha P J, Ravich W J, Hendrix T R et al 1995 Intrasphincteric botulinum toxin for the treatment of achalasia. New England Journal of Medicine 332: 774

Pearson D C, May G R, Fick G H et al 1995 Azathioprine and 6-mercaptopurine in Crohn's disease: a meta-analysis. Annals of Internal Medicine 122: 132-142

Report of meeting of physicians and scientists, Royal Free Hospital and School of Medicine, London 1995 Genetic diversity of hepatitis C virus: implications for pathogenesis, treatment, and prevention. Lancet 345: 562-567

Rickman A L, Freeman W R, Green W R et al 1995 Uveitis caused by *Tropheryma whippelii* (Whipple's bacillus). New England Journal of Medicine 332: 363-367

Rustgi A K 1994 Hereditary gastrointestinal polyposis and non-polyposis syndromes. New England Journal of Medicine 331: 1694-1703

Sandord N L, Kerlin P 1995 Current management of oesophageal varices. Australian and New Zealand Journal of Medicine 25: 528-534.

Scharschmidt B F 1995 Hepatitis E: a virus in waiting. Lancet 346: 519-520.

Skeens J, Semba C, Dake M 1996 Transjugular portosystemic shunts. Annual Review of Medicine 46: 95-102

Tait N, Little J M 1995 The treatment of gallstones. British Medical Journal 311: 99-105

Toribara N W and Sleisenger M H 1995 Current concepts: screening for colorectal cancer. New England Journal of Medicine 332: 861-868

Walsh J H, Peterson W L 1995 The treatment of *Helicobacter pylori* in the management of peptic ulcer disease. New England Journal of Medicine 333: 984-991

Williams R, Rizzi P 1996 Treating small hepatocellular carcinomas. New England Journal of Medicine 334: 728-729

EMERGENCY MEDICINE

Danzl D F, Pozos R S 1994 Accidental hypothermia. New England Journal of Medicine 331: 1756-1760

European Resuscitation Council guidelines 1992 (abridged) 1993 British Medical Journal 306: 1589-1593

Mouhaffel A H, Madu E C, Satmary W A et al 1995 Cardiovascular complications of cocaine. Chest 107: 1426-1434.

Vale J A, Proudfoot A T 1995 Paracetamol (acetaminophen) poisoning. Lancet 346: 547-552

Abbreviations

1,25 (OH) D	1,25 dihydroxy cholecalciferol
5-ASA	5-amino salicylic acid
25(OH) D	25 hydroxy cholecalciferol
A1	Adenosine 1 receptor
ACE	Angiotensin converting enzyme
ACTH	Adrenocorticotrophic hormone
ADP	Adenosine diphosphate
AF	Atrial fibrillation
AIDS	Acquired immunodeficiency syndrome
AMAN	Acute motor axonal neuropathy
AMI	Acute myocardial infarction
AP	Alkaline phosphatase
APC	Adenomatous polyposis gene
APKD	Adult polycystic kidney disease
APL	Acute promyelocytic leukaemia
AQP	Aquaporin
ARDS	Adult / acute respiratory distress syndrome
AT	Angiotensin
AT	Ataxia telangiectasia
ATP	Adenosine triphosphate
ATRA	All-trans retinoic acid
BCC	Basal cell carcinoma
bFGF	basic fibroblast growth factor
BMT	Bone marrow transplant
BP	Blood pressure
BTS	British Thoracic Society
C	Complement
Ca	Calcium
CABG	Coronary artery bypass grafting
cAMP	cyclic adenosine monophosphate
CD	Cluster of differentiation
cDNA	complimentary deoxyribonucleic acid
CFTR	Cystic fibrosis transmembrane regulator
cGMP	cyclic-guanosine monophosphate
CGRP	Calcitonin gene related peptide
CHOP	Cyclophosphamide, hydroxodaunorubicin, vincristine, prednisolone
CJD	Creutzfeldt-Jakob disease
CLL	Chronic lymphocytic leukaemia

CML	Chronic myeloid leukaemia
CMV	Cytomegalovirus
COPD	Chronic obstructive pulmonary disease
CPAP	Continuous positive airway pressure
CRH	Corticotrophin releasing hormone
CRP	C reactive protein
CSF	Cerebrospinal fluid
CSF	Colony stimulating factor
CT	Computed tomography
D1	Dopamine 1 receptor
D3	Cholecalciferol
DC	Direct current
DIC	Disseminated intravascular coagulation
DM	Diabetes mellitus
DNA	Deoxyribonucleic acid
DVLA	Driver and Vehicle Licensing Agency
DVT	Deep vein thrombosis
EBV	Epstein-Barr virus
ECG	Electrocardiogram
ECMO	Extracorporeal membrane oxygenation
EEG	Electroencephalogram
ELISA	Enzyme-linked immunosorbent assay
EMG	Electromyogram
EPI	Echo-planar imaging
ERCP	Endoscopic retrograde cholangiopancreatography
ESR	Erythrocyte sedimentation rate
ESRF	End-stage renal failure
FAP	Familial adenomatous polyposis
FDG	Fluorodeoxyglucose
FEV1	Forced expiratory volume in one second
FFP	Fresh frozen plasma
FLASH	Fast low angle shot
fMRI	functional magnetic resonance imaging
FSGS	Focal segmental glomerulosclerosis
GABA	Gamma-aminobutyric acid
GBS	Guillain-Barré syndrome
G-CSF	Granulocyte colony stimulating factor
GDP	Guanine diphosphate
Gla	Gamma-carboxyglutamate
GM-CSF	Granulocyte macrophage colony stimulating factor
gp	Glycoprotein
G protein	Guanine nucleotide binding protein
GTN	Glyceryl trinitrate
GTP	Guanine triphosphate
GVHD	Graft-versus-host disease
H2	Histamine 2 receptor
HAV	Hepatitis A virus
HBsAg	Hepatitis B surface antigen
HBV	Hepatitis B virus
HCG	Human chorionic gonadotrophin
HCM	Hypertrophic cardiomyopathy

HCV	Hepatitis C virus
HDL	High density lipoprotein
HHT	Hereditary haemorrhagic telangiectasia
HIV	Human immunodeficiency virus
HLA	Human leucocyte antigen
HMG-CoA	3-hydroxy-3-methyl glutaryl coenzyme A
HNPCC	Hereditary nonpolyposis colorectal cancer
HPV	Human papilloma virus
HUS	Haemolytic uraemic syndrome
HVPG	Hepatic venous wedge pressure gradient
ICAM	Intercellular adhesion molecule
ICD	International classification of diseases
IDDM	Insulin-dependent diabetes mellitus
IFÑ	Interferon
Ig	Immunoglobulin
IL	Interleukin
INR	International normalised ratio
K	Potassium
LDL	Low density lipoprotein
LOS	Lower oesophageal sphincter
MALT	Mucosa associated lymphoid tissue
MDR	Multidrug-resistance
MDRTB	Multidrug-resistant Tuberculosis
MEN	Multiple endocrine neoplasia
Mg	Magnesium
MHC	Major histocompatibility complex
MI	Myocardial infarction
MIP	Major intrinsic protein
MMR	Measles Mumps Rubella
MND	Motor neurone disease
MRC	Medical Research Council
MRCP	Member / membership of the Royal College of Physicians
MRI	Magnetic resonance imaging
mRNA	messenger ribonucleic acid
MS	Multiple sclerosis
Na	Sodium
NAC	N-acetyl cysteine
NIDDM	Non insulin-dependent diabetes mellitus
NIPPV	Nasal intermittent positive-pressure ventilation
NO	Nitric oxide
NSAID	Non-steroidal anti-inflammatory drug
OCP	Oral contraceptive pill
ODN	Oligodeoxynucleotide
OSA	Obstructive sleep apnoea
P	Probability
$PaCO_2$	Partial pressure of arterial carbon dioxide
PAF	Platelet activating factor
PaO_2	Partial pressure of arterial oxygen
PAS	Periodic acid schiff
PAVM	Pulmonary arteriovenous malformation
PCP	*Pneumocystis carinii* pneumonia

PCR	Polymerase chain reaction
PET	Positron emission tomography
PML	Progressive multifocal leucoencephalopathy
PMN	Polymorphonuclear leucocyte
PRP	Prion related protein
PSC	Primary sclerosing cholangitis
PTCA	Percutaneous transarterial coronary angioplasty
RNA	Ribonucleic acid
SAP	Serum amyloid protein
SCC	Squamous cell carcinoma
SLE	Systemic lupus erythematosus
SMR	Standardised mortality ratio
SOD	Superoxide dismutase
SPECT	Single-photon emission spectroscopy
SVT	Supra-ventricular tachycardia
T3	Triiodothyronine
T4	Thyroxine
TB	Tuberculosis
TGF	Transforming growth factor
TIA	Transient ischaemic attack
TIPS	Transjugular intrahepatic portosystemic shunt
TNF	Tumour necrosis factor
tPA	tissue plasminogen activator
tRNA	transfer ribonucleic acid
TSH	Thyroid stimulating hormone
TTP	Thrombotic thrombocytopenic purpura
VCAM	Vascular cell adhesion molecule
VDRL	Venereal diseases reference laboratory
VEGF	Vascular endothelial growth factor
VF	Ventricular fibrillation
VLDL	Very low density lipoprotein
VT	Ventricular tachycardia
VTE	Venous thromboembolism
WHO	World Health Organization

Index